2004
YEAR BOOK OF
NUCLEAR MEDICINE®

The 2004 Year Book Series

Year Book of Allergy, Asthma, and Clinical Immunology™: Drs Rosenwasser, Boguniewicz, Milgrom, Routes, and Spahn

Year Book of Anesthesiology and Pain Management™: Drs Chestnut, Abram, Black, Lang, Roizen, Trankina, and Wood

Year Book of Cardiology®: Drs Gersh, Cheitlin, Graham, Kaplan, Sundt, and Waldo

Year Book of Critical Care Medicine®: Drs Dellinger, Parrillo, Balk, Bekes, Dries, and Roberts

Year Book of Dentistry®: Drs Zakariasen, Boghosian, Burgess, Hatcher, Horswell, McIntyre, and Zakariasen

Year Book of Dermatology and Dermatologic Surgery™: Drs Thiers and Lang

Year Book of Diagnostic Radiology®: Drs Osborn, Birdwell, Dalinka, Gardiner, Groskin, Levy, Maynard, and Oestreich

Year Book of Emergency Medicine®: Drs Burdick, Cone, Cydulka, Hamilton, Handly, and Quintana

Year Book of Endocrinology®: Drs Mazzaferri, Becker, Kannan, Kennedy, Kreisberg, Meikle, Molitch, Osei, Poehlman, and Rogol

Year Book of Family Practice®: Drs Bowman, Apgar, Dexter, Miser, Neill, and Scherger

Year Book of Gastroenterology™: Drs Lichtenstein, Dempsey, Ginsberg, Katzka, Kochman, Morris, Nunes, Reddy, Rosato, and Stein

Year Book of Hand Surgery®: Drs Berger and Ladd

Year Book of Medicine®: Drs Barkin, Frishman, Klahr, Loehrer, Mazzaferri, Phillips, Pillinger, and Snydman

Year Book of Neonatal and Perinatal Medicine®: Drs Fanaroff, Maisels, and Stevenson

Year Book of Neurology and Neurosurgery®: Drs Gibbs and Verma

Year Book of Nuclear Medicine®: Drs Coleman, Blaufox, Royal, Strauss, and Zubal

Year Book of Obstetrics, Gynecology, and Women's Health®: Drs Mishell, Kirschbaum, and Miller

Year Book of Oncology®: Drs Loehrer, Arceci, Glatstein, Gordon, Morrow, Schiller, and Thigpen

Year Book of Ophthalmology®: Drs Rapuano, Cohen, Eagle, Grossman, Myers, Nelson, Penne, Regillo, Sergott, Shields, and Tipperman

Year Book of Orthopedics®: Drs Morrey, Beauchamp, Peterson, Swiontkowski, Trigg, and Yaszemski

Year Book of Otolaryngology-Head and Neck Surgery®: Drs Paparella, Keefe, and Otto

Year Book of Pathology and Laboratory Medicine®: Drs Raab, Grzybicki, Bejarano, Bissell, and Stanley

Year Book of Pediatrics®: Dr Stockman

Year Book of Plastic and Aesthetic Surgery™: Drs Miller, Bartlett, Garner, McKinney, Ruberg, Salisbury, and Smith

Year Book of Psychiatry and Applied Mental Health®: Drs Talbott, Ballenger, Frances, Jensen, Markowitz, Meltzer, and Simpson

Year Book of Pulmonary Disease®: Drs Phillips, Barker, Blanchard, Dunlap, Lewis, and Maurer

Year Book of Rheumatology, Arthritis, and Musculoskeletal Disease™: Drs Panush, Hadler, Hellmann, Hochberg, Lahita, and Seibold

Year Book of Sports Medicine®: Drs Shephard, Alexander, Cantu, Nieman, Sanborn, and Shrier

Year Book of Surgery®: Drs Copeland, Bland, Cerfolio, Daly, Eberlein, Howard, Luce, Mozingo, and Seeger

Year Book of Urology®: Drs Andriole and Coplen

Year Book of Vascular Surgery®: Dr Moneta

2004

The Year Book of NUCLEAR MEDICINE®

Editor in Chief
R. Edward Coleman, MD

Associate Editors
M. Donald Blaufox, MD, PhD
Henry D. Royal, MD
H. William Strauss, MD
I. George Zubal, PhD

Mosby

Mosby
Dedicated to Publishing Excellence

Vice President, Continuity Publishing: Timothy M. Griswold
Developmental Editor: Beth Martz
Senior Manager, Continuity Production: Idelle L. Winer
Issue Manager: Donna M. Skelton
Composition Specialist: Betty Dockins
Illustrations and Permissions Coordinator: Kimberly E. Hulett

2004 EDITION

Printed in the United States of America
Composition by Thomas Technology Solutions, Inc.
Printing/binding by Sheridan Books, Inc.

Editorial Office:
Elsevier
300 East
170 South Independence Mall West
Philadelphia, PA 19106-3399

International Standard Serial Number: 0084-3903
International Standard Book Number: 0-323-02073-9

Editorial Board

Table of Contents

JOURNALS REPRESENTED xi

INTRODUCTION xiii

1. **Physics, Instrumentation and Dosimetry** 1

Introduction 1

2. **Radiopharmaceutical** 33

Introduction 33

3. **Radiation** 49

Introduction 49

4. **Pulmonary** 75

Introduction 75

V/Q Imaging 75

Spiral CT 85

PET 90

Miscellaneous 99

5. **Gastrointestinal** 103

Introduction 103

6. **Cardiovascular** 123

Introduction 123

7. **Oncology** 167

Introduction 167

8. **Musculoskeletal** 215

Introduction 215

9. **Inflammation and Infection** 229

Introduction 229

10. **Endocrinology** 235

Introduction 235

11. **Renal** 265

Introduction 265

12. Vascular 287
Introduction 287
13. Central Nervous System 295
Introduction 295
SUBJECT INDEX. 305
AUTHOR INDEX 335

Journals Represented

Mosby and its editors survey approximately 500 journals for its abstract and commentary publications. From these journals, the editors select the articles to be abstracted. Journals represented in this YEAR BOOK are listed below.

Acta Paediatrica
American Journal of Cardiology
American Journal of Gastroenterology
American Journal of Kidney Diseases
American Journal of Medicine
American Journal of Neuroradiology
American Journal of Roentgenology
American Surgeon
Annals of Internal Medicine
Annals of Rheumatic Diseases
Annals of Surgery
Annals of Surgical Oncology
Archives of Environmental Health
Archives of Internal Medicine
British Journal of Radiology
British Journal of Urology International (WRONG)
British Medical Journal
Cancer
Chest
Circulation
Clinical Endocrinology (Oxford)
Clinical Nuclear Medicine
Clinical Physiology
Digestive Diseases and Sciences
Epilepsia
European Heart Journal
European Journal of Nuclear Medicine
European Journal of Nuclear Medicine and Molecular Imaging
European Journal of Surgical Oncology (London)
European Respiratory Journal
Gut
Gynecologic Oncology
Intensive Care Medicine
International Journal of Cancer
International Journal of Cardiology
Journal of Clinical Endocrinology and Metabolism
Journal of Clinical Oncology
Journal of Computer Assisted Tomography
Journal of Diabetes and Its Complications
Journal of Emergency Medicine
Journal of Neurology, Neurosurgery and Psychiatry
Journal of Neurosurgery
Journal of Nuclear Medicine
Journal of Rheumatology
Journal of Thoracic and Cardiovascular Surgery
Journal of Urology
Journal of the American College of Surgeons

Lancet
Mayo Clinic Proceedings
Medical Physics
Mutation Research
Nature
New England Journal of Medicine
Nuclear Medicine Communications
Otolaryngology-Head and Neck Surgery
Pediatric Emergency Care
Pediatric Radiology
Physics in Medicine and Biology
Proceedings of the National Academy of Sciences
Radiation Research
Radiology
Respiratory Medicine
Skeletal Radiology
Surgery
The Laryngoscope Journal
Thorax
Urology

Standard Abbreviations

The following terms are abbreviated in this edition: acquired immunodeficiency syndrome (AIDS), cardiopulmonary resuscitation (CPR), central nervous system (CNS), cerebrospinal fluid (CSF), computed tomography (CT), deoxyribonucleic acid (DNA), electrocardiography (ECG), [fluorine-18]-fluorodeoxyglucose (FDG), gadolinium-diethylenetriamine-pentaacetic acid (Gd-DTPA), health maintenance organization (HMO), human immunodeficiency virus (HIV), intensive care unit (ICU), intramuscular (IM), intravenous (IV), magnetic resonance (MR) imaging (MRI), nuclear magnetic resonance (NMR), positron emission tomography (PET), ribonucleic acid (RNA), single-photon emission CT (SPECT), ultrasound (US), and ultraviolet (UV).

Note

The Year Book of Nuclear Medicine is a literature survey service providing abstracts of articles published in the professional literature. Every effort is made to assure the accuracy of the information presented in these pages. Neither the editors nor the publisher of the Year Book of Nuclear Medicine can be responsible for errors in the original materials. The editors' comments are their own opinions. Mention of specific products within this publication does not constitute endorsement.

To facilitate the use of the Year Book of Nuclear Medicine as a reference tool, all illustrations and tables included in this publication are now identified as they appear in the original article. This change is meant to help the reader recognize that any illustration or table appearing in the Year Book of Nuclear Medicine may be only one of many in the original article. For this reason, figure and table numbers will often appear to be out of sequence within the Year Book of Nuclear Medicine.

Introduction

In my life as an academic physician, some aspects of what I do are more enjoyable than others. Meeting with the residents in radiology and nuclear medicine is an enjoyable part of my job. Reviewing and reporting clinical cases, reviewing cases from the weekend, and reviewing interesting cases from the last week provide an opportunity for me to teach residents what I have learned over the years, and for me to learn what they know about the disease and images. Reviewing the current literature to select articles to appear in the YEAR BOOK OF NUCLEAR MEDICINE is also quite enjoyable. When Alexander Gottschalk, MD, recruited me to participate in this endeavor, he noted the enjoyment that he received from reviewing the current literature and abstracting articles that he thought would be of interest to the nuclear medicine community. I concur with him that this is another aspect of my position that I find enjoyable. Dr Gottschalk was the Editor-in-Chief of the YEAR BOOK OF NUCLEAR MEDICINE for 9 years, and he has done an excellent job in leading an effort to provide abstracts of the current literature with appropriate commentary to the literature. He has set a standard that the associate editors and myself will attempt to maintain.

CHALLENGES FROM PET/CT

In this YEAR BOOK OF NUCLEAR MEDICINE, we continue to see an increasing number of articles devoted to PET imaging. PET is obviously becoming an increasingly important modality in nuclear medicine. Most nuclear examinations are interpreted by diagnostic radiologists. In the private practice of diagnostic radiology, diagnostic radiologists generally do the nuclear medicine because they are qualified by the six months of training that they receive during the four-year diagnostic radiology training program. FDG-PET is now being introduced into many private practices of radiology, and these individuals are now interpreting FDG-PET scans with minimal, if any, training in PET. Some individuals are attending a two- or three-day course, or possibly a five-day visiting fellowship, and then are interpreting FDG-PET scans.

Although FDG-PET is a fantastic modality, the studies are not easy to interpret. For those of us who have been interpreting FDG-PET images for many years, we realize that there is a marked physiologic variability in the uptake of FDG. I have now interpreted more than 15,000 PET scans, and every day I see a normal variant that I have not previously seen. Unfortunately, for the uninitiated, these normal variants frequently become described as pathology. Several of my clinical colleagues at Duke University Medical Center are quite concerned about the misinterpretation of PET scans that they are seeing from institutions that do not have adequate experience in performing and interpreting PET scans.

PET-CT brings new challenges in the performance and interpretation of both PET and CT scans. Before the introduction of the combined devices, we spent a lot of time reviewing the CT scan with the PET scan results. Some centers found registration of the anatomic information from the CT with the metabolic information from PET helpful in that correlation. The registration techniques have been demonstrated to work well in the brain, but they do have more limitations elsewhere in the body. Many of these limitations are overcome with the combined PET-CT device. With the introduction of PET-CT, diagnostic radiologists have become even more interested in interpreting the PET scans with little, if any, training, similar to what had been seen with PET-only devices. Because of the CT information, these diagnostic radiologists feel more comfortable interpreting these scans with the FDG being perceived as a "contrast" for CT.

Furthermore, nuclear medicine physicians who have been well trained in nuclear medicine and PET frequently have not had adequate training in CT to interpret the CT portion of the PET-CT study. These physicians are feeling disenfranchised because the modality that was developed and initially used in nuclear medicine is being usurped by diagnostic radiology.

The American College of Radiology and the Society of Nuclear Medicine have seen the problems associated with performing and interpreting PET-CT scans. They have developed a working group to provide guidelines for performance and interpretation of PET-CT scans. Dr Dominique Delbeke from Vanderbilt University and I are co-chairing that working group. Our challenge is to provide a document to describe the additional training that diagnostic radiologists would need in interpreting PET scans and that nuclear medicine physicians would need in interpreting CT scans as part of a PET-CT scan. These guidelines are expected to be completed by the summer of 2004. The development of these guidelines will not be an easy task. Fortunately, the working group consists of experienced radiologists and nuclear medicine physicians. We anticipate being able to form a consensus for the additional training needed for interpreting PET-CT scans.

R. Edward Coleman, MD

1 Physics, Instrumentation and Dosimetry

Introduction

It should come as no surprise that the hottest topic regarding instrumentation this year deals with the recent introduction of combined PET and CT scanners into a unified metabolism and anatomy diagnostic camera. As I look around to my colleagues' institutions, these new PET/CT units are being installed at an astounding rate. The popularity of these instruments goes hand-in-hand with an overwhelming number of publications covering the performance and characteristics of these cameras. Over half of the technical articles arriving to my desk for review covered PET/CT scanners, and more than half of the selected articles for this chapter reflect this trend.

Some interesting new questions are being posed due to the advent of these new machines. First, "What about respiratory motion?" The first two articles demonstrate that although combined PET/CT scanners seem to be the perfect solution for registering function with anatomy, the simple fact that the patient breathes causes a major technical difficulty. These articles take a close look at this problem.

Another interesting question is "Can we register function and anatomy well enough without having to purchase a combined PET/CT scanner?" If you have followed the development of image processing algorithms in nuclear medicine over the past years, you would know that registering function with anatomy has been around since the 1980s. In that decade, software algorithms were developed to take independently acquired SPECT or PET and CT or MRI scans and register them by matching surfaces. Due to the popularity of PET/CT scanners (which accomplish this more directly through mechanical means), many investigators have revitalized their software algorithms and are improving such post-hoc registrations. The next three articles in the chapter look at some of these software methods.

One topic that is always central to nuclear medicine technology is the constant effort to improve reconstruction algorithms. The next four articles direct this recurring theme at these new combined scanners. Iterative reconstruction methods continue to gain acceptance and the easily obtainable registered anatomic image makes for improved attenuation corrections.

And finally, concerning PET/CT scanners, three more articles look at extending the established designs of these clinical devices by investigating newer detector materials (GSO, LSO) and miniaturizing the geometry for imaging rodents. These developments have proceeded so quickly over the last few years, that GSO- and LSO-based PET/CT scanners and small animal units can be considered to be state-of-the-art commercially available devices.

Other interesting developments reported this past year include a dynamic phantom which simulates the beating heart so as to make comparisons between cameras or institutions more objective. This reflects the constant trend in nuclear cardiology to become more quantitative when reporting cardiac function.

Pinhole SPECT seems to have found a good niche in mammography. The very high spatial resolution afforded by this technique will hopefully make scintigraphic mammography more widespread and diagnostically more sensitive.

CdZnTe continues to be one of the newest detector systems with the highest potential in nuclear medicine. Until some of the difficulties in its production are worked out, we see in this 15th article of the chapter, that small hand-held gamma cameras using this semiconductor may be a good testbed for evaluating its performance characteristics.

Two of the next three dosimetry papers reporting new radiopharmaceuticals are labeled with F-18 (reemphasizing the focus on PET). However, more interestingly, all three of the new investigational radiopharmaceuticals described here are neuroreceptor imaging agents. I believe this reflects the steady development of moving past perfusion and metabolism imaging in the brain toward the more intriguing imaging of neuroreceptor densities and affinities in humans. I believe that soon new reconstruction and quantification methods will be developed for analyzing this next exciting class of functional nuclear medicine images.

The last article reminds us that amidst all the new technology and instrumentation, paying close attention to radiation doses is one of our central responsibilities. This investigation, which looks at age dependent estimated doses, reports on one of the more important duties we have to our patients.

I. George Zubal, PhD

Dual-Modality PET/CT Imaging: The Effect of Respiratory Motion on Combined Image Quality in Clinical Oncology

Beyer T, Antoch G, Blodgett T, et al (Univ Hosp Essen, Germany; Univ of Pittsburgh, Pa; Mem Sloan Kettering Cancer Ctr, New York)

Eur J Nucl Med Mol Imaging 30:588-596, 2003 1–1

Introduction.—To diminish potential misregistration from differences in the breathing pattern between 2 complementary PET and CT data sets, pa-

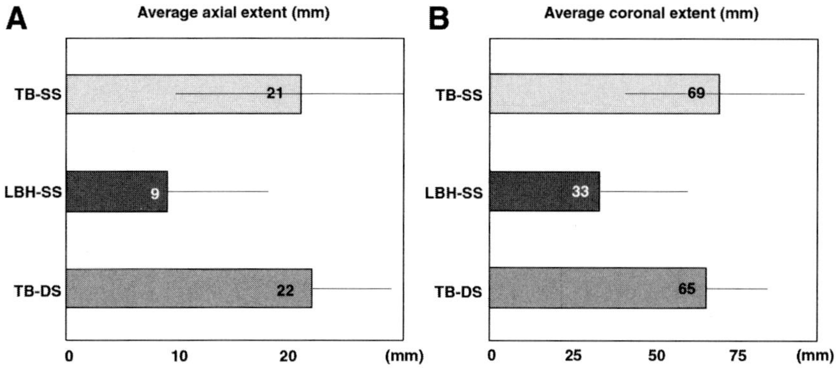

FIGURE 7.—Average spatial extent (**A**) axial, (**B**) coronal of respiration artifacts in CT images of 62 patients, according to the acquisition protocol used. (Courtesy of Beyer T, Antoch G, Blodgett T, et al: Dual-modality PET/CT imaging: The effect of respiratory motion on combined image quality in clinical oncology. *Eur J Nucl Med Mol Imaging* 30:588-596, 2003.)

tients are usually permitted to breathe quietly during a dual-modality scan using a combined PET/CT. Often, local misregistration between the CT and PET is seen. Respiration artifacts may occur in most cases if no respiration protocol is used. The appearance, magnitude, and frequency of respiration-induced artifacts were assessed in CT images of dual-modality PET/CT studies of 62 patients who were referred by their oncology physicians from 3 clinical sites.

Methods.—Three variants of CT scan acquisition were assessed as part of the PET/CT acquisition protocols: single-slice CT during tidal breathing (TB-SS); single-slice CT and limited breath-hold (LBH-SS) technique in which patients were asked to hold their breath during normal respiration for as long as the spiral CT covered the lower thorax and the liver; and dual-slice CT during tidal breathing (TB-DS). All participants were injected with about 370 MBq of FDG; PET/CT scanning was initiated 1 hour after injection. The CT images were reconstructed and, after appropriate scaling, they were used for on-line attenuation correction of the PET emission data.

Results.—When applying the limited breath-hold method, the rate of severe artifacts in the area of the diaphragm was diminished by half and the spatial extent of respiration-induced artifacts was diminished by a minimum of 40%, compared with that of acquisition protocols without any breathing instructions. The spatial extent of respiration-induced artifacts varied widely in the TB-SS, LBH-SS, and TB-DS groups (Fig 7).

Conclusion.—Special breathing protocols are effective and should be used for CT scans as part of combined imaging protocols using dual-modality PET/CT imaging. These findings can also be applied to multislice CT to potentially diminish further breathing artifacts in PET/CT imaging and to improve overall image quality.

► Registration of functional and anatomical images is of course complicated by the fact that the patient moves; respiration is probably the major contributor to this registration error and introduces image artifacts. This article provides color images demonstrating these artifacts and provides quantitative evaluation of how large (in mm) these excursions are (see figure).

I. G. Zubal, PhD

Respiratory Motion Artifacts on PET Emission Images Obtained Using CT Attenuation Correction on PET-CT

Osman MM, Cohade C, Nakamoto Y, et al (Johns Hopkins Univ, Baltimore, Md; St Louis Univ)

Eur J Nucl Med Mol Imaging 30:603-606, 2003 1–2

Introduction.—Artifacts originating from the use of CT data for attenuation correction (CTAC), rather than germanium-68 transmission data (Ge AC), have yet to be well characterized. Translation of the patient's body between PET and CT is a possible source of misalignment, and physiologic activities, including breathing, may cause artifacts. Images for 50 consecutive patients with known or suspected cancer were analyzed for possible respiratory motion artifacts (RMA) in PET images, attenuation corrected with CT from PET-CT.

Methods.—The PET-CT scans were performed using a Discovery LS PET-CT system in 23 men and 27 women with a mean age of 58.2 years. Both CTAC and Ge AC transmission data acquired during free tidal breathing were used to correct PET emission images. Cold artifacts at the interface of the lungs and diaphragm, considered to be due to RMA, were observed on CTAC images but not on Ge AC images. These were assessed qualitatively

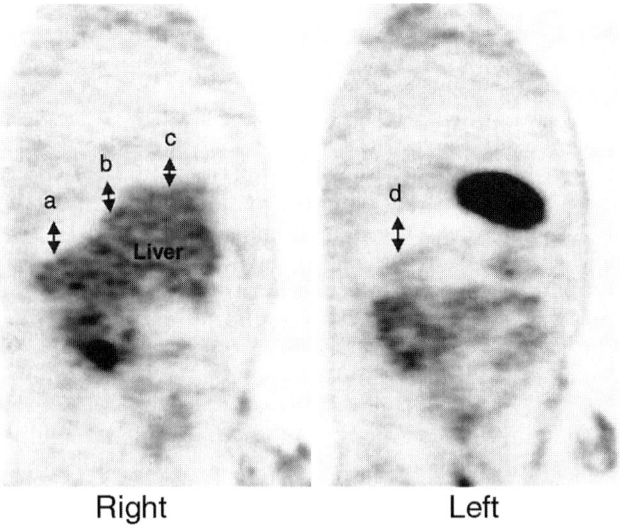

FIGURE 2.—Examples of quantitative assessment of RMA. In the right lung: **a**, posterior; **b**, middle; **c**, anterior; in the left lung: **d**, posterior. *Abbreviation: RMA*, Respiratory motion artifact. (Courtesy of Osmann MM, Cohade C, Nakamoto Y, et al: Respiratory motion artifacts on PET emission images obtained using CT attenuation correction on PET-CT. *Eur J Nucl med Mol Imaging* 30:603-606, 2003.)

on a 4-point scale (0, no artifact; 1, mild artifact; 3, moderate artifact; 3 severe artifact). The RMA was measured for height.

Results.—Curvilinear cold artifacts paralleling the dome of the diaphragm at the lung-diaphragm interface were observed on 84% of PET/CT image acquisitions (Fig 2) but were not observed on the ^{68}Ge-corrected images. These artifacts were rarely severe.

Conclusion.—Respiratory motion artifacts of varying magnitude were observed in most patients as a curvilinear cold area at the lung-diaphragm interface. They were not diagnostically problematic.

▶ This article echoes the concerns of the previous one, but includes such a vivid, obvious example of a respiratory artifact (see figure), that it was worth reproducing here.

I. G. Zubal, PhD

Automated 3-Dimensional Registration of Stand-Alone ^{18}F FDG Whole-Body PET With CT

Slomka PJ, Dey D, Przetak C, et al (Univ of Western Ontario, London, Canada; Cedars-Sinai Med Ctr, Los Angeles; Zentralklinik Bad Berka, Germany)

J Nucl Med 44:1156-1167, 2003 1–3

Introduction.—PET is used increasingly in the diagnosis and follow-up of patients with cancer. A combined interpretation of stand-alone PET and CT images is often required to optimize patient diagnosis or therapy. Image registration and fusion of whole-body ^{18}F-FDG PET with thoracic CT would permit combination of anatomic detail from CT with functional PET information, which could lead to improved diagnosis or PET-based radiotherapy planning. Software algorithms were developed for thoracic PET/CT image registration that would permit robust, rapid, fully automated, and retrospective fusion of images obtained with stand-alone PET and CT machines.

Methods.—A set of 18 PET and CT patient datasets was evaluated by a practical and fully automated algorithm for the elastic 3-dimensional image registration of whole-body PET and CT images, which compensates for the nonlinear deformation caused by breath-hold CT imaging. Initially, a 9-parameter linear registration is performed by maximizing the mutual information–based cost function, between the CT and the combination of emission and transmission PET volumes, by using progressively increasing matrix sizes to enhance speed and offer better convergence. Subsequently, lung contours on transmission maps and corresponding contours on CT volumes are automatically identified. A large number (few hundreds) of corresponding point pairs are automatically obtained, defining a thin-plate-spline elastic transformation of PET emission and transmission scans to match the CT scan.

Results.—In all 18 participants, the automatic linear registration with multiresolution converged close to the final alignment. In 10 cases, the nonlinear difference in the diaphragm position and chest wall remained clearly

TABLE 1.—Reproducibility of Transmission Data (*TR*), Emission Data (*EM*), and TR + EM Image Registration

Data	Translation	Scaling	Rotation
TR + EM	0.3 ± 0.5	1.1 ± 1.6	0.3 ± 0.2
TR	0.3 ± 0.4	1.1 ± 1.5	0.2 ± 0.5
EM	0.3 ± 0.4	1.8 ± 2.2	0.4 ± 0.4

Units of reproducibility are pixels for translations, % for scaling, and degrees for rotation.

(Reprinted by permission of the Society of Nuclear Medicine, from Slomka PJ, Dey D, Przetak C, et al: Automated 3-dimensional registration of stand-alone ^{18}F-FDG whole-body PET with CT. *J Nucl Med* 44:1156-1167, 2003.)

visible. The nonlinear adjustment, which was in the order of 40 to 75 mm, significantly improved the alignment between breath-hold CT and PET, particularly in the areas of the diaphragm. Lung volumes determined from transmission and CT scans closely match after the warping has been implemented. The average computation time is less than 40 seconds and less than 30 seconds for the linear and nonlinear components, respectively, for a typical PET scan with 4 to 6 bed positions. The reproducibility error of the registrations for transmission data (TR), emission data (EM), and TR + EM were evaluated quantitatively (Table 1).

Conclusion.—A technique has been established for automatic nonlinear registration of CT and PET whole-body images to common spatial coordinates. This method may be applied for automatic fusion of PET and CT obtained on stand-alone scanners during normal breathing or breath-hold data acquisition.

► If you operate a stand-alone PET scanner, and a combined PET/CT scanner is not in your hospital budget, there is hope. The investigators here have developed a robust registration program for combining separate PET and CT scans. As documented in Table 1, the translation, scaling, and rotation errors of approximately 3 pixels, 10%, and 0.4° appear completely adequate for clinical interpretation. One would hope that suppliers of stand-alone PET instruments would be able to supply software packages like these as part of their operational system.

I. G. Zubal, PhD

PET-MR Image Fusion in Soft Tissue Sarcoma: Accuracy, Reliability and Practicality of Interactive Point-Based and Automated Mutual Information Techniques

Somer EJR, Marsden PK, Benatar NA, et al (Kings College, London; Guy's and St Thomas' Hosp, London)

Eur J Nucl Med 30:54-62, 2003 1–4

Introduction.—The advantages of a multidisciplinary and multimodality approach to the management of soft-tissue sarcoma are well established.

The combining of the registration and fusion of PET with MRI or CT images allows accurate tumor localization and clearer boundary demarcation and is useful in differentiating between tumor and inflammatory tissue. Soft-tissue image fusion using PET-MRI is complicated by a lack of conspicuous anatomical characteristics and by deviation from the rigid-body model. The practicality, reliability, and accuracy of a point-based external marker technique was compared with those of an automated mutual information algorithm when applied to the evaluation of soft-tissue sarcoma.

Methods.—Ten patients with suspected sarcoma in the knee, thigh, groin, flank, or back underwent MR and PET scanning after the attachment of 9 external fiducial markers. In evaluation of the point-based technique, 3 error measures were considered: fiducial localization error (FLE), fiducial registration error (FRE), and target registration error (TRE). The FLE represents the accuracy with which the fiducial points can be localized and is linked to the FRE, minimized by the registration algorithm. The registration accuracy is best portrayed by the TRE, which is the distance between corresponding points in each image space after registration. In the absence of salient characteristics within the target volume, the TRE can be measured at fiducials excluded from the registration process. To assess the mutual information technique, PET data obtained after physically removing the markers were reconstructed in various ways and registered with MRI. After applying the transform suggested by the algorithm to the PET scan obtained before the markers were removed, the residual distance between PET and MR marker-pairs was measured.

Results.—The manual point-based technique provided the best results (root-mean-square [RMS] TRE = 8.3, max = 22.4 mm, min = 1.7 mm) and performed better than the automated algorithm (RMS TRE = 20.0 mm, max = 30.5 mm, min = 7.7 mm) when registering filtered back-projection PET images to MRI (Table 3). Images reconstructed using an iterative algo-

TABLE 3.—Summary of Errors

	>	Fiducial Registration Error (mm)			Target Registration Error (mm)		
		RMS	Min	Max	RMS	Min	Max
Manual	MR1 to MR1	1.4	0.9	1.8	1.8	0.2	3.5
	MR2 to MR1 (n=6)	1.4	1.2	1.4	2.0	0.4	3.3
	MR3 to MR1 (n=8)	2.7	2.1	4.5	5.0	0.3	19.1
	FBP PET to MR1	3.6	1.8	5.2	8.3	1.7	22.4
Automatic	MR2 to MR1	—	—	—	2.2	0.0	5.0
	MR3 to MR1	—	—	—	6.2	0.0	15.0
	FBP PET to MR	—	—	—	20.0	7.7	30.5
	AWOSEM PET to MR	—	—	—	51.0	5.8	137.3
	Transmission (TR) to MR	—	—	—	29.3	9.9	73.0
	FBP nAC PET to MR	—	—	—	131.3	8.6	219.0
	80% FBP PET + 20% TR to MR	—	—	—	20.9	5.6	39.5

(Courtesy of Somer EJR, Marsden PK, Benatar NA, et al: PET-MR image fusion in soft tissue sarcoma: Accuracy, reliability, and practicality of interactive point-based and automated mutual information techniques. *Eur J Nucl Med* 30:54-62, 2003. Copyright, Springer-Verlag.)

rithm or registration of a composite emission-transmission image did not enhance the overall accuracy of the registration process.

Conclusion.—Point-based PET-MRI registration using external markers is practical, reliable, and accurate to within about 5 mm toward the fiducial centroid. The automated algorithm was not as accurate or reliable.

▶ This article goes further to document registration differences between manual and automatic techniques. It also incorporates different reconstruction methods for PET scans (emission and transmission) to see how they affect the registration error. The comparison of separate MRI scans can be seen as a "gold standard," which, in certain respects, demonstrates the best accuracy that could be expected.

I. G. Zubal, PhD

SPET/CT Image Co-Registration in the Abdomen With a Simple and Cost-Effective Tool

Förster GJ, Laumann C, Nickel O, et al (Johannes Gutenberg Univ Hosp Mainz, Germany)

Eur J Nucl Med 30:32-39, 2003 1–5

Introduction.—The fusion of morphology and function improves the diagnostic accuracy of several clinical situations. The interpretation of these images in the abdomen is particularly difficult because of the absence of readily identifiable anatomical structures. Multimodality image coregistration can be accomplished by several techniques using external markers or internal markers. Instruments that combine CT with PET or SPET are currently on the market, but they are expensive, are available in only a few centers, and are limited to the combination of 2 modalities. An alternative strategy may be the use of a vacuum cushion as a tool to fix the patient's body position and the use of a simple coregistration tool for image fusion. The effectiveness of this cheap and commonly applicable approach in a diagnostic situation demanding high diagnostic accuracy was determined.

Methods.—Fourteen fusion investigations were performed in 10 patients, 39 to 68 years old (3 male, 7 female; mean age, 54.9 years), with a neuroendocrine tumor (8 intestinal carcinoids, 1 neuroendocrine pancreatic tumor, and 1 neuroendocrine gastrointestinal tumor in multiple endocrine neoplasia type I) with liver metastases. At 5 hours after injection of 100 MBq ^{111}In-DTPA-ocreotide, 14 patients were fixed in a vacuum cushion and underwent helical CT in a mid-inspiration position. Directly after the CT, a SPET study (SPET1) of the abdominal region was performed without changing the patient's position. A second SPET study (SPET2), 24 hours after injection, was obtained after repositioning the patient in his or her individual molded vacuum cushion. Nine markers appropriate for imaging with CT and SPET were fixed on a cushion. Datasets were fused via internal landmarks (metastases or margin of abdominal organs) or by external markers. Image fusion

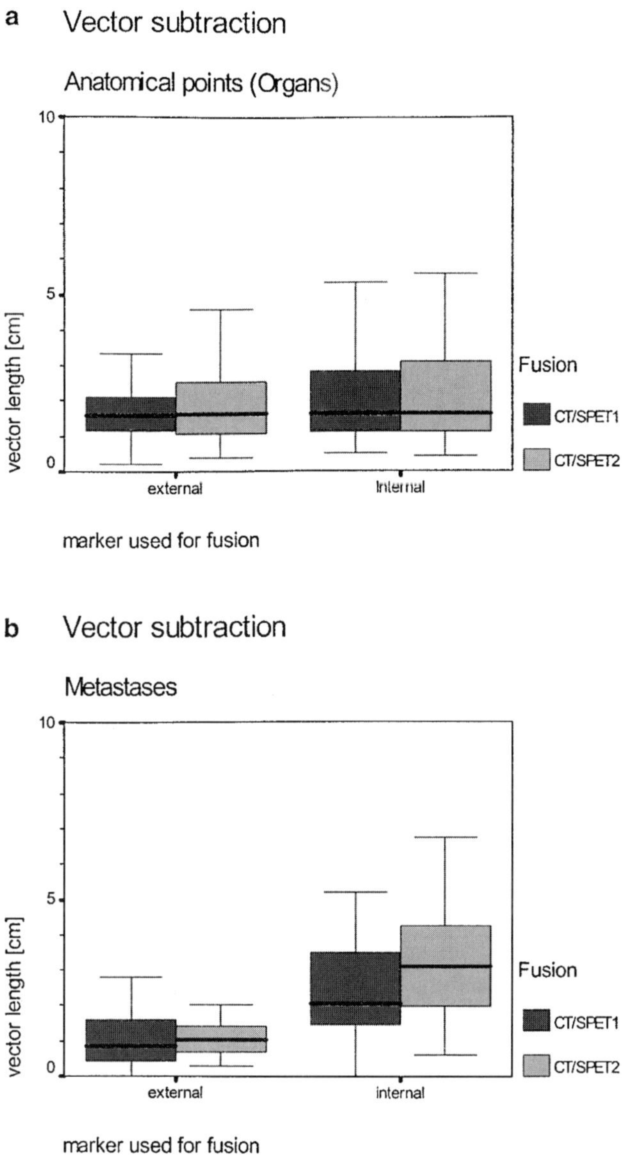

FIGURE 5.—Vector length subtraction of corresponding anatomical points (**a**) and metastases (**b**) in CT and re-sampled SPET datasets. The difference in vector lengths reflect the accuracy of the image fusion. (Courtesy of Forster GJ, Laumann C, Nickel O, et al: SPET-CT image co-registration in the abdomen with a simple and cost-effective tool. *Eur J Nucl Med* 30:32-39, 2003. Copyright Springer-Verlag.)

using external markers was fast and simple to handle, compared with that using internal landmarks.

Results.—Using SPET/CT image coregistration in the abdomen, all 28 lesions identifiable by SPET appeared precisely superimposed on the respective CT morphology by visual inspection. Image fusion of CT/SPET1 and CT/SPET2 revealed a mean deviation of the external markers that in the former instance was smaller than the pixel size of 4.67 mm: mean, 4.17 for CT/SPET1 and 5.52 mm for CT/SPET2, respectively. Using internal landmarks, the mean deviation of the chosen landmarks for CT/SPET1 and CT/SPET2 was 6.47 mm and 7.78 mm, respectively. Vector subtraction of corresponding anatomical points of the CT and the resampled SPET volume data sets produced a similar accuracy. Vector subtraction of the metastases revealed a significantly less accurate superimposition when internal landmarks were used ($P < .001$) (Fig 5). The vacuum cushion did not alter the image quality of CT and SPET.

Conclusion.—It is possible to acquire reasonably accurate anatomical fusion images of CT and SPET in the abdominal region using a simple device to ensure a fixed patient position and realignment on the basis of identification of fiducial markers, attached to the fixation device rather than on the patient's skin. The proposed technique is an easy and cost-effective method for generating abdominal data sets suitable for image fusion.

▶ This method is probably the original, tried and true (human-based observer) method for determining the best registration between function and anatomy. It was originally developed when function (nuclear medicine) and anatomy (CT, MRI) images were acquired on separate cameras, usually on separate days. The fact that humans are part of the registration process has, of course, advantages and disadvantages. The main advantage is that they can make changes to improve the final, accepted registration. Automated registrations could occasionally give incorrect superpositions that, at times, were difficult to fix.

It is very interesting to look at the tabulated registration errors, which in this case can be more than 5 mm; however even the more modern combined PET/CT scanners may not have registration accuracies better than this (because of patient motion).

I. G. Zubal, PhD

▶ Functional/anatomic imaging is likely to become the standard for imaging in the future. Ten years from now, I expect that most nuclear medicine imaging devices will be coupled with CT for anatomic localization. Perhaps unintentionally, this study paper indicates the difficulties of co-registering images that are obtained on separate devices. First, they used fiducial markers. Fiducial markers are not routinely used in anatomic imaging studies, so some method to reliably identify patients whose images were going to be co-registered would have to be developed. Second, the images that gave the best results were obtained on the same day. Images obtained on different days by using a molded vacuum cushion had larger registration errors. Coupled devices also provide attenuation correction. An example of co-registration is shown in Fig 3 in the original article.

H. D. Royal, MD

ROC Analysis for Assessment of Lesion Detection Performance in 3D PET: Influence of Reconstruction Algorithms

Glatting G, Werner C, Reske SN, et al (Univ of Ulm, Germany; Univ of Applied Sciences, Jena, Germany)

Med Phys 30:2315-2319, 2003 1–6

Introduction.—Image quality in PET may be evaluated with physical parameters, including spatial resolution and signal-to-noise ratio. Psychophysical approaches may also be used and include observer performance and the considered task (receiver operating characteristic [ROC] analysis). For PET in oncology, the reliable identification of small hot lesions is an important and representative task. The lesion identification performance due to sufficient modeling of the scanner and the measurement process in the image reconstruction process were examined.

Methods.—The standard ordered-subsets expectation-maximization software of the manufacturer was compared with a sophisticated fully 3-dimensional iterative reconstruction method (USC MAP). A rectangular phantom with 6 oblique line sources in a homogeneous background (2.5 kBq/mL ^{18}F) was imaged dynamically using an ECAT EXACT HR+ scanner in 3-dimensional mode. Reconstructed activity ranged between 15 and 0, as the line sources were filled with ^{11}C (3.2 MBq/mL). Measured attenuation and standard randoms, dead time, and scatter corrections of the manufacturer were utilized.

For the ROC analysis, a software tool presented a cutout of the phantom (15 × 15 pixels) to 2 investigators who rated them (5 classes). The area A_z

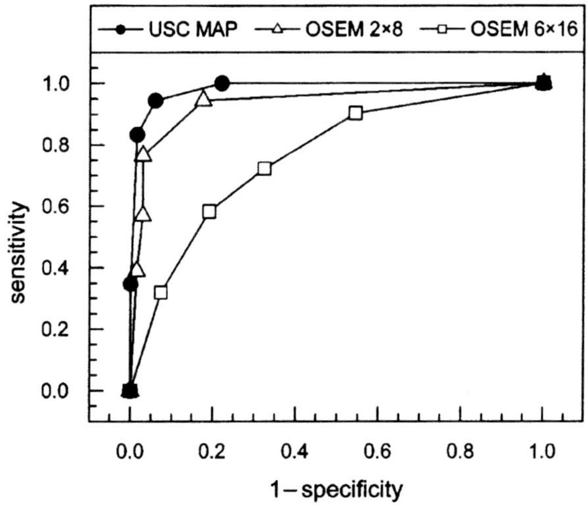

FIGURE 3.—Examples of receiver operating characteristic curves for the 3 evaluated image reconstruction algorithms for the measured frames 19-21. *Abbreviation: OSEM,* Ordered-subsets expectation-maximization. (Courtesy of Glatting G, Werner C, Reske SN, et al: ROC analysis for assessment of lesion detection performance in 3D PET: Influence of reconstruction algorithms. *Med Phys* 30:2315-2319, 2003.)

under the ROC curve was ascertained as a measure of detection performance.

Results.—The improvement for A_z with USC MAP compared to the ordered-subsets expectation-maximization reconstructions ranged between 0.02 and 0.23 for signal-to-noise ratios of the background between 2.8 to 3.1 and lesion contrast between 2.1 and 4.2. The areas under the ROC curves of the USC MAP reconstructions were greater (Fig 3) by a factor of 1.05 versus the OSEM 2 × 8 reconstructions.

Conclusion.—Adequate modeling of the measurement process in the reconstruction algorithm greatly enhanced the identification of small hot lesions.

► This article repeats the important, obvious fact that given the instrument characteristics, the images are only as good as the reconstruction algorithm we use. This article takes a good scientific view of applying different reconstruction algorithms to the same phantom data. It is interesting to note that by changing the subset parameters for ordered-subsets expectation-maximization reconstructions, the ROC performance characteristics change appreciably, and by implementing MAP reconstructions, the resulting images become incrementally better. We applaud the investigators in that they show the comparison of reconstruction algorithms by way of ROC graphs, since ultimately it is the visual interpretation of images that is most often used for patient diagnosis.

I. G. Zubal, PhD

PET Instrumentation and Reconstruction Algorithms in Whole-Body Applications

Tarantola G, Zito F, Gerundini P (Istituto di Ricovero e Cura a Carattere Scientifico, Milano, Italy)

J Nucl Med 44:756-769, 2003 1–7

Introduction.—PET for clinical diagnoses is being used increasingly, even in centers that do not have a cyclotron, thanks to the distribution of ^{18}F-FDG produced in licensed sites that are located within a reasonable distance of the imaging center. Scanners with various performance features have been developed (including the hybrid gamma cameras and partial or full-ring dedicated tomographs) that work in 2-dimensional (2D) or 3-dimensional (3D) mode to achieve different requirements and variable clinical workloads. The recent introduction of new scintillation crystals (lutetium oxyorthosilicate [LSO] and gadolinium orthosilicate [GSO]) and the combined PET-CT systems can enhance the scanner's technical performance and, at the same time, increase the clinical effectiveness of PET imaging. A comparison of state-of-the-art dedicated PET systems available on the market is presented.

Overview.—The use of ^{18}F-FDG PET imaging is quickly increasing along with the number and variety of coincidence detection systems. To improve the diagnostic accuracy of PET and allow effective anatomical integration to

TABLE 3.—State-of-the Art PET Scanners: Physical Performance (Factory Data)

Performance	ALLEGRO (Philips-ADAC)	C-PET (Philips-ADAC)	ECAT ART (CTI-Siemens	ECAT EXACT (CTI-Siemens)	ECAT EXACT HR+ (CTI-Siemens)	ECAT ACCEL (CTI-Siemens)	ADVANCE/ADVANCE Nxi (General Electric)
Transaxial resolution							
FWHM (mm) at 1 cm	4.8*	5.0*	6.2	6.0 (2D/3D)	4.6 (2D) 4.5 (3D)*	6.2 (2D) 6.3 (3D)*	4.8 (2D/3D)
FWHM (mm) at 10 cm	5.9*	6.4*	6.9	6.7 (2D/3D)	5.4 (2D) 5.6 (3D)*	6.7 (2D) 7.4 (3D)*	5.4 (2D/3D)
Axial resolution							
FWHM (mm) at 0 cm	5.4*	5.5*	4.9	4.5 (2D) 4.6 (3D)	4.2 (2D) 4.2 (3D)*	4.3 (2D) 5.8 (3D)*	4.0 (2D) 4.7 (3D)
FWHM (mm) at 10 cm	6.5*	5.9*	6.6	5.9 (2D) 6.5 (3D)	5.0 (2D) 5.7 (3D)*	6.0 (2D) 7.1 (3D)*	5.4 (2D) 6.3 (3D)
System sensitivity (net trues) (cps/Bq/mL)	19.0*	12.1*	7.3	4.9 (2D) 21.1 (3D)	5.4 (2D) 24.3 (3D)	5.4 (2D) 27.0 (3D)	5.4 (2D)† 31.0 (3D)‡
Scatter fraction (%)	25	25	36	16 (2D) 36 (3D)	17 (2D) 36 (3D)	16 (2D) 36 (3D)	10 (2D) 35 (3D)

Note: All parameters were measured following NEMA NU 2-1994 whenever not specified.
*Assessed according to NEMA NU 2-2001.
†Measured at 300 keV LLD in high sensitivity mode.
‡Measured at 300-keV LLD.
Abbreviations: FWHM, Full width at half maximum; *LLD*, lower-level energy discriminator.
(Reprinted by permission of the Society of Nuclear Medicine from Tarantola G, Zito F, Gerundini P: PET instrumentation and reconstruction algorithm in whole-body applications. *J Nucl Med* 44:756-769, 2003.)

functional data, attention needs to be focused on sensitivity, spatial resolution, dead time, noise equivalent counting rate, and scatter fraction (Table 3). In a comparison of various scanners, full-ring systems should be preferred for their higher sensitivity in contrast with partial-ring or coincidence cameras, despite the higher cost, to take advantage of potential spatial resolution and to speed up patient throughput in departments with high clinical workload. The new faster LSO and GSO systems, because of their improved counting-rate capability, appear promising for full 3D PET application. High-performance 3D reconstruction algorithms and scatter correction procedures along with powerful workstations are needed to transfer these systems into clinical routine. The PET-CT technology is capable of improving ^{18}F-FDG PET diagnostic accuracy for oncologic patients by contributing high-resolution anatomical references to corresponding lower-resolution metabolic images of body tissues.

Conclusion.—The new PET scanners have good potential for improving the accuracy and image quality of ^{18}F-FDG PET whole-body studies. New developments are in progress to optimize acquisition procedures and reconstruction algorithms.

▶ The essence of my comments for this article is quite short: "If you want to know about state-of-the-art PET instrumentation, read this article!!" I have found no better article that incorporates technical features, physical performance, reconstruction options, transmission scans, in fact, all fundamental characteristics of each currently available scanner into such an easily referenced and understandable presentation. In addition to the table reproduced here, numerous other tables, graphs, and figures make this article one of the most valuable references on state-of-the-art PET instruments.

I. G. Zubal, PhD

Implementation and Evaluation of an Ordered Subsets Reconstruction Algorithm for Transmission PET Studies Using Median Root Prior and Inter-Update Median Filtering

Bettinardi V, Alenius S, Numminen P, et al (Univ of Milano-Bicocca, Milan, Italy; Tampere Univ of Technology, Finland; Turku Univ, Finland)

Eur J Nucl Med 30:222-231, 2003 1–8

Background.—PET has become an important modality for staging cancer. Several technical aspects have contributed to the success of PET in this setting. In this study, an ordered subsets (OS) reconstruction algorithm based on the median root prior (MRP) and inter-update median filtering was used to reconstruct low count statistics transmission (TR) scans.

Methods.—The OS-MRP-TR algorithm was assessed with the use of an experimental phantom, simulating PET whole-body studies, and patient data. Various experimental conditions were used. The performance of the algorithm was determined by comparing the mean value of attenuation coefficient (MVAC) of known tissue types with the coefficient of variation for low-count TR images, reconstructed with the OS-MRP-TR algorithm.

Reference values were obtained from high-count TR images reconstructed with a filtered back-projection algorithm. Reconstructed OS-MRP-TR images were then used to correct attenuation of the corresponding emission (EM) data. Emission images reconstructed with attenuation correction produced by OS-MRP-TR images of low-count statistics were compared with EM images corrected for attenuation using reference, (high statistics) TR data.

Findings.—In the experimental conditions, the OS-MRP-TR algorithm demonstrated a tendency toward a stable solution with MGAC (Fig 2). In addition, there was a difference in MVAC of within 5% for a TR scan or 1 minute reconstructed with the OS-MRP-TR and a TR scan of 1-hour reconstructed with the filtered back-projection algorithm. Noise reduction was effective, especially for low-count statistics data. There was a difference of within 3% between the mean counts in the EM images attenuation corrected using the OS-MRP-TR images of 1 minute and the average counts in the EM images attenuation corrected using the OS-MRP-TR images of 1 hour. Good image quality was preserved in both TR and EM reconstructed images.

Conclusion.—The OS-MRP-TR algorithm is especially appropriate for whole body PET studies. This approach allows the acquisition of a very

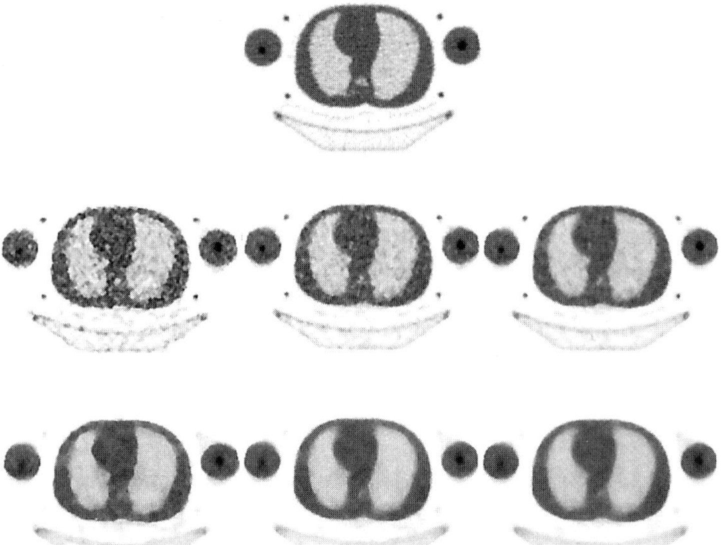

FIGURE 2.—Rando Alderson phantom. A representative transmission (*TR*) image of the Rando Alderson phantom reconstructed by: **top row**, filtered back-projection (FBP)-TR(1 hour); **middle row** from left to right, ordered subset (OS)-median root prior $(MRP)_{\beta(0.3)M(3)}$-TR(1 minute), $OS\text{-}MRP_{\beta(0.3)M(3)3DPMF}$-TR(1 minute), $OS\text{-}MRP_{\beta(0.3)M(3)DIMF}$-TR(1 minute); **bottom row** from left to right, $OS\text{-}MRP_{\beta(0.9)M(5)}$-TR(1 minute), $OS\text{-}MRP_{\beta(0.9)M(5)3DPMF}$-TR(1 minute), $OS\text{-}MRP_{\beta(0.9)M(5)3DIMF}$-TR(1 minute). All the OS-MRP-TR images were obtained after 10 full iterations. (Courtesy of Bettinardi V, Alenius S, Numminen P, et al: Implementation and evaluation of an ordered subsets reconstruction algorithm for transmission PET studies using median root prior and inter-update median filtering. *Eur J Nucl Med* 30:222-231, 2003. Copyright Springer-Verlag.)

short TR scan (within 1 minute), reconstruction of TR data in low-noise TR images, and the use of reconstructed OS-MRP-TR images to correct attenuation of corresponding EM data.

▶ I believe one could generally say that iterative reconstructions (OSEM) are replacing filtered back projection (FBP) methods in nuclear medicine. Clearly, FBP is still used extensively, but the momentum is in the direction of the methods of OSEM implementation. The figure included here shows several results using OSEM with various parameters and demonstrates the various qualities of the resulting image. In order to appreciate the improved characteristics of OSEM images, one still relies on comparing them to the FBP image shown on top.

I. G. Zubal, PhD

CT-Based Attenuation Correction in the Calculation of Semi-Quantitative Indices of [^{18}F]FDG Uptake in PET

Visvikis D, Costa DC, Croasdale I, et al (Royal Free and Univ College, London; GE Med Systems, Slough, England)

Eur J Nucl Med 30:344-353, 2003 1–9

Background.—The numerous advantages of combined PET/CT include the utilization of CT images for PET attenuation correction (AC). The accuracy of CT attenuation corrected (CTAC) was investigated, along with the resulting bias and signal-to-noise ratio in image-derived semi-quantitative update indexes.

Methods.—Using a combined PET/CT system and different sized phantoms containing variable density components, the authors assessed the inherent accuracy of a bilinear transformation in converting CT images to 511-keV attenuation maps. A phantom study was then performed simulating tumor imaging conditions, with a tumor-to-background ratio of 5:1. Contrast agents at different concentrations was administered. A CT scan was obtained, followed by 5-minute emission with 1- and 3-hour transmission frames. In addition, clinical data on 50 patients were studied.

The patients had had a CT scan under normal breathing conditions ($CTAC_{nb}$) or breath-hold with inspiration ($CTACT_{insp}$) or expiration ($CTAC_{exp}$). This was followed by a PET scan of 5 and 3 minutes per bed position for the emission and transmission scans, respectively. Segmented AC (SAC) and CTAC were used to reconstruct phantom and patient studies. Measured AC was done in the phantom studies with the 1-hour transmission frame.

Findings.—When the attenuation coefficients from the CT- and rod source–based attenuation maps were compared (Fig 4), there were differences of 3% and less than 6% before and after segmentation of the measured transmission maps, respectively. Differences of up to 6% and 8% were documented in the mean density (SUV_{avg}) between phantom images reconstructed with measured AC and those reconstructed with CTAC and SAC,

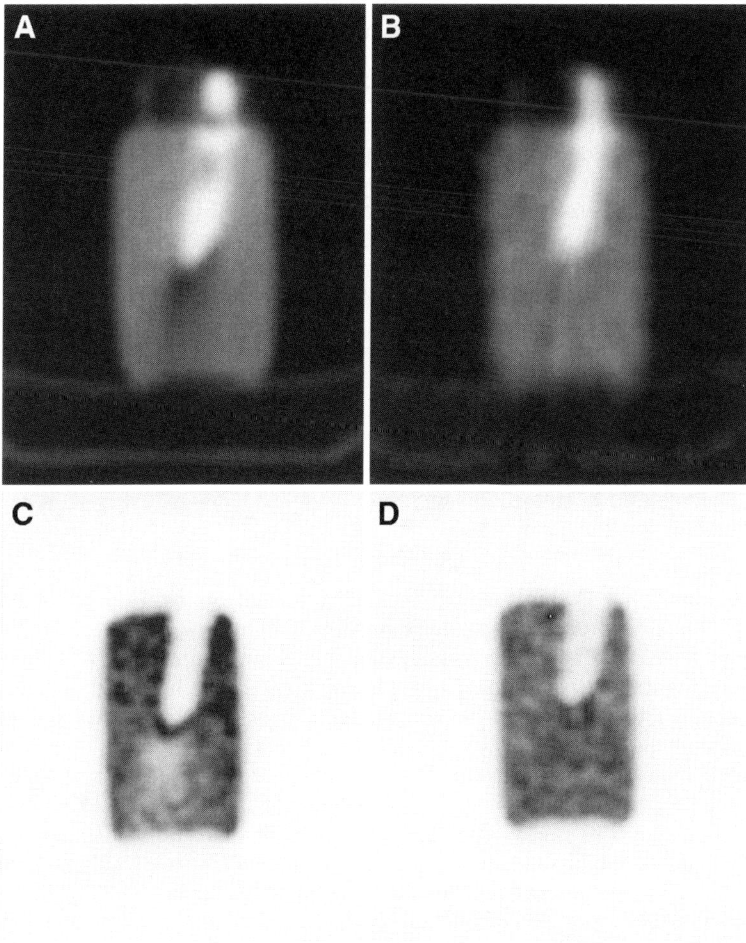

FIGURE 4.—A-D. A slice from the images of the phantom with the titanium alloy prosthesis present. **A**, CT attenuation map; **B**, segmented attenuation map; **C**, emission image reconstructed with CT attenuation correction; and **D**, emission image reconstructed with segmented attenuation correction. (Courtesy of Visvikis D, Costa DC, Croasdale I, et al: CT-based attenuation correction in the calculation of semi-quantitative indices of [^{18}F] FDG uptake in PET. *Eur J Nucl Med* 30:344-353, 2003. Copyright Spring-Verlag.)

respectively. With CTAC, the difference increased up to 27% with the presence of contrast agent. When metallic implants were present, the surrounding SUV_{avg} was underestimated, and increasing nonuniformity in the proximity of the implant was noted.

In the patient study, no significant differences in the SUV_{avg} emerged between either $CTAC_{nb}$ or $CTAC_{exp}$ and SAC-reconstructed images. Greater differences were recorded in the lung. Both the phantom and patient studies showed a mean increase of about 25% in the signal-to-noise ratio for the CTAC-reconstructed emission images compared with SAC-reconstructed images.

Conclusion.—These data suggest that, in whole-body studies, $CTAC_{nb}$ or $CTAC_{exp}$ is a viable alternative to SAC. When using CTAC, clinicians need to carefully consider the interpretation of images and the use of SUVs with oral contrast and in the proximity of metallic implants.

► This article takes an interesting close look at how CT-based AC for combined PET/CT scanners can influence the emission image. The image of the phantom shown here demonstrates changes in the PET image influenced by whichever method of AC is used. Using such simple phantoms is always educational for fundamentally understanding such effects and allows us to apply such knowledge to clinical patient images.

I. G. Zubal, PhD

Performance of a Brain PET Camera Based on Anger-Logic Gadolinium Oxyorthosilicate Detectors

Karp JS, Surti S, Daube-Witherspoon ME, et al (Univ of Pennsylvania, Philadelphia; Philips Med Systems, Philadelphia)

J Nucl Med 44:1340-1349, 2003 1–10

Introduction.—A high-sensitivity, high-resolution brain PET scanner (G-PET) has been developed that is similar in geometry to a previous brain scanner developed at the University of Pennsylvania, the HEAD Penn-PET. Improvements in detector technology and electronics have enhanced performance. The design and performance of the G-PET scanner were described.

Methods.—The G-PET scanner has a detector ring diameter of 42.0 cm with a patient aperture of 30.0 cm and an axial field of view of 25.6 cm. It is composed of a continuous light-guide that couples 18,560 (320 × 58 array) 4 × 4 × 10 mm^3 gadolinium oxyorthosilicate crystals to 288 (36 × 8 array) 39-mm photomultiplier tubes in a hexagonal arrangement.

The scanner operates only in 3-dimensional mode since there are no interplane septa. Performance measurements on the G-PET scanner were performed following National Electrical Manufacturers Association NU 2-2001 procedures for most measurements. The NU 2 1994 procedures were used when considered more pertinent for a brain scanner (eg, scatter fraction and counting-rate performance measurements).

Results.—The transverse and axial resolutions for the G-PET scanner near the center are 4.0 and 5.0 mm, respectively. At a radial offset of 10 cm, these numbers deteriorate by about 0.5 mm. The absolute sensitivity, measured by a 70-cm long line source, is 4.79 counts/s/kBq. The scatter fraction determined with a line source in a 20-cm-diameter × 19-cm-long cylinder is 39% (for a lower energy threshold of 410 keV).

For this cylinder, the peak noise equivalent counting rate is 60 kcps at an activity concentration of 7.4 kBq/mL (0.20 μCi/mL). Images from the Hoffman brain phantom, along with ^{18}F-FDG patient scans, demonstrate the high quality of image acquired on the G-PET scanner.

Conclusion.—The Ge-PET scanner achieves the goal of high performance for brain imaging by the use of the Anger-logic gadolinium oxyorthosilicate detector design with continuous optical coupling. This detector design allows good energy resolution, which is required in 3-dimensional imaging to minimize scatter and random coincidences.

► LSO has perhaps recently received the most attention; however, another new scintillator, GSO, is making its way into PET camera designs. Although GSO is not as fast (does not emit its light as quickly) as LSO, it delivers better energy resolution. When comparing the brain images shown here to the images in the previous abstract (Abstract 1–9), we realize that whether employing LSO or GSO in these new state-of-the-art camera systems, the images are of such high quality that they appear to be approaching the limits of PET imaging physics.

I. G. Zubal, PhD

Characterization of a Single LSO Crystal Layer High Resolution Research Tomograph

Boellaard R, Buijs F, de Jong HWAM, et al (VU Univ, Amsterdam; CTI PET Systems, Knoxville, Tenn)

Phys Med Biol 48:429-448, 2003 1–11

Introduction.—The single-layer High Resolution Research Tomograph (HRRT; a high-resolution PET scanner designed for human brain and small animal imaging that consists of 8 panel detectors, which have one layer of 2.1 × 2.1 × 7.5-mm thick lutetium oxy-orthosilicate [LSO] crystals) has a lower sensitivity than the dual scanner because of the smaller amount of crystal material, yet it does not have the potential difficulties linked with depth of interaction and significantly decreases the cost of the scanner. Only LSO is used in the single layer scanner. The LSO crystal has a high light yield and short scintillation rise and decay time, permitting a short coincidence time window and minimal dead time losses. Because of the good scintillator properties of LSO, a single crystal layer of 7.5-mm thickness combined with fully 3-dimensional (3D) data acquisition may result in adequate sensitivity and noise equivalent count rate (NECR) performance for both human and small animal studies. The performance of a single LSO crystal layer HRRT PET scanner was examined.

Methods.—Several phantom studies were conducted to ascertain scanner characteristics, including resolution, scatter fraction, count rate, and NECR. The NECR curves were calculated according to both NEMA NU2-1994 and NU2-2001 for 3 different energy windows (ie, lower level discriminators [lld] of 350, 400, and 450 keV and an upper level discriminator [uld] of 650 keV). Accuracy of scatter and single-photon attenuation corrections were assessed according to NU2-1994. Data were obtained by using a ring difference of 67 and a span of 9. Reconstructions were performed by using FORE + 2D FBP or OSEM.

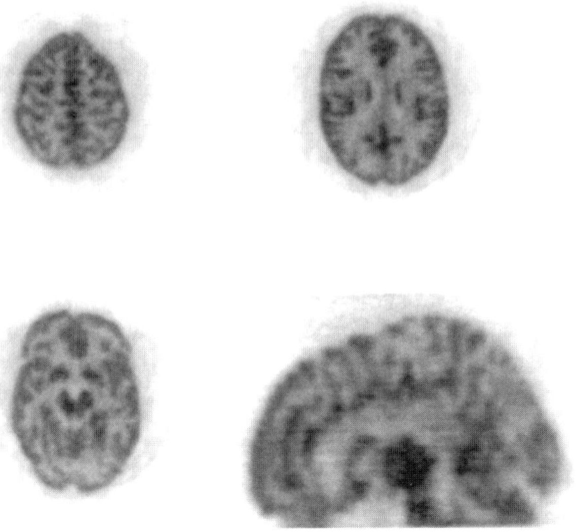

FIGURE 11.—Axial and coronal slices of a high quality scan of the 3D brain phantom. (Courtesy of Boellaard R, Buijs F, de Jong HWAM, et al: Characterization of a single LSO crystal layer High Resolution Research Tomograph. *Phys Med Biol* 48:429-448, 2003.)

Results.—Transaxial resolution varied from 2.7 to 2.9 mm FWHM between 1 and 10 cm off center locations. The axial resolution varied from 3.2 to 4.4 mm FWHM. Scatter fractions, according to NU2-1994, equaled 0.31, 0.42, and 0.54 for lld of 450, 400, and 350 keV, respectively. The NECR data were highest for lld of 400 keV and demonstrated a maximum of 46 kcps at 38 kBq cm^{-3}. Lower NECR values were seen according to NU2-2001, yet were still optimal for an lld of 400 keV. After undergoing scatter and attenuation corrections, pixel values within water, air, and teflon inserts of the NU2-1994 phantom were 14%, 4%, and 35% of the background activity, respectively.

Conclusion.—The single-layer LSO HRRT scanner demonstrated excellent spatial resolution, making it appropriate for small animal studies (Fig 11). The low count rate performance, resulting from the small amount of LSO, prohibits investigation of the human brain, but it is adequate for studies in small laboratory animals.

► In stride with the very high level of interest and engineering revolving around combined PET/CT scanners, we also currently see the advent of LSO crystals. If you want to gain a better understanding of all the characteristics that favor the use of LSO crystals, this article does a very good job of explaining LSO's performance and reporting measurements from one example instrument.

I. G. Zubal, PhD

Performance Evaluation of the MicroPET R4 PET Scanner for Rodents

Knoess C, Siegel S, Smith A, et al (Max-Planck-Institute for Neurological Research, Cologne, Germany; Concorde Microsystems Inc, Knoxville, Tenn; Ctr of Molecular Medicine, Cologne, Germany; et al)

Eur J Nucl Med Mol Imaging 30:737-747, 2003 1–12

Introduction.—The microPET R4 scanner is a dedicated PET for investigating rodents. A number of microPET R4 parameters were assessed within the scope of rodent studies to characterize the performance of this system in practice.

Findings.—In the center of the field of view, a maximal sensitivity of 43.66 cps/kBq for a centered point source was determined from a measurement

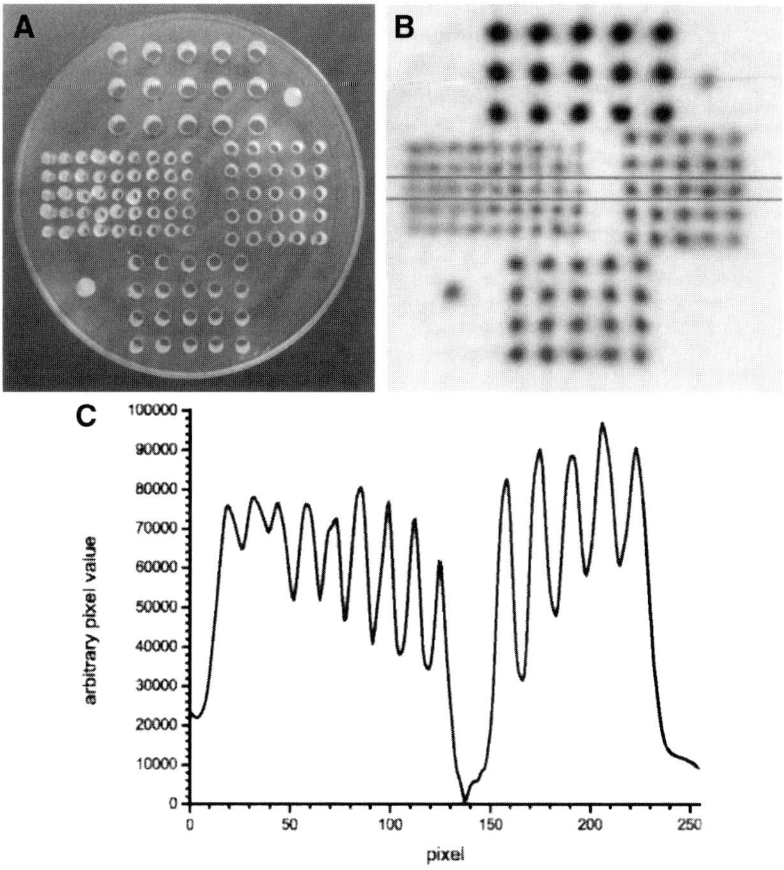

FIGURE 10.—A, The high resolution phantom with holes of different diameter and center-to-center spacing. B, Image of the high-resolution phantom as measured with the microPET R4 and reconstructed with FORE + 2D-FBP. The phantom was placed vertically and centered in the field of view. The *lines* indicate the position of the profile shown in C. (Courtesy of Knoess C, Siegel S, Smith A, et al: Performance evaluation of the microPET R4 PET scanner for rodents. *Eur J Nucl Med Mol Imaging* 30:737-747, 2003.)

with a germanium-68 line source within an energy window of 250 to 750 keV. A spatial resolution of 1.85 mm full-width at half-maximum in the axial direction and 1.66 mm full-width at half-maximum in the transaxial direction was determined in the center with a 1-mm–diameter sodium-22 point source.

Within the inner 20 mm of the field of view, the volumetric resolution exceeded 15.6 µl, which corresponds to a linear resolution of below 2.5 mm in all 3 dimensions. Images of a high-resolution phantom and those from rat and mice investigations demonstrate the good performance of the scanner. A maximal noise equivalent count rate was achieved at 174 kcps for a mouse phantom and at 93 kcps for a rat phantom (energy window 250-750 keV).

Scatter fractions were observed between 0.30 and 0.42 of an energy window of 250 to 750 keV and phantom diameters similar to rats and mice. All hot spots in the 4-hole configurations were clearly resolved, even the 2-mm holes, in the FORE+2D−FBP image of the high-resolution phantom (Fig 10). A comparison with the microPET P4 model for primates demonstrated the gain in sensitivity due to a smaller detector ring diameter and changes in noise equivalent count rate.

Conclusion.—Several scanner parameters—including spatial resolution, sensitivity, scatter, and count rate performance—have been determined, demonstrating that the microPET R4 is an appropriate PET scanner for rats and mice.

► New radiopharmaceuticals are, of course, first tested in animals, and small rodents are usually the animal model of choice. Several manufacturers are now offering miniaturized PET instruments, and the one described here is representative of the sensitivities and resolutions achieved by these scanners. The smallest holes and spacing of this multi-whole phantom is 2 mm, which are resolved quite well (and compares to similar instruments developed by others). This article additionally does a very good job of covering virtually all important characteristics of such animal-dedicated cameras, including: energy resolution, sensitivity, scatter components, count rate performance, and noise equivalent counts for various geometries. This makes it a good reference article for understanding small animal PET scanners in general.

I. G. Zubal, PhD

Validation of Gated Blood-Pool SPECT Cardiac Measurements Tested Using a Biventricular Dynamic Physical Phantom

De Bondt P, Nichols K, Vandenberghe S, et al (Ghent Univ Hosp, Belgium; Columbia Univ, New York; Ghent Univ, Belgium)

J Nucl Med 44:967-972, 2003 1–13

Introduction.—Gated blood-pool (GBP) SPECT offers many potential advantages over conventional equilibrium radionuclide angiography. A biventricular dynamic physical cardiac phantom was created to test GBP SPECT image-processing algorithms. These phantoms provide absolute values against which to evaluate the accuracy of both right and left computed ventricular volume and ejection fraction (EF) measurements.

Methods.—Two silicon-rubber chambers driven by 2 piston pumps simulated crescent-shaped right ventricles wrapped partially around ellipsoid left ventricles (Fig 1). Twenty experiments were performed, for which right- and left-ventricular true volume were 66 to 275 mL and 55 to 165 mL, respectively, and EF ranges, right and left ventricular, were 7% to 49% and 12% to 69%, respectively. The resulting 64 × 64 simulated GBP SPECT images acquired at 16 frames per R-R interval were analyzed by 2 independent observers who were unaware of the true values. Algorithms automatically divided right ventricular activity volumetrically from left ventricular activity. Automated valve planes, mid-ventricular planes, and segmentation regions were made available to the observers, who accepted these choices or modified them as needed. One observer repeated measurements more than 1 month later without reference to earlier determinations.

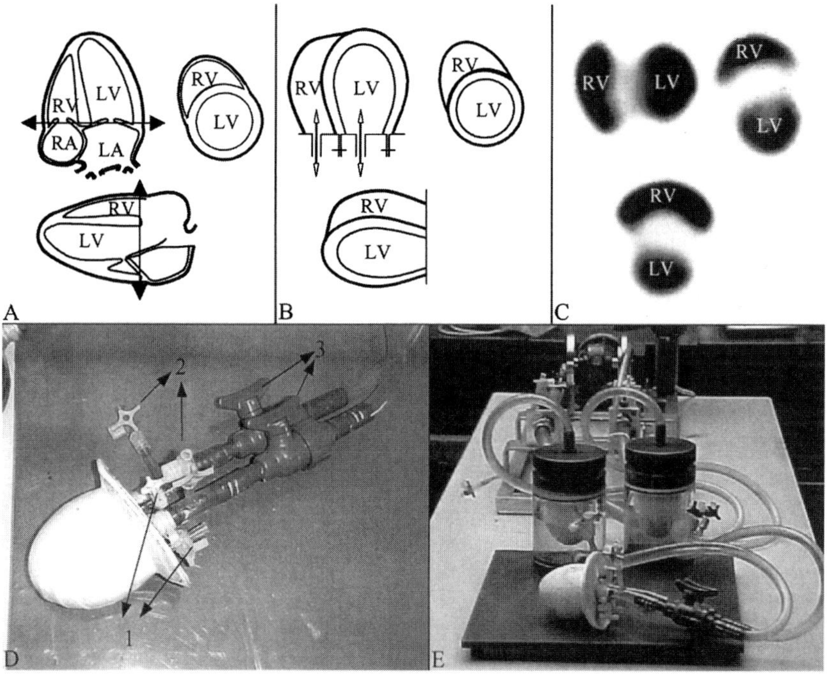

FIGURE 1.—Development and description of phantom. (**A**) Ventricles were cut off at atrioventricular border. (**B**) Single-walled RV was attached to double-walled LV. (**C**) Horizontal long-axis slice (**top left**), short axis slice (**top right**), and ventricle long-axis slice (**bottom**) of activity distribution in phantom. (**D**) Detail of biventricular model. Valves 1 are used to fill septal wall with gel; valves 2 are used to deaerate tubings, to inject tracer, and to empty ventricles for volume measurement. Valves 3 are in- and outgoing tubes to ventricles. (**E**) Overview of experimental model, with piston pump in back, membranes in middle, and ventricular model at front. (Reprinted by permission of the Society of Nuclear Medicine from De Bondt P, Nichols K, Vanderberghe S, et al: Validation of gated blood-pool SPECT cardiac measurements tested using a biventricular dynamic physical phantom. *J Nucl Med* 44:967-972, 2003.)

Results.—The linear correlation coefficients (r) of the mean of the 3 GBP SPECT images versus true values for right and left ventricles were 0.80 and 0.94 for EF and 0.94 and 0.95 for volumes, respectively. The correlations for right and left ventricles were 0.97 and 0.97 for EF and 0.96 and 0.89 for volumes, respectively, for interobserver agreement and 0.97 and 0.98 for EF and 0.96 and 0.90 for volumes, respectively, for intraobserver agreement. No trends were observed, but volumes and right ventricular EFs were significantly higher than the true values.

Conclusion.—Overall, GBP SPECT measurements were strongly correlated with true values. The phantom evaluated demonstrates considerable promise for helping to guide algorithm developments for improved GBP SPECT accuracy.

► Years ago, I remember reading about "ejection fraction phantoms," which could be used for calibrating clinical analysis programs for planar cardiac imaging. I believe that this fully 3-dimensional anthropomorphic phantom demonstrates that SPECT imaging has emerged as an established clinical method for evaluating cardiac function. Since many institutions rely on their own in-house database to determine normal versus abnormal EF ranges, this phantom finally permits these ranges to be tested for accuracy and allows for comparisons between institutions.

I. G. Zubal, PhD

Mammotomography With Pinhole Incomplete Circular Orbit SPECT

Tornai MP, Bowsher JE, Jaszczak RJ, et al (Duke Univ, Durham, NC)

J Nucl Med 44:583-593, 2003 1–14

Background.—The use of ^{99m}Tc-labeled compounds for detecting breast malignancy has prompted the development of different approaches to radionuclide breast cancer imaging. Enhanced 3-dimensional imaging with very high stopping power apertures may enable the use of improved sensitivities for detecting lesions in the breast. This study assessed dedicated mammotomography with pinhole incomplete circular orbit (PICO) SPECT imaging of an uncompressed pendant breast with small, very high stopping power pinhole apertures.

Methods.—A pendulous, uncompressed breast phantom in planar and PICO-SPECT modes was studied. Spherical lesions 0.6 to 1 cm in diameter were imaged using pinhole collimators made of high-density and high atomic number ^{184}W or depleted ^{238}U, with aperture diameters from 1 to 4 mm (Fig 2).

Findings.—Small differences in measured counting rate sensitivity and lesion contrast were documented overall for PICO-SPECT imaging, with greater signal-to-noise ratios (SNRs) between tungsten and depleted uranium pinhole materials at this energy and these lesion sizes. Because of the rapid sensitivity falloff for pinhole apertures, backgrounds from simulated myocardial uptake contributed in a minor fashion to all reconstructed image

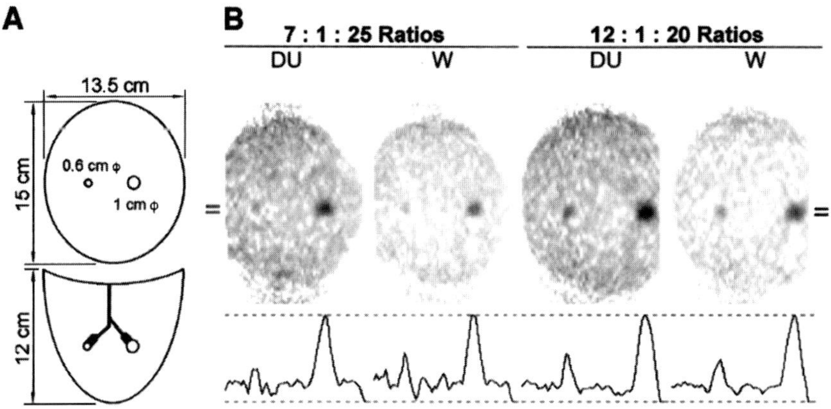

FIGURE 2.—A, Schematic diagram of breast phantom with approximate locations of lesions, with sizes indicated (φ = diameter). Coronal view (**top**) with lesions and sagittal view (**bottom**) illustrate how lesions were held in place. Materials are made of acrylic. **B**, Coronal views of reconstructed images obtained with 3 mm depleted ^{238}U (*DU*) and tungsten pinholes at indicated lesion, breast and body, and myocardial activity concentrations. PICO-SPECT data were acquired with trajectory along vertical dimension. Profiles at **bottom** are obtained from indicated regions through images. (Reprinted by permission of the Society of Nuclear Medicine from Tornai MP, Bowsher JE, Jaszczak RJ, et al: Mammotomography with pinhole incomplete circular orbit SPECT. *J Nucl Med* 44:583-593, 2003.)

volumes. The optimal aperture diameter determined from peak SNR was between 2 and 3 mm. These aperture sizes may perform best in the assessment of lesions as small as 0.6 cm in diameter, with activity concentration ratios of ^{99m}Tc similar to those currently observed in patients. Both lesions were visualized better with PICO-SPECT than with planar pinhole imaging. Respective contrast improvements were more than 20 times the values obtained from planar imaging for the same pinholes.

Conclusion.—In small lesion identification with PICO-SPECT, the enhanced spatial resolution of smaller apertures seems to outweigh the loss in sensitivity. Dedicated PICO-SPECT of the breast appears to have advantages over conventional planar pinhole scintimammography. It provides enhanced contrast and SNR for imaging small lesions with high-resolution pinhole apertures along with 3-dimensional lesion localization.

► In years past, this chapter has reported on interesting applications of pinhole SPECT, and here is another use for this interesting imaging method. The results shown here clearly demonstrate that a 6-mm nodule can clearly be imaged. It would have been interesting to show the same phantom image using parallel hole or fan beam collimator SPECT. I would assume that the small nodule would not be visualized using more conventional collimators.

I. G. Zubal, PhD

Performance Evaluation of a Hand-Held, Semiconductor (CdZnTe)-Based Gamma Camera

Abe A, Takahashi N, Lee J, et al (Yokohama CIty Univ, Japan; Anzai Med Ctr Ltd, Japan)

Eur J Nucl Med Mol Imaging 30:805-811, 2003 1–15

Introduction.—A small field of view gamma camera, the eZ SCOPE, has been developed and is based on utilization of a CdZnTe semiconductor. The device uses proprietary signal processing technology and an interface to a computer-based imaging system. The performance of the eZ scope was compared with currently used gamma camera technology.

Methods.—The detector consists of a single wafer of 5-mm-thick CdZnTe that is divided into a 16 × 16 array (256 pixels), with the sensitive area being a square of dimension 3.2 cm (Table 1). The system is equipped with 2 parallel-hole collimators that have a matching (256 hole) pattern to the CdZnTe detector array: a low-energy, high-resolution parallel-hole (LEHR) collimator fabricated of lead and a low-energy, high-sensitivity parallel hole (LEHS) collimator fabricated of tungsten.

Performance measurements and the data analysis were done according to the procedures of the NEMA standard. The long-term stability of the system was evaluated with continuous use and variations in ambient temperature.

Results.—Intrinsic energy resolution was 8.6% FWHM at 141 keV. Linearity was excellent between photopeaks and the known gamma ray energies for the given isotopes. For the central field of view, the integral uniformity and the differential uniformity were, respectively, 1.6% and 1.3% for the LEHR collimator; for the LEHS collimator, these rates were 1.9% and 1.2%.

The full-width at half-maximum measurements taken at the surface of the collimator were 2.2 mm for LEHR and 2.9 mm for LEHS. The average S/N ratios (counts in the irradiated pixel divided by counts in surrounding pixels) for the inner ring pixels (8)/outer ring pixels (16) were 3.2%/0.2% using the LEHS collimator and 3.7%/0.3% for the LEHR collimator. It was not possible to ascertain the maximum count rate and the 20% loss count rate from these data since the plateau was not reached while using the solutions measured.

TABLE 1.—eZ SCOPE Specifications

Outer Dimensions	77 mm H×73 mm W×212 mm L
Detector	CdZnTe (thickness 5 mm)
Weight	820 g
Total no. of pixels	256 (16×16 array)
Pixel size	1.85×1.85 mm
Field of view	32×32 mm
Measuring source	γ-ray
Energy Range measured	71 (^{201}Tl)~364 (^{131}I) keV

(Courtesy of Abe A, Takahashi N, Lee J, et al: Performance evaluation of a hand-held, semiconductor (CdZnTe)-based gamma camera. *Eur J Nucl Med Mol Imaging* 30:805-811, 2003.)

Average acquisitions were 11,052 cpm/MBq (LEHR) and 28,590 cpm/MBq (LEHS). The system exhibited minimum corresponding shift in cps with temperature changes in the measured temperature range.

Conclusion.—The basic performance of this camera compared favorably with gamma camera technology used today. The most important differences include spatial resolution, sensitivity, high count rate characteristics, and energy resolution. This device should be useful in several clinical applications, including sentinel node detection and radio-pharmaceutical–guided surgery.

► Semiconductors continue to hold the promise of replacing scintillator crystals with photomultiplier tube readout. However, disappointingly few cameras have actually been built utilizing these potentially new-generation detector systems. This article does a good job of covering all of the important characteristics required of an imaging camera and how CdZnTe excels compared to scintillator-based cameras. This helps us to keep our hopes up that in the future, semiconductor nuclear medicine cameras may be commonplace.

I. G. Zubal, PhD

Dosimetry of the Dopamine Transporter Radioligand ^{18}F-FPCIT in Human Subjects

Robeson W, Dhawan V, Belakhlef A, et al (North Shore Univ Hosp, Manhasset, NY)

J Nucl Med 44:961-966, 2003 1–16

Background.—N-(3-^{18}F-fluoropropyl-2β-carbomethoxy-3β-(4-iodophenyl)nortropane (^{18}F-FPCIT) is a new dopamine transporter radioligand de-

TABLE 4.—Radiation Dose Estimates for Reference Adult

Target Organ	Total Dose mGy/MBq	rad/mCi	Primary Contributor	(%)	Secondary Contributor	(%)
Urinary bladder wall	5.86E-02	2.17E-01	Urinary bladder	97.2	Remainder of body	2.8
Lungs	1.92E-02	7.09E-02	Lungs	100		
Liver	1.86E-02	6.89E-02	Liver	100		
Small intestine	1.84E-02	6.82E-02	Small intestine	91.1	Remainder of body	8.9
ULI wall	1.84E-02	6.82E-02	ULI	91.1	Remainder of body	8.9
Spleen	1.02E-02	3.78E-02	Spleen	100		
Heart wall	8.20E-03	3.03E-02	Heart wall	100		
Brain	8.11E-03	3.00E-02	Brain	100		
Bone surfaces	6.74E-03	2.49E-02	Trabecular bone	72.8	Remainder of body	27.2
LLI wall	6.63E-03	2.45E-02	LLI	75.2	Remainder of body	24.8
Red marrow	5.11E-03	1.89E-02	Trabecular bone	50.7	Remainder of body	49.3
Kidneys	4.82E-03	1.78E-02	Kidneys	100		
Ovaries	3.29E-03	1.22E-02	Remainder of body	100		
Testes	3.29E-03	1.22E-02	Remainder of body	100		
Total body	4.40E-03	1.63E-02	Remainder of body	68.0	Liver	11.0
Effective dose	mSv/MBq	rem/mCi				
equivalent	1.20E-02	4.44E-02	Remainder of body	62.2	Lungs	19.2

Abbreviations: ULI, Upper large intestine; *LLI*, lower large intestine.

(Reprinted by permission of the Society of Nuclear Medicine from Robeson W, Dhawan V, Belakhlef A, et al: Dosimetry of the dopamine transporter radioligand ^{18}F-FPCIT in human subjects. *J Nucl Med* 44:961-966, 2003.)

veloped to study dopaminergic function. The radiation dosimetry of this new radiopharmaceutical was determined for humans.

Methods.—Six subjects underwent dynamic PET scans of the urinary bladder. Two had brain scans, and 5 had thoracic or abdominal scans. To obtain time-activity curves, the regions of interest were placed over composite images of each organ for which activity was visualized.

Findings.—The urinary bladder wall was the critical organ for dosimetry, with a mean dose of 0.0586 mGy/MBq. The dose resulted mainly from activity in the urinary bladder contents. This dose was lower than any of the other agents commonly used in PET to evaluate dopaminergic function. The effective dose equivalent was 0.0120 mGy/MBq, which was also lower than comparable compounds (Table 4).

Conclusion.—Compared with other agents used to assess dopaminergic function, ^{18}F-FPCIT has a favorable dosimetry. Adults may be given doses as high as 853 MBq and these doses remain within accepted guidelines.

▶ Here again we see the estimated doses for a fluorinated neuroreceptor ligand, this time for the dopamine transporter. Again, as in Abstract 1–17 the urinary bladder wall appears as the critical organ. This reminds us again that we should always instruct patients to drink plenty of liquids, which helps to lower the absorbed dose to this (and other) organs.

I. G. Zubal, PhD

Biodistribution and Radiation Dosimetry of ^{18}F-Fluoro-A-85380 in Healthy Volunteers

Bottlaender M, Valette H, Roumenov D, et al (French Atomic Agency, Orsay, France; Institut Gustave Roussy, Villejuif, France)

J Nucl Med 44:596-601, 2003 1–17

Background.—Several neurodegenerative diseases are characterized by degeneration of cells containing nicotinic acetylcholine receptors (nAChRs). Developing radiolabeled tracers appropriate as PET ligands for imagin nAChRs is therefore an important goal. The biodistribution and radiation dosimetry of ^{18}F-fluoro-A-85380, a promising radioligand for imaging of central nAChRs, were reported.

Methods.—Three healthy men volunteered for the study. Whole-body scans were performed up to 2 hours after IV injection of 137 to 238 Mbq ^{18}F-fluoro-A-85380. Transmission scans in 2-dimensional mode were used subsequently to correct attenuation of emission scans. Emission scans were obtained over 2 hours. Venous blood samples were obtained and urine was collected freely up to 2 hours after radiotracer injection.

The percentage of injected activity measured in regions of interest in brain, intestine, stomach, bladder, kidneys, and liver was fitted to a monoexponential model as an uptake phase followed by a monoexponential washout, or to a biexponential model to produce time-activity curves for each volunteer.

TABLE 3.—Mean Radiation Absorbed Dose Estimates (mGy/MBq) for ^{18}F-Fluoro-A-85380

Target Organ	Subject 1	Subject 2	Subject 3	Mean ± SD
Adrenals	1.49E-02	1.37E-02	1.60E-02	1.49E-02 ± 1.15E-03
Brain	1.29E-02	1.13E-02	1.43E-02	1.28E-02 ± 1.50E-03
Gallbladder wall	1.82E-02	1.62E-02	1.89E-02	1.78E-02 ± 1.40E-03
LLI wall	3.67E-02	3.24E-02	2.95E-02	3.29E-02 ± 3.62E-03
Small intestine	3.69E-02	2.49E-02	2.37E-02	2.85E-02 ± 7.30E-03
Stomach	1.22E-02	1.19E-02	1.35E-02	1.25E-02 ± 8.50E-04
ULI wall	4.01E-02	2.85E-02	2.77E-02	3.21E-02 ± 6.94E-03
Heart wall	1.11E-02	1.12E-02	1.30E-02	1.18E-02 ± 1.07E-03
Kidneys	5.25E-02	3.90E-02	4.75E-02	4.63E-02 ± 6.83E-03
Liver	3.90E-02	3.07E-02	4.06E-02	3.68E-02 ± 5.31E-03
Lungs	9.99E-03	9.99E-03	1.16E-02	1.05E-02 ± 9.30E-04
Muscle	1.00E-02	1.06E-02	1.12E-02	1.06E-02 ± 6.00E-04
Pancreas	1.45E-02	1.37E-02	1.58E-02	1.47E-02 ± 1.06E-03
Red marrow	2.74E-02	2.02E-02	2.06E-02	2.27E-02 ± 4.05E-03
Bone surfaces	1.95E-02	1.58E-02	1.68E-02	1.74E-02 ± 1.91E-03
Skin	7.28E-03	7.71E-03	8.55E-03	7.85E-03 ± 6.46E-04
Spleen	2.18E-02	1.82E-02	2.11E-02	2.04E-02 ± 1.91E-03
Testes	9.27E-03	1.13E-02	1.07E-02	1.04E-02 ± 1.04E-03
Thyroid	8.85E-03	9.34E-03	1.07E-02	9.63E-03 ± 9.58E-04
Urine bladder wall	6.16E-02	1.39E-01	4.49E-02	8.18E-02 ± 5.02E-02
Total body	1.19E-02	1.17E-02	1.26E-02	1.21E-02 ± 4.73E-04

Note: Figures are in milligrays per megabecquerel.

Abbreviations: LLI, Lower large intestine; *ULI,* upper large intestine.

(Reprinted by permission of the Society of Nuclear Medicine from Bottlaender M, Valette H, Roumenov D, et al: Biodistribution and radiation dosimetry of ^{18}F-fluoro-A-85380 in healthy volunteers. *J Nucl Med* 44:596-601, 2003.)

Radiation-absorbed doses for body organs were estimated considering 10 source organs.

Findings.—The volunteers tolerated ^{18}F-fluoro-A-85380 injection well. Blood and urine parameters did not change significantly. The main routes of clearance were renal and intestinal. Activity was high in the bladder, kidneys, and liver 10 minutes after injection. Uptake was slow in the brain. The highest absorbed dose was documented in the liver. The estimated mean effective ^{18}F-fluoro-A-85380 dose was 0.0194 mSv/MBq (Table 3).

Conclusions.—These data suggest that ^{18}F-fluoro-A-85380 is a safe tracer clinically and biologically. The biodistribution of this agent showed high, stable brain uptake. The dosimetry of ^{18}F-fluoro-A-85380 appears favorable for clinical PET imaging. This tracer is now ready for testing on patients with neurodegenerative disease.

► Clearly, brain imaging has moved from perfusion and metabolism imaging into a more exciting direction of neuroreceptor imaging. Often new tracers are first developed for PET imaging. From the dosimetry point of view, this agent for imaging the nAChR shows the similarity with FDG in that the urine bladder wall is the critical organ.

I. G. Zubal, PhD

Biodistribution and Radiation Dosimetry of [^{123}I]ADAM in Healthy Human Subjects: Preliminary Results

Kauppinen TA, Bergström KA, Heikman P, et al (Helsinki Univ; MAP Med Technologies Oy, Helsinki)

Eur J Nucl Med 30:132-136, 2003 1–18

Background.—[^{123}I]ADAM, with a high specificity for serotonin transporters (SERT), is a very promising imaging ligand for detecting these transporters. To date, [^{123}I]ADAM has been studied only in animal models. Its radiation dosimetry and biodistribution were investigated in a study of healthy human volunteers.

Methods.—Eleven subjects underwent serial whole-body imaging up to 24 hours following administration of 157 to 220 MBq [^{123}I]ADAM. Absorbed radiation disease for body organs was estimated, with 12 source organs under consideration.

Findings.—The greatest absorbed organ doses were to the lower large intestine wall, at 8.3×10^{-2} mGy/MBq; the kidneys, at 5.2×10^{-2} mGy/MBq; the urinary bladder wall, at 4.9×10^{-2} mGy/MBq; and the thyroid, at 4.3×10^{-2} mGy/MBq. The estimated effective dose was 2.2×10^{-2} mGy/MBq (Table 2).

Conclusion.—These data show that [^{123}I]ADAM may be a useful tracer for SPECT of serotonin receptors in humans. The dosimetry is acceptable, and brain uptake is high.

► Here we see a SPECT agent for imaging serotonin receptors, demonstrating that development of SPECT-based neuroreceptor agents continues to be an active subfield in nuclear medicine and that SPECT brain imaging can hold its own compared to PET.

I. G. Zubal, PhD

TABLE 2.—Radiation Dose Estimates for [^{123}I]ADAM: Absorbed Doses for Different Target Organs

Organ	Radiation Dose [mean±SD (mGy/MBq)]
Brain	$(4.02\pm0.77)\cdot10^{-3}$
Gallbladder wall	$(3.06\pm2.09)\cdot10^{-2}$
LLI wall	$(8.30\pm8.86)\cdot10^{-2}$
Small intestine	$(1.18\pm0.76)\cdot10^{-2}$
ULI wall	$(3.31\pm2.52)\cdot10^{-2}$
Heart wall	$(1.25\pm0.72)\cdot10^{-2}$
Kidneys	$(5.15\pm0.88)\cdot10^{-2}$
Liver	$(7.00\pm3.82)\cdot10^{-3}$
Lungs	$(2.71\pm0.52)\cdot10^{-2}$
Thyroid	$(4.28\pm3.22)\cdot10^{-2}$
Urinary bladder wall	$(4.91\pm0.64)\cdot10^{-2}$
Total body	$(3.89\pm0.69)\cdot10^{-3}$

Abbreviations: LLI, Lower large intestine; *ULI*, upper large intestine.

(Courtesy of Kauppinen T, Bergström KA, Heikman P, et al: Biodistribution and radiation dosimetry of [^{123}I]ADAM in healthy human subjects: Preliminary results. *Eur J Nucl Med* 30:132-136, 2003. Copyright Springer-Verlag.)

MIRD Pamphlet No 19: Absorbed Fractions and Radionuclide S Values for Six Age-Dependent Multiregion Models of the Kidney

Bouchet LG, Bolch WE, Blanco HP, et al (Univ of Florida, Gainesville; Case Western Reserve Univ, Cleveland, Ohio; Nuclear Physics Enterprises, Cherry Hill, NJ; et al)

J Nucl Med 44:1113-1147, 2003 1–19

Introduction.—Since the kidneys act as the major excretory organ of the body, radioactivity uptake and local tissue irradiation are consistently seen in this organ. The liver and spleen concentrate radioactive materials fairly uniformly at the macroscopic level. Because of their unique physiology, the kidneys appear to concentrate radioactivity nonuniformly. Current single-region dosimetric models of the kidneys force the assumption of a uniform distribution of radioactivity across the entire organ. The average absorbed dose to the kidneys predicted by these models may misrepresent local regional doses to specific substructures. To assist in suborgan dosimetry for the kidneys, 6 new age-dependent multiregion kidney models were discussed.

Methods.—The outer dimensions of the models conform to those currently used in single-region kidney models. Interior structures are defined for the renal cortex, the medullary pyramids with papillae (2 vertical and 3 horizontal), and the renal pelvis. Absorbed fractions of energy were determined for both photon and electron sources (10keV to 4 MeV) located in each source region within the 6 age-dependent models. The absorbed fractions were used to construct S values for radionuclides of potential interest in suborgan kidney dosimetry.

Results.—In adults, the absorbed dose to the renal cortex for ^{90}Y-labeled compounds retained within that subregion is approximately 1.3 times that predicted by the single-region kidney model; the medullary dose is 26% of that same single-region value. For compounds that are rapidly filtered in the kidneys, the renal cortex dose is about one half of that predicted under the single-region model. The tissues of the medullary pyramids receive an absorbed dose 1.5 to 1.8 times greater.

Conclusion.—The multiregion model described allows estimates of regional kidney doses not previously supported by the current single-region models. Full utilization of the new model necessitates serial imaging of the kidneys with regions of interest assigned to the renal cortex and medulla.

▶ The encouraging trend in dose estimations in nuclear medicine is to be more patient specific and realistic when modeling the geometry of internal organs. The mathematical model illustrated here closely approximates the important internal substructures of the kidneys and therefore gives a very important update on expected radiation burdens associated with various radiotracers. This article contains 24 pages tabulating S values of the major renal substructures for adults and children of various ages. I photocopied these pages and added them to my copy of NM/MIRD Pamphlet No 11. It is truly an important and useful update.

I. G. Zubal, PhD

2 Radiopharmaceutical

Introduction

Although instruments are critical to imaging, it is the radiopharmaceutical that allows us to look at pathophysiology. Advances are made when the kinetics of molecules designed to fit into specific receptors are studied. This year there have been a number of new agents described. The following sections highlight a few of the major advances that have been made.

Villegagne and colleagues describe the presence of opioid receptors in human myocardium. The specific role of these receptors in the myocardium is unknown. However in other systems, these agents alter the production of cytokines and modify the response of inflammatory cells. If the receptors play a similar role in the myocardium the opioid system may play an important role in myocarditis, transplant rejection, heart failure, or even the apoptosis associated with myocardial infarction.

Experiments with tracer adenosine provided an unexpected outcome, identifying the distribution of perfusion with this tracer. It is interesting to consider the potential of using this agent for imaging. The rapid catabolism of the molecule would require immediate imaging. However, the rapid catabolism could be helpful, because the myocardial concentration returns to 'background' levels quickly. This would allow multiple determinations of perfusion in the course of a single stress test. Multiple measurements would allow determination of the site(s) of onset of ischemia and the pattern of propagation in the myocardium.

The discussion of two glucose analogs, C-11 glucose and FDG provides a striking contrast in kinetics. The concentration of C-11 glucose in the cell is constantly changing, as the molecule traverses the multitude of pathways available for glucose catabolism. C-11 glucose requires dynamic imaging and metabolic models to use the information effectively. FDG, on the other hand, is straightforward to image, and is most useful to define the putative utilization of glucose by the tissue. Although many assumptions are made about the meaning of FDG concentration in tissue, the quality of the images and relative simplicity of data acquisition make the imaging extremely valuable.

Specific imaging of hypoxia is a major area of interest because of the role of low oxygen tension in tissue viability. In the brain and heart, identifying ischemic but viable tissue is important to define specific treatment regimens to reduce tissue oxygen requirements while restoring adequate oxygen supplies to the tissue. In tumors, identifying hypoxia is important because of the resistance of hypoxic tissue to therapy. Detection of hypoxia is complicated by the difficulty delivering the tracers to sites of low perfusion. The quality of images recorded with generator produced Copper ATSM, however, appear significantly better than those recorded with other agents.

Therapy is a growing area of nuclear medicine. Although many agents are available to treat patients with painful bone metastasis, they all require patients to have an acceptable platelet count before treatment. An agent that minimized marrow exposure is desirable, because it would allow offer a greater safety margin. Bone seeking alpha emitting nuclides distributing primarily in bone mineral, sparing adjacent marrow. Radium 223, with its cascade decay, is under investigation for this purpose.

H. W. Strauss, MD

PET Imaging of Human Cardiac Opioid Receptors

Villemagne PSR, Dannals RF, Ravert HT, et al (Johns Hopkins Univ, Baltimore, Md)

Eur J Nucl Med 29:1385-1388, 2002 2–1

Background.—Endogenous opioids affect cardiac function by direct interaction with different types of opioid receptors and by way of their inhibitory effects on autonomic traffic at increased cardiac work. Previous studies in the mammalian heart have shown that these opioids modulate myocardial contraction and action potentials and have a role in heart failure, ischemic preconditioning, reperfusion arrhythmias, and myocardial ischemia. The purpose of the present study was to image μ and δ opioid receptors in the human heart using PET.

Methods.—PET scanning of the chest was performed in 3 women and 2 men with a median age of 65 ±8 years. Scanning was performed with ^{11}C-carfentanil (CFN) and ^{11}C-*N*-methyl-naltrindole (MeNTI), and the images were analyzed for indications of opioid receptor binding in the heart. Either ^{11}C-CFN or ^{11}C-MeNTI (20 mCi) was injected IV, and dynamic images were obtained over 90 minutes. For the blocking studies, either 0.2 mg/kg or 1 mg/kg of naloxone was injected 5 minutes before the injection of ^{11}C-CFN and ^{11}C-MeNTI, respectively. Regions of interest were indicated over the left ventricle, left ventricular chamber, lung, and skeletal muscle.

Results.—Graphical analysis demonstrated average baseline myocardial binding potentials of 4.37 ±0.91 with ^{11}C-CFN and 3.86 ±0.60 with ^{11}C-MeNTI. The administration of 0.2 mg/kg of naloxone before injection of ^{11}C-CFN produced a 25% reduction in binding potentials in 1 patient compared with baseline values, and a 19% decrease in myocardial distribution volume. The administration of 1 mg/kg of naloxone before ^{11}C-MeNTI in another subject produced a 14% decrease in binding potentials and a 21% decrease in the myocardial distribution volume.

Conclusion.—The μ and δ opioid receptors can be imaged in vivo with PET. PET imaging of cardiac opioid receptors may facilitate a greater understanding of their involvement in cardiovascular pathophysiology and how heart function is affected by the abuse of opioids and drugs.

► This is intriguing work, suggesting the presence of opioid receptors in the heart. Future studies need to be done to define the importance of these receptors in the myocardium and the relation of changes in myocardial uptake to traditional hemodynamic parameters such as heart rate and blood pressure.

H. W. Strauss, MD

An Artifical Amino Acid, 4-Iodo-L-*meta*-Tyrosine: Biodistribution and Excretion via Kidney

Shikano N, Kawai K, Flores LG II, et al (Ibaraki Prefectural Univ, Japan; Kanazawa Univ, Ishikawa, Japan; Miyazaki Med College, Japan; et al)
J Nucl Med 44:625-631, 2003 2–2

Purpose.—Various diseases are associated with alterations of amino acid transport. Tyrosine derivatives have been investigated as tracers for clinical and research purposes. Radiolabeled 4-iodo-L-*meta*-tyrosine was assessed as a new amino acid transport marker. The pharmacologic characteristics of this compound, particularly the biodistribution and excretion, were investigated by performing in vivo and in vitro studies with 4-^{125}I-iodo-L-*meta*-tyrosine (4-^{125}I-*m*Tyr, Fig 1).

Methods.—In vivo biodistribution and excretion studies of 4-^{125}I-*m*Tyr were performed in male ddY mice. The findings were compared with those of L-^{14}C-Tyr and 3-^{125}I-iodo-α-methyl-L-tyrosine (^{125}I-IMT).

Results.—The new tracer showed good pancreatic and renal accumulation, with brain uptake similar to that of ^{125}I-IMT (Table 1). However, 4-^{125}I-*m*Tyr was cleared from the blood significantly faster than ^{125}I-IMT. More than 70% of 4-^{125}I-*m*Tyr was excreted in urine within 3 hours, with less than 5% detected in feces. On autoradiography, the renal cortex showed only moderate accumulation of 4-^{125}I-*m*Tyr, compared with high accumulation of ^{125}I-IMT. Renal accumulation and excretion of both tracers were significantly reduced by probenecid. Thirty minutes after injection, intact free 4-^{125}I-*m*Tyr accounted for more than 98% of the total amount of tracer in the kid-

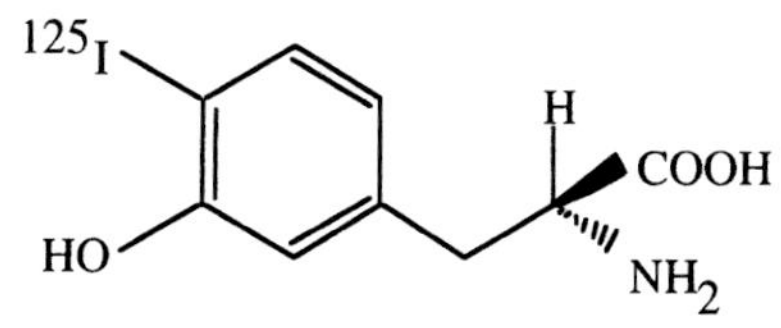

4-[^{125}I]iodo-L-*meta*-tyrosine (4-^{125}I-*m*Tyr)

FIGURE 1.—Chemical structure of 4-^{125}I-*m*Tyr. (Reprinted by permission of the Society of Nuclear Medicine, courtesy of Shikano N, Kawai K, Flores LG II, et al: An artificial amino acid, 4-iodo-L-*meta*-tyrosine: Biodistribution and excretion via kidney. *J Nucl Med* 44:625-631, 2003.)

TABLE 1.—Biodistribution of 4-^{125}I-*m*Tyr in Male ddY Mice

Biodistribution	5 Min	15 Min	30 Min
Blood*	3.72 ± 0.40	1.56 ± 0.36	0.45 ± 0.09
Brain	0.61 ± 0.16	0.47 ± 0.07	0.32 ± 0.08
Pancreas	25.44 ± 1.85	14.03 ± 3.69	2.00 ± 0.57
Liver	4.31 ± 0.51	1.80 ± 0.42	0.64 ± 0.16
Stomach	1.24 ± 0.22	1.05 ± 0.37	2.82 ± 2.27
Intestine	2.26 ± 0.29	1.03 ± 0.26	0.56 ± 0.06
Kidney	23.77 ± 4.89	12.89 ± 9.53	4.24 ± 1.92
Heart	2.51 ± 0.33	1.42 ± 0.34	0.92 ± 0.36
Lung	3.76 ± 0.52	1.90 ± 0.41	0.74 ± 0.14
Spleen	4.04 ± 0.64	2.35 ± 1.05	0.54 ± 0.17

All data except blood are expressed as %ID/g tissue, mean ± 1 SD.
*%ID/mL blood (n = 5 mice).
(Reprinted by permission of the Society of Nuclear Medicine, courtesy of Shikano N, Kawai K, Flores LG II, et al: An artificial amino acid, 4-iodo-L-*meta*-tyrosine: Biodistribution and excretion via kidney. *J Nucl Med* 44:625-631, 2003.)

ney and more than 96% in the urine, with no evidence of protein incorporation.

In in vitro studies, 4-^{125}I-*m*Tyr uptake by LLC-PK$_1$ cell monolayers was reduced significantly by 5 mmol/L L-Tyr and incubation at 4°C, but reduced by half in the presence of 5 mmol/L D-Tyr. A similar pattern was observed for the 2 comparison tracers, although 0.1 mmol/L 2,4-dinitrophenol—which inhibits generation of energy-rich phosphates—significantly increased ^{125}I-IMT uptake.

Conclusions.—An artificial amino acid transport marker, 4-^{125}I-*m*Tyr, shows good metabolic stability with rapid blood clearance, fast excretion in urine, and biodistribution similar to that of other radiolabeled L-Tyr analoguess. The renal handling of 4-^{125}I-*m*Tyr may make it particularly useful as an amino acid transport marker.

► Nuclear medicine needs tracers of amino acid metabolism to characterize neoplasms and myocardial hypertrophy. Institutions with a radiochemistry program can often synthesize carbon-11–labeled analogues of amino acids. An agent with a longer half-life, however, will be easier to use, and potentially provide higher quality images. The initial distribution of 4-iodo-L-*meta*-tyrosine appears very promising. The rapid concentration of this agent in the kidneys, however, will limit the utility of this agent in the abdomen. The agent may, however, have great potential for characterizing amino acid incorporation in the brain and heart.

H. W. Strauss, MD

Percutaneous Ethanol Injection Plus Radioiodine Versus Radioiodine Alone in the Treatment of Large Toxic Thyroid Nodules

Zingrillo M, Modoni S, Conte M, et al (Scientific Inst "Casa Sollievo della Sofferenza," San Giovanni Rotondo, Italy; Centro di Riferimento Oncologico Regionale della Basilicata, Rionero in Vulture, Italy; Istituto di Clinica Medica Università di Foggia, Italy; et al)

J Nucl Med 44:207-210, 2003 2–3

Introduction.—The treatment modalities for toxic thyroid nodules (TTNs) are thyroidectomy, radioiodine (RAI) ablation, and percutaneous ethanol injection (PEI). Surgery is usually considered in patients with TTNs larger than 4 cm. Some patients may be at high surgical risk. The efficacy of RAI and PEI for TTNs larger than 4 cm in patients for whom surgery may be high risk was examined in a prospective, randomized trial.

Methods.—Twenty-two patients with TTNs larger than 4 cm were randomly assigned to receive 1 of 2 treatments: (1) RAI at a dose of 12,580 kBq/mL of nodular volume (NV) that was corrected for 100% 24-hour ^{131}I uptake (RAIU) (subgroup A), or (2) 2 to 4 sessions of PEI (ethanol injected = 30% NV) followed at 2 months by 24-hour RAIU and RAI dosing (subgroup B). The inclusion criteria were clinical and biochemical hyperthyroidism; a single palpable, hot nodule at ^{99m}Tc scintigraphy; and high surgical risk or refusal to have surgery. Patients provided informed consent. Local symptoms were assessed by a previously validated score (symptom score [SYS]).

Results.—Both RAI and PEI were well tolerated. Subgroup B had a significant decrease in NV at 2 months after PEI (33.6 mL vs 60.8 mL, $P < .05$). The 24-hour RAIU in subgroup B was similar to that of subgroup A (53.9% vs 61.8%). The administration of RAI dose was significantly lower for subgroup B (730 MBq) versus subgroup A (1048 MBq). At 12 months after RAI, subgroup B had a higher decrease in NV and a lower SYS, compared with subgroup A. One patient in subgroup A had subclinical hyperthyroidism, 2 had slightly increased levels of thyroid-stimulating hormone, and 1 was clinically hypothyroid. One patient in subgroup B had a slightly increased level of thyroid-stimulating hormone.

Conclusion.—RAI alone or with PEI can be used as a valid alternative for TTNs larger than 4 cm when surgery is either refused or contraindicated. Also, PEI plus RAI can be used when substantial shrinkage of a nodule is necessary or when reduction of the RAI dose can prevent hospitalization.

▶ The major difference between RAI therapy alone and RAI therapy plus PEI was a difference in nodule size at 12 months. There was greater shrinkage with the combined therapy. This may be helpful in some patients, and the addition of ethanol should be considered when the nodules are large and the patient is not a candidate for surgery.

H. W. Strauss, MD

^{99m}Tc-Aprotinin Scintigraphy in Amyloidosis

Schaadt BK, Hendel HW, Gimsing P, et al (Copenhagen Univ Hosp; Hillerød Sygehus, Denmark; Danish Medicines Agency, Copenhagen)

J Nucl Med 44:177-183, 2003 2–4

Background.—Amyloidosis is a disorder of protein metabolism in which autologous proteins are deposited extracellularly in a characteristic fibrillar manner, resulting in organ impairment that ranges from an initially asymptomatic state to later progressive organ failure and death. Amyloidosis may be focal, localized, or systemic, and the disease may be hereditary or acquired. There is great variation in the rate of progression among patients and in different organs in the same patient. Changes in the amount and distribution of amyloid lesions have been difficult to monitor because they usually are only demonstrable by evident symptoms or by biopsy. Progress in the treatment of amyloidosis in recent years has underscored the need for an early diagnosis of this disease as well as the need for noninvasive monitoring

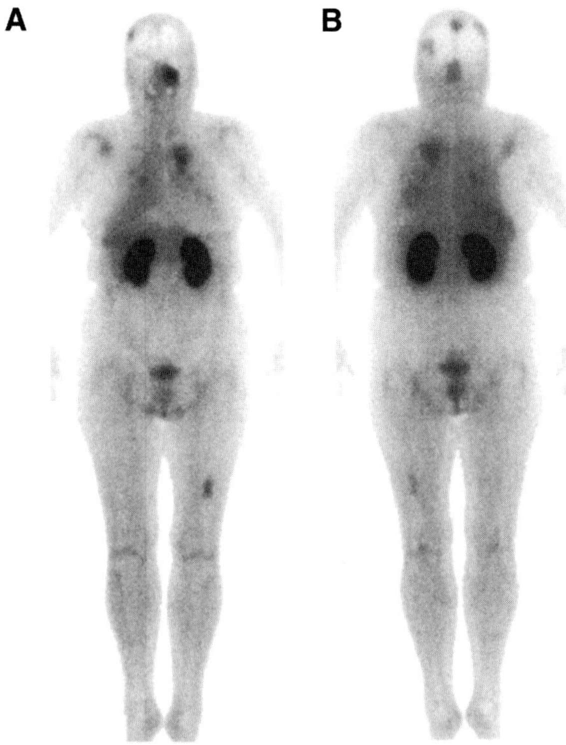

FIGURE 4.—Whole-body scintigram shows pathologic uptake in left maxillary sinus in 78-y-old woman (patient 6) with plasmacytoma. Several accumulations in calvarium, lungs or pleura, left femur, and shoulder are also revealed. Patient had no symptoms from these sites, but physical examination of calvarium revealed palpable masses and biopsy confirmed amyloid. **A**, Anterior view. **B**, Posterior view. (Reprinted by permission of the Society of Nuclear Medicine, from Schaadt BK, Hendel HW, Gimsing P, et al: ^{99m}Tc-aprotinin scintigraphy in amyloidosis. *J Nucl Med* 44:177-183, 2003.)

during treatment. The ability of ^{99m}Tc-aprotinin scintigraphy to determine the extent of amyloid deposits in various organs was determined in patients with known or suspected amyloidosis.

Methods.—^{99m}Tc-aprotinin was injected IV in 23 consecutive patients with known or suspected amyloidosis. Whole-body scans, regional images, and SPECT tomograms were obtained 90 minutes after tracer injection.

Results.—Focal accumulations of ^{99m}Tc-aprotinin were observed in different organs in 22 of 23 patients with a total of 90 lesions, of which 20 lesions were confirmed by biopsy or autopsy (Fig 4). Scintigraphy revealed "silent" amyloid deposits in at least 5 patients in whom clinical symptoms later developed. Physiologic uptake or excretion in the liver and kidneys could not be differentiated from pathologic lesions in these organs.

Conclusions.—^{99m}Tc-aprotinin scintigraphy appears to be an adequately sensitive and specific noninvasive diagnostic technique for patients with suspected amyloidosis. This procedure is minimally stressful to the patient and has the capacity to detect a wide range of lesions.

► This is a very interesting agent. However, the investigators did not do 2 key control studies that would make this work very compelling. First, it would be helpful to know the distribution of the agent in subjects without amyloid. Second, it would be helpful to understand whether other small radiolabeled proteins, such as albumin, also leak into these lesions. The results of both of these controls would help establish the specific value of aprotinin imaging.

H. W. Strauss, MD

Evaluation of ^{18}F–FA-4 and ^{11}C–pipzA-4 as Radioligands for the In Vivo Evaluation of the High-Affinity Choline Uptake System

Gilissen C, de Groot TJ, Bronfman F, et al (Katholieke Universiteit Leuven, Belgium; KULeuven–Campus Gasthuisberg, Leuven, Belgium)

J Nucl Med 44:269-275, 2003 2–5

Background.—The sodium-dependent high-affinity choline uptake (HACU) system is a marker of the functional status of the cholinergic presynaptic terminals. It has been found to be upregulated in the brains of patients with Parkinson disease, whereas the brains of patients with Alzheimer disease have been reported to show both upregulation and downregulation of the HACU system. However, the latter observation may be explained by the observation that activity-related changes in the choline uptake undergo a rapid reversal in postmortem tissues. The gold standard for the study of the HACU system in vitro is hemicholinium-3 (HC-3), a reversible and competitive inhibitor of HACU. However, HC-3 is a quaternary ammonium salt and so cannot cross the blood-brain barrier, and radiolabeled quarternary ammonium HC-3 derivatives cannot be used for in vivo visualization of the HACU transporter. ^{18}F–FA-4 and ^{11}C–pipzA-4 were evaluated as potential in vivo tracers for the HACU system.

Methods.—The biodistribution of ^{18}F–FA-4 and ^{11}C–pipzA-4 was determined in mice, and the intracerebral distribution of both compounds was visualized by ex vivo and in vitro autoradiography. The in vitro affinity of ^{18}F–FA-4 and ^{11}C–pipzA-4 was determined by a displacement study with ^{3}H–HC-3 on mice brain slices.

Results.—Both tracers showed a high and persistent uptake in the mouse brain. In vitro autoradiography showed binding to the striatum, whereas ex vivo autoradiography showed homogeneous binding throughout the brain. ^{18}F–FA-4 and ^{11}C–pipzA-4 inhibited the ^{3}H–HC-3 binding with a 50% inhibitory concentration of 57 nmol/L and 320 nmol/L, respectively.

Conclusions.—These 2 compounds, ^{18}F–FA-4 and ^{11}C–pipzA-4, demonstrated affinity for HACU and showed high uptake in the brain. In vitro binding of the compounds to the striatum cannot be inhibited by the presence of HC-3, and binding of HC-3 is inhibited by the presence of both FA-4 and pipzA-4, which suggests allosteric binding.

► There is a growing need for radiopharmaceuticals to evaluate specific signaling pathways in the brain. This is particularly true for the cholinergic system. It appears that these 2 agents may offer an opportunity to image this system with microPET.

H. W. Strauss, MD

Long-term Efficacy of High-Activity ^{111}In-Pentetreotide Therapy in Patients With Disseminated Neuroendocrine Tumors

Buscombe JR, Caplin ME, Hilson AJW (Royal Free Hosp, London)

J Nucl Med 44:1-6, 2003 2–6

Background.—It has been possible to treat disseminated neuroendocrine tumors (NETs) with targeted therapy by using ^{131}I-metaiodobenzylguanidine (^{131}I-MIBG), which has been shown to have some clinical activity in the 60% of patients who have expression of the amine uptake gene. However, ^{131}I-MIBG therapy cannot be used in patients in whom there is poor uptake or no uptake of ^{131}I-MIBG in the tumor. Patients with progressive metastatic NETs have few therapeutic options. Chemotherapy is toxic and has limited efficacy, and interferon by itself has no tumorcidal properties. There may some benefit to interferon in combination with Sandostatin, but possibly at the cost of significant morbidity. Hepatic artery embolization is reserved for patients with large liver metastases but will not affect extrahepatic disease. Recent studies have shown that ^{111}In-pentetreotide can be administered in activities of up to 5 GBq with minimal toxicity. The efficacy of high-activity ^{111}In-pentetreotide as a therapy for metastatic NETs was investigated retrospectively.

Methods.—The case records of 16 patients who had received high activities of ^{111}In-pentetreotide (with cumulative activities as high as 36.6 GBq) during a 2.5-year period were reviewed. The 8 female and 8 male patients ranged in age from 32 to 76 years. Ten patients had carcinoid tumors, 2 had medullary cell carcinomas of the thyroid, and 1 each had a glucagonoma, gastrinoma, fibrolamellar cancer, and malignant histiocytoma. The minimum number of treatments was one in 2 patients (with activities of 3.1 and 7 GBq), and the maximum was 10 treatments (total, 36.6 GBq). Treatment was administered by an infusion pump and repeated at 4- to 12-week intervals. Patients received an average of 6 treatments per patient. Therapeutic response was determined by changes in the size of the tumor on CT with the use of the response evaluation criteria in solid tumors. Toxicity was determined by means of blood and urine tests of renal, hepatic, thyroid, and bone marrow function. The mean and median time from the last treatment to progression of disease and death (if applicable) was also calculated.

Results.—There was no significant or long-lasting toxicity in any of the patients. At 6 months after the last treatment, 5 patients (30%) had progression of disease, 2 had complete responses, and 3 had partial responses. At 12 months after their last treatment, 9 patients (56%) had disease progression, and at 18 months after the last treatment, 11 patients (69%) had disease progression. The mean progression-free survival was 12.25 months. For patients who survived 6 months after their last treatment, the mean survival was 15.75 months. At the 6-month assessment point, there had been 3 deaths (19%), 1 of which was not related to cancer. There was 1 additional death at 12 months and 3 additional deaths at 18 months, 1 of which was not related to the patient's carcinoid tumor but to a second coexistent cancer. Seven patients (44%) had died by the end of the 18-month assessment period (Table 2).

Conclusions.—In patients with disseminated NETs, treatment with high-activity ^{111}In-pentreotide provided some benefit in 70% of patients for at

TABLE 2.—Results of Treatment

Patient No.	Tumor Type	Total Activity (GBq)	Response (RECIST)	Progression-Free Period (mo)	Death (mo)
1	MCT	11.4	CR	None	Alive
2	Carcinoid	15.2	DS	8	10
3	Carcinoid	36.6	DS	18	Alive
4	Carcinoid	18.1	DS	12	18
5	Carcinoid	33.6	PR	None	Alive
6	Carcinoid	3.1	DP	1	1*
7	Carcinoid	16.7	DP	2	3
8	Gastrinoma	12.5	DS	16	Alive
9	Carcinoid	24.4	DS	8	14*
10	Carcinoid	21.1	PR	None	Alive
11	MCT	10.5	CR	None	Alive
12	Carcinoid	14.8	DP	2	4
13	Glucagonoma	11.6	DS	8	Alive
14	Carcinoid	23.0	DS	None	Alive
15	Fibrolamellar	12.2	DP	2	15
16	Malignant histiocytoma	7	PR	14	Alive

*Patients died from cause other than tumor for which they were being treated.

Abbreviations: RECIST, Response evaluation criteria in solid tumors; *MCT*, medullary carcinoma of the thyroid; *CR*, complete response; *DS*, disease stability; *PR*, partial response; *DP*, disease progression.

(Reprinted by permission of the Society of Nuclear Medicine, from Buscombe JR, Caplin ME, Hilson AJW: Long-term efficacy of high-activity ^{111}In-pentetreotide therapy in patients with disseminated neuroendocrine tumors. *J Nucl Med* 44:1-6, 2003.)

least 6 months after the end of treatment. However, 31% of patients will obtain a sustained benefit at 18 months from this treatment without significant toxicity.

▶ This is a good step forward, but not necessarily the best that can be done. Other radiolabels, such as yttrium, may be better suited for therapy. In addition, if an approach could be found to effectively block the kidneys, the administered dose can be increased.

H. W. Strauss, MD

In Vivo Detection of Cell Death in the Area at Risk in Acute Myocardial Infarction

Thimister PWL, Hofstra L, Liem IH, et al (Univ Hosp Maastricht, The Netherlands)

J Nucl Med 44:391-396, 2003 2–7

Background.—Annexin A5, a phospholipid-binding protein with high affinity for phosphatidyl serine, is externalized by cells undergoing programmed cell death. After myocardial infarction (MI), programmed cell death rates in the heart are increased. Annexin A5 uptake in vivo was localized, and the area at risk in humans with acute MI was determined.

Methods.—Nine patients participated in the study. ^{99m}Tc-sestamibi was injected IV before reperfusion, and myocardial ^{99m}Tc-sestamibi perfusion scintigraphy was done after reperfusion. ^{99m}Tc-labeled annexin A5 was then given IV, and scintigraphic images of the heart were obtained. One to 3 weeks after the onset of MI, myocardial ^{99m}Tc-sestamibi scintigraphy was repeated. In 2 patients, ^{99m}Tc-annexin uptake was assessed in the subacute MI phase.

Findings.—Perfusion defects on ^{99m}Tc-sestamibi scintigraphy concordant with the infarct location were evident in all patients. All patients also demonstrated ^{99m}Tc-annexin A5 accumulation at the infarct site, indicating the presence of cardiomyocytes with externalized phosphatidyl serine in the infarct area. The ^{99m}Tc-sestamibi defects seen 1 to 3 weeks after the onset of MI were significantly smaller than those seen in the acute phase. The 2 patients assessed in the subacute phase showed no ^{99m}Tc-annexin uptake.

Conclusions.—Increased programmed cell death in acute MI can be localized correctly in vivo in the area at risk. The decrease seen in ^{99m}Tc-sestamibi defect size in the subacute phase of the MI further suggests that reversible myocardial damage, instead of necrosis, is present in cardiomyocytes in parts of the at-risk area.

▶ A new "hot spot" agent. Although there are relatively few infarcts that are not detectable by enzymes or troponin, "seeing" the site and extent of the lesion may be helpful in selecting patients for specific therapies.

H. W. Strauss, MD

Targeting of Osseous Sites With α-Emitting ^{223}Ra: Comparison With the β-Emitter ^{89}Sr in Mice

Henriksen G, Fisher DR, Roeske JC, et al (Univ of Oslo, Norway; Anticancer Therapeutic Inventions AS, Oslo, Norway; Pacific Northwest Natl Lab, Richland, Wash; et al)

J Nucl Med 44:252-259, 2003 2–8

Background.—Bone-targeting pharmaceuticals, such as the β-emitters ^{32}P orthophosphate and ^{89}Sr (as strontium chloride), are widely used for the relief of bone pain in patients with metastatic lesions in the skeleton. However, toxicity to the normal bone marrow cells is a major dose-limiting factor with this therapeutic approach. Preclinical animal studies and radiation dose estimates indicate that α-particle radiation should be excellent for the treatment of metastatic cancers. The bone-seeking property and the potential exposure of red marrow by the α-emitter ^{223}Ra were compared with those of the β-emitter ^{89}Sr in mice.

Methods.—The biodistributions of ^{223}Ra and ^{89}Sr were studied in young male BALB/c mice. The animals were killed, and tissue uptake was determined at 1 and 6 hours, 1 day, 3 days, and 14 days after IV administration, and radiation-absorbed doses were calculated for soft tissues and bone. In addition, multicellular-level doses were estimated for bone marrow cavities.

Results.—Both ^{89}Sr and ^{223}Ra selectively concentrated on bone surfaces relative to soft tissues. However, ^{223}Ra showed slightly higher bone uptake than that of ^{89}Sr. At 24 hours, the femur uptake of ^{223}Ra was 40.1% ± 7.7% of the administered activity per gram of tissue. ^{223}Ra uptake in the spleen and most other soft tissues was higher than uptake of ^{89}Sr. Predominant clearance of ^{223}Ra was observed from the soft tissues within the first 24 hours, but the bone uptake of ^{223}Ra, which was not significantly different from maximum after only 1 hour, was not significantly reduced during the 14 days. In addition, there was little redistribution of ^{223}Ra daughter products away from bone. Estimates of the dose to marrow cavities showed that the ^{223}Ra α-emitter might have a marrow-sparing advantage in comparison with β-emitters for targeting of osteoid surfaces, because the short-range α-particles irradiate a significantly lower fraction of the marrow volumes, while the bone surfaces receive a therapeutically effective dose of radiation.

Conclusions.—^{223}Ra is a promising candidate for high-linear-energy transfer α-particle irradiation of cancer cells on bone surfaces. Together with its daughter radionuclides, ^{223}Ra can deliver an intense and highly localized radiation dose to the bone surfaces with significantly less irradiation of healthy bone marrow in comparison with standard bone-seeking β-emitting radiopharmaceuticals.

► Radium is a bone-seeking nuclide. The dosimetry from α-radiation should be far more effective than β-radiation, and have much less marrow toxicity. The early renal uptake, however, may limit the utility of this agent.

H. W. Strauss, MD

Tracer Adenosine: A Novel Myocardial Flow Marker

Lauer T, Loncar R, Deussen A (Heinrich-Heine-Universität, Düsseldorf, Germany; TU Dresden, Germany)

J Nucl Med 44:641-648, 2003 2–9

Introduction.—The direct assessment of regional myocardial blood flow is of great importance in both experimental and clinical settings, but there is a lack of useful flow markers. Findings of animal studies suggest that tracer amounts of labeled adenosine may serve as a powerful flow marker. The hypothesis that the local deposition density of labeled adenosine within the heart reflects local myocardial blood flow was tested in an experimental study.

Methods.—Tracer microspheres, the standard for local blood flow measurement, were injected and compared with simultaneously injected adenosine in tracer concentration. The tracers were injected into the left atrium of 7 anesthetized beagle dogs. Myocardial deposition densities were determined through β-scintillation and γ-counting measurements in samples of an average wet mass of 487 mg. In 3 experiments, alprostadil was infused into the left circumflex artery to challenge local myocardial blood flow.

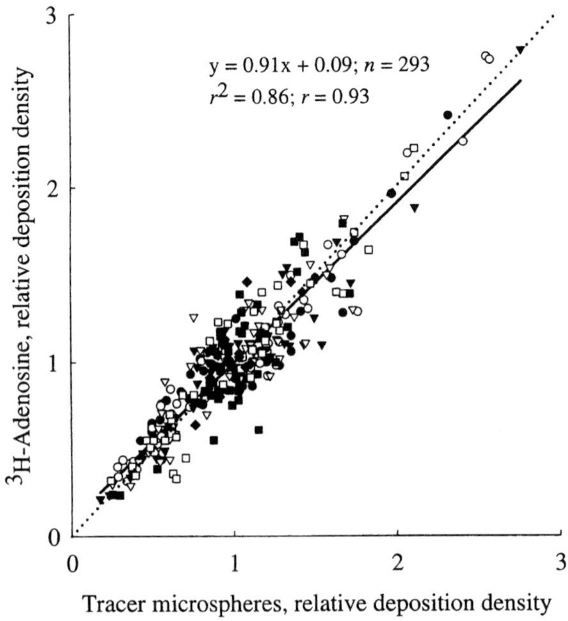

FIGURE 2.—Relationship between relative deposition densities of coinjected tracer microspheres and ^{3}H-adenosine in left ventricular free wall during either control conditions, EHNA infusion, or alprostadil infusion. To facilitate comparison of different experiments, absolute flow values were normalized with respect to average deposition densities. Linear regression analysis was performed for all data points (*solid line*). *Dotted line* is line of identity. *Abbreviation: EHNA*, Erythro-9-hydroxy-nonyl-adenine. (Reprinted by permission of the Society of Nuclear Medicine, from Lauer T, Loncar R, Deussen A: Tracer adenosine: A novel myocardial flow marker. *J Nucl Med* 44:641-648, 2003.)

Erythro-9-hydroxy-nonyl-adenine (EHNA) was infused in 2 other experiments to inhibit degradation of injected adenosine to inosine.

Results.—At the doses applied, systemic vasoactive effects were not produced by the injection of labeled microspheres, adenosine, or EHNA. Tracer adenosine and microspheres were both almost completely extracted from blood within 2 minutes and locally retained in the tissue. The deposition densities of tracer adenosine and microspheres were closely correlated in the experiments over a wide range of local myocardial blood flows (Fig 2).

Conclusion.—Because of its ability to explain local blood flow as measured with the tracer microsphere with 86% probability, adenosine was a reliable myocardial flow marker in dog myocardium. First-pass extraction of adenosine is nearly complete, and therefore a sophisticated mathematic-model analysis is not required for assessment of regional blood flow. In addition, adenosine may be labeled with various stable isotopes or radioisotopes and used with a variety of imaging techniques.

► This is a marvelous and unexpected result. Although there are transporters of adenosine, which result in adenosine uptake in myocardium, there are also significant concentrations of circulating adenosine deaminase, and a substantial "sink" where adenosine is concentrated in red blood cells, both of which could lead to rapid loss of the agent before presentation to the myocardium. However, the data in this study demonstrate striking myocardial uptake.

H. W. Strauss, MD

Comparison of 1-^{11}C-Glucose and ^{18}F-FDG for Quantifying Myocardial Glucose Use With PET

Herrero P, Sharp TL, Dence C, et al (Washington Univ, St Louis)

J Nucl Med 43:1530-1541, 2002 2–10

Background.—Quantification of the rate of myocardial glucose use (rMGU) is essential to a better understanding of normal cardiac development and physiology as well as a variety of cardiac disease processes such as myocardial ischemia, left ventricular hypertrophy, and cardiomyopathy. ^{18}F-FDG PET has been the most commonly used method for noninvasive quantification of rMGU. A previous study by this group reported that rMGU could be quantified by using PET with glucose radiolabeled in the 1-carbon position with ^{11}C (1-^{11}C-glucose). The accuracy of the rate of rMGU measured by using PET and 1-^{11}C-glucose was compared with the rate measured by using PET and the more conventional tracer ^{18}F-FDG.

Methods.—PET measurements of myocardial tracer uptake (K, in mL/g/min) and rMGU (in nmol/g/min) were obtained in 21 dogs with ^{18}F-FDG (using kinetic modeling) and 1-^{11}C-glucose (using the Patlak graphical method). Eighteen of the dogs were studied during hyperinsulinemic-euglycemic clamp performed either at rest or combined with phenylephrine, dobutamine, intralipid infusion, or intralipid infusion and dobutamine. The remaining 3 dogs were studied during intralipid infusion alone under resting conditions. Arterial–coronary sinus sampling measured the K of both tracers in 14 dogs, and the rMGU by the Fick method in 21 dogs.

Results.—The PET-derived values for K from either 1-^{11}C-glucose or ^{18}F-FDG were closely correlated with directly measured tracer K values. However, correlation with K values of unlabeled glucose measured directly was better for 1-^{11}C-glucose than for ^{18}F-FDG. Thus, PET-derived values for rMGU were more closely correlated with Fick-derived measurements of unlabeled glucose using 1-^{11}C-glucose than with ^{18}F-FDG.

Conclusions.—PET-derived measurements of rMGU are more accurate when obtained with 1-^{11}C-glucose than with ^{18}F-FDG.

▶ The results are very striking. However, 1-^{11}C-glucose is fully metabolized, which requires continuous imaging to record the metabolic data. Although the data are more precise, FDG will perform well for most clinical indications.

H. W. Strauss, MD

Delineation of Hypoxia in Canine Myocardium Using PET and Copper(II)-Diacetyl-*bis*(*N*^{4}-Methylthiosemicarbazone)

Lewis JS, Herrero P, Sharp TL, et al (Washington Univ, St Louis; Fukui Med Univ, Japan)

J Nucl Med 43:1557-1569, 2002 2–11

Background.—The primary role of ischemia and resultant tissue hypoxia in the pathophysiology of coronary artery disease is well known. Noninvasive techniques for detecting myocardial ischemia currently measure either the level of myocardial oxygen supply or the downstream effects of myocardial hypoxia, such as altered mechanical function or electric instability. There is a need for the development of imaging agents with the capacity to delineate hypoxia in tissue. Copper(II)-diacetyl-*bis*(*N*^{4}-methylthiosemicarbazone) (Cu-ATSM) is a hypoxia-avid tracer for the selective identification of hypoxic tissue. This study reports on findings with the use of Cu-ATSM (which is defined as ^{60}Cu, ^{61}Cu, or ^{64}Cu) for the delineation of ischemic and hypoxic myocardium in a canine model.

Methods.—Three protocols were used. In protocol I, myocardial hypoxia was induced by global hypoxia in 3 dogs. In protocol II, myocardial ischemia was induced by the occlusion of the left anterior descending coronary artery in 9 dogs. In protocol III, coronary artery stenosis was generated by a stenosis in the left anterior descending coronary artery in 4 dogs. PET dynamic data were obtained immediately after tracer injection. Tracer retention kinetics were analyzed with either monoexponential analysis ($1/k_{mono}$) or a simple 2-compartment model ($1/k_4$).

Results.—In the first protocol, tracer retention in the hypoxic myocardium was 2-fold greater than in normal myocardium, despite a 7-fold increase in blood flow. In protocol II, at about 3 hours after occlusion the retention of Cu-ATSM within 20 minutes was greater in ischemic regions of the myocardium than in normal tissue. In some of the dogs, there was a decrease in tracer retention at 24 hours, which suggests the development of necrosis without subsequent retention of Cu-ATSM. In the third protocol, dobutamine infusion after placement of a stenosis resulted in increased tracer retention, which was consistent with hypoxia in the damaged regions.

Conclusion.—These findings in 3 canine models of hypoxia show that Cu-ATSM PET demonstrates quantitative selective uptake in hypoxic myocardium within 20 minutes of tracer administration.

► This study documents the relationship of myocardial Cu-ATSM distribution to decreased myocardial pO_2. The study also identified the relationship of viable tissue to tracer retention, since necrotic tissue did not trap Cu-ATSM. It is unclear, however, what role this tracer could play in the management of patients with ischemic heart disease. Since ischemia is the most common cause of decreased tissue oxygen levels, perfusion tracers can usually identify and characterize most clinical disease. On the other hand, as indicated by the authors in the Discussion section, if hypoxic markers injected prior to a stress test are retained in areas of ischemia, the tracer could become very valuable clinically. As these agents enter clinical trials, we will learn whether they can replace perfusion imaging as a means of identifying ischemia.

H. W. Strauss, MD

3 Radiation

Introduction

I am pleased that Dr Coleman accepted my suggestion to add a section on radiation safety to the YEAR BOOK. In my other life, I have been very involved with the radiation protection community. I was co-team leader of the health effects portion of the IAEA's International Chernobyl Project; I served on the Presidential Advisory Committee on Human Radiation Experiments (ACHRE) and several other National Academy of Sciences committees. I am currently on the Board of Directors of the National Council on Radiation Protection and Measurements (NCRP), chair of an NCRP committee writing a report on the effects of radiation (including I-131) on the thyroid, scientific chair of the Veterans Advisory Committee on Environmental Hazards (VACEH), and a member of the US delegation to the United Nations Scientific Committee on the Effects of Atomic Radiation (UNSCEAR).

Given this background, you can imagine that I have some opinions regarding radiation safety and radiation effects. For example, as documented in the first 2 articles of this section, health care workers, including radiologists and nuclear medicine physicians, are remarkably ignorant about radiation doses (and radiation effects). Admittedly the issues are often complex but there should be an incentive to gain an understanding of the basic concepts given the public and patient interest in this mostly misunderstood topic. Hopefully this yearly review will provide a useful overview of major concepts and developments.

Henry D. Royal, MD

Do Physicians Correctly Estimate Radiation Risks From Medical Imaging?

Finestone A, Richter E, Schlesinger T, et al (Central Orthopedic Clinic, Zerifin, Israel; Hebrew Univ, Jerusalem; Soreq Nuclear Research Ctr, Yavneh, Israel; et al)

Arch Environ Health 58:59-61, 2003 3–1

Background.—Physicians ordering imaging studies for their patients must balance the expected benefits of the test against its possible risks. A sur-

TABLE 1.—Number and Percentage of Responses Comparing Radiation From 1 Bone Scan to an Equivalent Exposure

Equivalent Exposure	Responses *n*	%
A trans-Atlantic flight*	51	24.1
1 chest x-ray	93	43.9
10 chest x-rays	41	19.3
80 chest x-rays	14	6.6
200 chest x-rays†	3	1.4
1,000 chest x-rays	1	0.5
No reply	9	4.2
Total	212	100

*Comparable with 1 to 2 chest x-rays.
†Correct response.
(Courtesy of Finestone A, Richter E, Schlesinger T, et al: Do physicians correctly estimate radiation risks from medical imaging? *Arch Environ Health* 58:59-61, 2003. Reprinted with permission of the Helen Dwight Reid Educational Foundation. Published by Heldref Publications, 1319 Eighteenth St, NW, Washington, DC 20036-1802. Copyright 2003.)

vey was taken to assess orthopedists' awareness of the radiation hazards associated with bone scans.

Methods.—Attendees at an annual meeting of the Israeli Orthopedic Society were asked to anonymously complete a 4-question survey. Respondents were asked to estimate the radiation dose from 1 bone scan relative to the radiation dose from 1 standard chest x-ray study and to estimate the mortality risk due to the potential carcinogenic effect of 1 bone scan.

Results.—In all, 309 physicians were asked to participate, and 198 (64%) returned a completed questionnaire. Orthopedists constituted 60% of the responders, while 39% were residents. About two thirds (68%) indicated that the radiation exposure from 1 bone scan is equivalent to that from 1

TABLE 2.—Number and Percentage of Responses Identifying Mortality Risk From a Bone Scan

Mortality Risk	Responses *n*	%
1/5,000*	9	4.5
1/10,000	6	3.0
1/40,000	3	1.5
1/100,000	9	4.5
1/400,000	9	4.5
1/1,000,000	31	15.7
1/4,000,000	12	6.1
1/10,000,000	25	12.6
1/40,000,000	18	9.1
1/100,000,000	76	38.4
No reply	14	6.6
Total	212	100

*Correct response.
(Courtesy of Finestone A, Richter E, Schlesinger T, et al: Do physicians correctly estimate radiation risks from medical imaging? *Arch Environ Health* 58:59-61, 2003. Reprinted with permission of the Helen Dwight Reid Educational Foundation. Published by Heldref Publications, 1319 Eighteenth St, NW, Washington, DC 20036-1802. Copyright 2003.)

chest x-ray or 1 trans-Atlantic flight (Table 1). Only 3 respondents (1.4%) identified the correct answer (200 chest x-ray tests). About one third (38.4%) said that the mortality risk associated with bone scans was 1/100 million scans (Table 2). Only 9 respondents (4.5%) identified the correct answer (1/5000). Senior physicians were significantly more likely to underestimate the mortality risk than were residents.

Conclusion.—These respondents grossly underestimated the potential radiation risks associated with bone scans. Physicians should know not only the costs of and indications for these imaging tests but their associated radiation hazards as well.

► The authors' choices and the answers from the respondents for "equivalent exposures" to the exposure from 1 bone scan are listed in Table 1. Presumably by "equivalent exposures" they mean "effective dose equivalent." They used 0.05 mSv as the dose of a chest x-ray and 0.42 mRem (sic) as the dose from a bone scan. When converting dose to radiation risk (Table 2), they used a risk coefficient of 4%/Sv. This risk coefficient applies to the general population but, for reasons cited below, does not apply to medical exposures.

Physicians are often criticized for not knowing the radiation doses of the studies that they order or perform. This criticism is overly harsh for a number of reasons. The issues are more complicated than they first appear. For example, the term "dose" is an extremely ambiguous term that can refer to skin dose, bone marrow dose, organ dose, effective dose, etc. In addition, "dose" is used as a surrogate for "risk." Risk is determined by additional important factors such as the age at the time of the exposure and the life expectancy of the patient. Surveys that calculate the per capita radiation dose due to medical exposures rarely take into account these important factors.

When I am asked about the dose of a nuclear medicine study, I generally will ask the patient what it is that they are concerned about and try to address that concern. The most common concern about the exposure to radiation is that it will cause cancer in the future. Although I think it is prudent not to needlessly expose individuals to even small amounts of radiation, radiation is a weak carcinogen. I generally reassure patients that there is no measurable increase in the risk of cancer following diagnostic nuclear medicine studies.

I do think it is important for nuclear medicine professionals and radiologists to have a basic understanding of radiation biology. It always troubles me when I hear someone say that having a myocardial perfusion study (EDE about 650 mrem) is like having a chest x-ray (EDE about 10 mrem).

H. D. Royal, MD

Doctors' Knowledge of Radiation Exposure: Questionnaire Study

Shiralkar S, Rennie A, Snow M, et al (Russells Hall Hosp, Dudley, England; Royal Berkshire Hosp, Reading, England)

BMJ 327:371-372, 2003 3–2

Background.—Each year, an estimated 100 to 250 people in the United Kingdom die of cancers directly related to medical exposure to radiation.

TABLE.—Equivalent Number of Doses of Radiation for Most Commonly Requested Investigations

Radiological Investigation	Equivalent No of Chest X Rays	No of Correct Answers (n=130)
Abdominal x ray	75	2 (1.5)
Lumbar spine x ray	120	3 (2)
Thoracic spine x ray	50	4 (3)
Barium swallow	100	6 (5)
Peroperative cholangiogram	65	3 (2)
Fixation of fractured neck of femur	45	10 (8)
Ultrasound of abdomen	0	124 (95)
CT of abdomen	400	8 (6)
Spiral CT of abdomen	300	9 (7)
MRI of abdomen	0	119 (92)
MRI of knee	0	119 (92)
MRI of spine	0	119 (92)
Leg arteriogram	400	0
Renal arteriogram	80	1 (1)
Thyroid isotope scan	50	8 (6)
White cell scan	150	2 (1.5)

Note: Doses for chest x-ray used as single unit dose of radiation. Figures are numbers (percentages) of doctors with correct answer

(Courtesy of Shiralkar S, Rennie A, Snow M, et al: Doctors' knowledge of radiation exposure: Questionnaire study. *BMJ* 327:371-372, 2003. With permission from the BMJ Publishing Group.)

Physicians' knowledge regarding the radiation doses delivered during commonly requested imaging studies was examined.

Methods.—One hundred thirty physicians at 2 hospitals were interviewed and asked to identify the average dose of radiation delivered during a standard chest x-ray. Each respondent (40 senior house officers, 40 specialist registrars, 40 consultants, and 10 consultant radiologists) then used this response to estimate the equivalent doses of radiation delivered during 16 common imaging tests. Answers within 20% above or below the correct answer were scored as correct.

Results.—None of the respondents knew the approximate dose of radiation received during a single chest x-ray (0.02 mSv) or even how this exposure is measured. Estimated radiation doses for the 16 common imaging tests were greatly underestimated (Table), on average by a factor of 6. The proportion of correct answers by each physician ranged from 0% to 59%. Additionally, 5% of respondents did not know that US does not involve ionizing radiation, and 8% did not know that MRI does not involve ionizing radiation.

Conclusion.—Few of the physicians in this convenience sample knew the radiation doses to which their patients are exposed during imaging.

▶ It is a bit embarrassing that physicians know so little about radiation exposure due to medical procedures. In this study, 8% of the physicians apparently did not know that MRI does not involve the use of radiation.

The lack of sophistication of the authors is apparent from the table. The authors never make it clear what dose (effective dose, organ dose, etc) they are using in their table. In order to be given credit for the "correct value," the respondent had to give an answer that was within 20% of the "correct value." The reality is that the "correct" value can easily vary by 100%, depending on technical factors. For thyroid scans and white cell scans, the radionuclide used is not indicated.

H. D. Royal, MD

Analysis of Dose Distribution for Heavily Exposed Workers in the First Criticality Accident in Japan

Endo A, Yamaguchi Y (Japan Atomic Energy Research Inst, Tokai, Naka, Japan)
Radiat Res 159:535-542, 2003 3–3

Background.—Japan's first criticality accident occurred on September 30, 1999. At a uranium processing plant in Tokai-mura, a large amount of enriched uranyl nitrate solution (18.8% ^{235}U by mass) was poured into a tank designed for use in processing crude U_3O_8. The resultant chain reaction exposed 3 workers to neutrons and γ-rays. The 2 workers who had been at the tank had massive exposures and died on December 21, 1999 and April 27, 2000. The dose distributions for these 2 workers were estimated to correlate exposure with their clinical course.

Methods.—The authors used mathematical human models and Monte Carlo radiation transport programs to estimate the skin dose distributions, depth dose distributions inside the trunk, and neutron-to-γ ray dose ratios in the 2 workers who died of radiation exposure.

Results.—Dose distributions from neutrons and γ rays varied greatly depending on the part of the body and the workers' postures. After the accident, the estimated ^{24}Na-specific activities in workers A and B were 8.91 and 5.23 Bq/g, respectively.

Estimated absorbed doses of neutrons were 5.40 and 3.19 Gy, respectively. Estimated absorbed doses of γ rays produced by nuclear fission and secondary γ rays in the uranium solution for workers A and B were 11.57 and 5.36 Gy, respectively; estimated absorbed γ-ray doses produced inside the body (ie, from secondary γ rays produced by the interaction of neutrons with the body elements) were 1.10 and 0.68 Gy, respectively. Dose distributions in the skin were as high as 66.9 Gy in worker A.

Dose distributions in the trunk depended mainly on the depth of the body surface facing the tank and on the height of the worker's trunk (areas close to the height of the uranium solution in the tank had the greatest exposure). The neutron-to–γ ray dose ratios in the trunk also varied according to the depth from the front to the back. The neutron dose was more affected than the γ rays by elastic scattering of nuclei within the body elements, and thus the neutron dose decreased to a greater extent as the neutrons penetrated the body.

Clinically, one of the major causes of worker A's death was gastrointestinal bleeding. The estimated absorbed doses around the small intestine (5-10 cm from the front) were 12–5 Gy for neutrons and 22–15 Gy for γ rays.

Other reports indicate that absorbed whole-body γ-ray doses of more than 8 Gy cause heavy diarrhea within 1 hour and death within 2 weeks. In this patient, however, heavy diarrhea did not develop until 4 weeks after exposure, and death did not occur until 82 days after the accident. This prolonged survival reflects our improved understanding of the effects of intense radiation exposure and more effective clinical interventions (eg, bone marrow transplantation, cytokine therapy).

Conclusion.—Detailed dose analysis of radiation exposure levels is critical for understanding the biological consequences of high-dose neutron and γ ray exposures and for assessing the efficacy of treatments for these patients.

▶ Radiation accidents usually only occur when someone does something incredibly stupid. The criticality accident in Tokai-mura, Japan on September 30, 1999 was such an accident. The workers were refining uranium fuel for an experimental fast breeder reactor. The refining process had been designed for dissolving, refining, and purifying crude U_3O_8. The process was not safe for redissolving highly purified uranium (18.8% ^{235}U). The mass limit for the refining process was 2.4 kg; however, at the time of the accident, the amount of ^{235}U in the tank reached 16.6 kg. This amount of uranium resulted in a criticality excursion that exposed 2 individuals to a lethal dose of radiation. A third worker had a smaller exposure and survived. The chain reaction continued intermittently for about 20 hours.

Without treatment, the whole-body radiation dose that will kill approximately 50% of healthy exposed individuals is about 350 rem. With medical treatment, the LD50 is about 650 rem. In an accident situation, doses are usually quite nonuniform, making predictions of the ultimate clinical course of the victims difficult. In this accident, determining the biological consequences of the victims was further complicated by the fact that the exposure was largely due to neutrons.

Despite average whole-body doses in the 1000 to 2000 rem range (with some local areas of much higher doses), the 2 workers did not die until 92 and 210 days following the accident. Their prolonged survival was due to medical advances that have increased our ability to treat patients with depressed bone marrows. Unfortunately, these patients ultimately died from multiorgan failure. It is unlikely that medical advances in the near future will provide effective treatment for multiorgan failure.

H. D. Royal, MD

Mortality After Radiological Investigation With Radioactive Thorotrast: A Follow-up Study of Up to Fifty Years in Portugal

dos Santos Silva I, Malveiro F, Jones ME, et al (London School of Hygiene and Tropical Medicine; Instituto de Higiene e Medicina Tropical, Lisboa, Portugal)

Radiat Res 159:521-534, 2003 3–4

Background.—Cerebral angiography with Thorotrast, a radioactive 20% to 25% colloidal solution of $^{232}ThO_2$, was pioneered in Portugal in the 1920s. This medium is retained by the reticuloendothelial system for life and has a half-life of several hundred years. Once the clinical effects of this lifelong exposure to internal radiation were realized, Thorotrast use was stopped in most countries by the 1950s. Follow-up results from Portuguese patients treated with Thorotrast from 1928 to 1959 were presented.

Methods.—Cancer-specific mortality rates were compared for 1096 patients with systemic exposure to Thorotrast (or 59% of those identified as receiving systemic exposure), 240 patients with local exposure (48% of those identified), and 1014 patients with exposure to nonradioactive contrast agents (46% of those identified) who could be followed up through the end of 1996. In about 80% of cases, systemic Thorotrast was administered for cerebral angiography, while local administration was used exclusively to visualize the perinasal sinuses.

Results.—Compared with patients unexposed to Thorotrast, patients with systemic exposure had significantly higher mortality for all causes (relative risk [RR], 2.63), all neoplasms (RR, 6.72), liver cancer (RR, 42.4), chronic liver disease (RR, 5.12), other nonneoplastic diseases of the digestive system (RR, 4.87), neoplastic hematologic disorders (RR, 21.9), nonneoplastic hematologic disorders (RR, 6.00), and nonneoplastic diseases of the respiratory system (RR, 4.31). In most of these conditions, the risk increased significantly with time since dosing and with the cumulative radiation dose of α particles, indicating that this increased risk was due to the contrast agent.

Mortality rates were also significantly higher for nonneoplastic disorders of the nervous system (RR, 12.7) and ill-defined conditions (RR, 3.74), but because these risks declined significantly with time or radiation dose, they probably reflect the initial diagnosis and are not due to Thorotrast exposure. Compared with patients unexposed to Thorotrast, patients with local exposure were not at significantly elevated risk of death from oropharyngeal or nasal cancers or from any other cause. Also, no clear trend for increased risk with time since exposure could be identified in patients with local Thorotrast exposure.

Conclusion.—The risks for many types of cancer remain high in patients with systemic (but not local) exposure to Thorotrast. In particular, the risk of liver disease with systemic Thorotrast increases steadily and significantly with the time since exposure.

► Thorotrast, a contrast medium containing $^{232}ThO_2$, an alpha emitter, was used until the 1950s in many European countries. Follow-up studies on these patients provide useful data on the effects of internal exposure. Internal exposures are very different than external exposures in that the doses are often much less uniform and the dose rates are usually much lower.

The radiation dose to the liver is very high following the systemic administration of Thorotrast because it is a colloidal solution. The radiation dose to the liver following a 25-mL injection is estimated to be 40 cGy (rad) per year. Cumulative doses would be 1200 to 2000 rad (12-20 Gy) over 30 to 50 years. Compared to x-rays or gamma rays, α (high LET) radiation has 20 times the biological effect of γ rays or x-rays (low LET); therefore, these cumulative doses would correspond to 24,000 to 40,000 rem. The increased liver cancer rate (RR, 42.4) observed in this study is consistent with these very large doses.

H. D. Royal, MD

Joint Effects of Radiation and Smoking on Lung Cancer Risk Among Atomic Bomb Survivors

Pierce DA, Sharp GB, Mabuchi K (Radiation Effects Research Found, Hiroshima, Japan; Natl Cancer Inst, Bethesda, Md)

Radiat Res 159:511-520, 2003 3–5

Background.—It is unclear whether the joint effects of radiation exposure and cigarette smoking on the risk of lung cancer are additive or multiplicative. Data from A-bomb survivors were examined to answer this question.

Methods.—The subjects were 45,113 persons in the Radiation Effects Research Foundation registry of A-bomb survivors. Subjects were followed up from 1958 through 1994 to determine the incidence of lung cancer and smoking status (none, moderate, heavy). The joint effect of radiation exposure and smoking on lung cancer risk was examined via 2 models. In an additive model, the risk of cancer due to radiation is added to the baseline risk of cancer due to smoking. In a multiplicative model, the risk of cancer due to radiation is estimated as a proportion of the baseline risk of cancer due to smoking.

Results.—During follow-up, 592 subjects (1.3%) developed primary lung cancer. The relative risk of lung cancer due to smoking had been low in previous studies of this cohort, probably because cigarettes were scarce in Japan before and after World War II. The smoking relative risk at last follow-up, however, was similar to that found in Western populations. The radiation and smoking effects on lung cancer were quite consistent with an additive model and significantly lower than those estimated by a multiplicative model.

After adjusting for smoking, the radiation-related risk relative to the background risks of nonsmokers was similar to those of other solid cancers: The sex-averaged excess relative risk per Sievert (ERR/Sv) for subjects 60 to 70 years old was about 0.9, and did not vary significantly with sex or age at exposure. The ERR/Sv did, however, decrease significantly with increasing smoking level.

Conclusion.—The joint effects of smoking and radiation on lung cancer are additive rather than multiplicative. These findings offer a means for computing lifetime risk estimates for acute single radiation exposures.

► An important problem in radiation biology is how to transfer radiation risks that are measured in 1 population to another population that has a different baseline cancer rate. The 2 simplest models are the additive and the multiplicative models. With the additive model, the risk from radiation is simply added to the baseline cancer rate. With the multiplicative model, the radiation risk is proportional to the baseline cancer risk.

The difference in these 2 models can be seen in Table 1 in the original journal article. The first column illustrates that smoking is a potent carcinogen. The relative risk for lung cancer is 10 for moderate smokers and 20 for heavy smokers. In contrast, the first row illustrates that radiation is a relatively weak carcinogen. The relative risk for lung cancer of 1.25 for moderate radiation exposure and 1.5 for heavy exposure. Possible ways in which these 2 risks may interact is shown in the last 2 columns and last 2 (4) rows of this table. The first entry for each level of smoking is an estimate of what would happen with the additive model, whereas the second entry is an example of what would happen with a multiplicative model. Examination of this table shows that a multiplicative model predicts a higher number of lung cancers than an additive model.

In this article, the authors used data from follow-up of the atomic bomb survivors to determine whether or not the effects of smoking and radiation are additive or multiplicative. Based on their analysis, the authors determined that in the A-bomb survivors, smoking and radiation is largely additive and almost certainly not multiplicative. One of the reasons why it has been difficult to sort out these effects using data on the atomic bomb survivors is that cigarettes were quite scarce during and after the war, so initially there was little effect of smoking on cancer rates. The authors note that the apparent additive effects of smoking and radiation for the A-bomb survivors cannot be generalized to the setting of radon exposure in homes.

H. D. Royal, MD

Studies of Mortality of Atomic Bomb Survivors: Report 13: Solid Cancer and Noncancer Disease Mortality: 1950-1997

Preston DL, Shimizu Y, Pierce DA, et al (Radiation Effects Research Found, Hiroshima, Japan; Radiation Effects Research Found, Nagasaki, Japan; Natl Cancer Inst, Bethesda, Md)

Radiat Res 160:381-407, 2003 3–6

Background.—Cancer and noncancer mortality rates among A-bomb survivors from 1950 through 1997 were reviewed.

Methods.—Data from 86,572 A-bomb survivors who have been followed up through 1997 in the Life Span Study of the Radiation Effects Research Foundation were presented. Individual dose estimates were available for all subjects, and 60% received doses of 5 $_{m}$Sv or greater. This report appeared 7 years after the previous one.

Results.—During 47 years of follow-up, 9335 subjects have died of solid cancer and 31,881 have died of diseases other than cancer. By comparing observed to expected deaths, it appears that only an estimated 440 (5%) of the solid cancer deaths and 250 (0.8%) of the noncancer deaths are related to the radiation exposure during the bombings. The excess solid cancer risks have increased with time within each age-at-exposure group and appear to be linear in dose, even for the lowest exposure level (0-150 mSv).

Still, the relative risks for A-bomb survivors have decreased as the subjects have aged, indicating that the age-related increase in excess cancer rates is less rapid in survivors than the age-related increase in excess cancer rates in the general population. The relative risk remains highest among people exposed as children (0-19 years of age). Neither the absolute nor the relative excess solid cancer risk differs significantly between Hiroshima and Nagasaki.

Overall, a useful benchmark for describing the effects of radiation in this cohort is that, for people exposed at age 30 years, the risk of solid cancer is 47% per Sievert higher at age 70 years. Men who were 30 years old and exposed to 0.1 Sv have an estimated 0.9% lifetime risk of radiation-related solid cancer death. Estimates of site-specific solid cancer risks differ according to the site and must be interpreted with caution as the number of deaths is small for many cancers. Radiation has also increased noncancer mortality in these subjects; they have significantly increased risks of heart disease, stroke, digestive diseases, and respiratory diseases. The estimated excess relative risk for noncancer death is 14% per Sievert.

The dose-response relationship for noncancer mortality may be nonlinear, but there is substantial uncertainty in the noncancer data. Doses of less than about 0.5 Sv appear to have no significant effect on noncancer mortality. Furthermore, noncancer relative risks do not change significantly with age, age at exposure, or sex. Yet the estimated lifetime risks of noncancer death for people exposed as adults are comparable to those seen for cancer-related mortality.

Conclusion.—At the end of the current study (1997), about half of the cohort was still alive. Excess mortality rates for cancer and noncancer deaths were highest for subjects exposed as children, and future studies are therefore likely to reveal higher excess rates of radiation-associated mortality in this cohort.

▶ Data from the atomic bomb survivors is the most important source of information that we have on the effects of radiation. Studies of this population are extremely important because of the large population that was exposed, the large range of doses, the fact that the exposure was a whole-body exposure, and the fact that the population contained all ages and was otherwise representative of a general population. This report is the most recent update of solid cancer and noncancer disease mortality in this cohort.

The key data from this article is shown in Figure 4 in the original journal article. The average excess relative risk for all solid tumors (exposure at age 30 and follow-up through age 70) is 47% per Sievert. This means that a there will be a 47% increase in mortality from all solid cancers for every 100 rem of radiation exposure. The normal risk of dying from cancer is about 22.5% so the expected cancer mortality following a 100-rem radiation exposure would be about 33%. Notice how great the uncertainty is for many individual cancers. This is because the numbers get to be very small when all solid cancers are divided into various subgroups. Table 7 in the original journal article lists the lifetime risk for solid cancer deaths for various ages of exposure. This table also includes an estimate of the years of life lost per excess death. This important factor needs to be taken into account when comparing risks because dying today is very different than dying 20 years from now.

One of the best kept secrets in radiation biology is that of the 9335 solid cancer deaths observed during the follow-up of the atomic bomb survivors, only about 440 (5%) can be attributed to radiation exposure. A new, interesting, and somewhat unexpected finding has been an increase in noncancer deaths associated with radiation exposure.[1] These deaths are due to diverse causes. It is uncertain at this time what the biological mechanism might be to cause this increase in such diverse diseases. In addition, it is unclear where a threshold exists for these noncancer effects.

This article uses the DS86 dosimetry. A more refined dosimetry system has recently been described (DS2002). It is unlikely that this new dosimetry system will significantly change risk estimates. Also of interest is that the latest BEIR report (BEIR VII) should be published by 2005. This new report should include a reanalysis of the atomic bomb survivor study data using DS2002.

H. D. Royal, MD

Reference

1. Shimizu, Y, et al: Studies of the mortality of atomic bomb survivors. Report 12, part II: Noncancer mortality: 1950-1990. *Radiat Res* 152:374-389, 1999.

Measuring Fast Neutrons in Hiroshima at Distances Relevant to Atomic-Bomb Survivors

Straume T, Rugel G, Marchetti AA, et al (Univ of Utah, Salt Lake City; Lawrence Livermore Natl Lab, Livermore, Calif; Technische Universität München, Germany; et al)

Nature 424:539-542, 2003 3–7

Background.—The 1986 reassessment of the atomic bomb radiation dosimetry for Hiroshima and Nagasaki (DS86) suggested that neutron doses may have been much larger than estimated. Measurements made within weeks of the bombing are considered valid only for about 700 m from the hypocenter. A new method based on detecting ^{63}Ni in copper samples provides an estimate of fast-neutron activation at distances further from the hypocenter.

Methods.—The authors developed a method for detecting trace amounts of ^{63}Ni in copper samples. In brief, copper samples from Hiroshima were electromechanically separated to remove the gross copper material, then the nickel was reacted with carbon monoxide to form nickel tetracarbonyl. This latter compound was thermally decomposed to nickel metal, which was then analyzed by accelerator mass spectrometry to detect ^{63}Ni atoms. About 95% of the ^{63}Ni in the copper samples from Hiroshima was produced by neutrons of more than 1.5 MeV. Samples were obtained from 380 to 1461 m from the hypocenter (which are the most relevant distances for A-bomb survivors), and their ^{63}Ni content was measured at least twice.

Results.—^{63}Ni measurements at distances between 300 and 1500 m correlate well with estimates from DS86. Measurements at 380 m are somewhat lower than the DS86 calculation, whereas measurements at 1500 m are somewhat higher. Overall, however, these estimates show close correlation with those from DS86.

Conclusion.—These data confirm previous estimates from DS86 regarding the neutron doses received by most survivors of the A-bomb (ie, those 380 to 1500 m from the hypocenter).

▶ This technical article described a method that has been used to better estimate the radiation dose to the atomic bomb survivors in Hiroshima. There has been concern that the neutron dose in Hiroshima has been underestimated in the past (this would result in an overestimation of the risk coefficients). Using a new technique (measurement of ^{63}Ni activation), the authors estimated the neutron dose. Their results (summarized in Fig 1 in the original article) indicate that DS86 overestimates the neutron dose at short distances from the hypocenter and underestimates the neutron dose at long distances from the hypocenter. These new data will be incorporated into the new dosimetry system (DS2002). The changes to past risk coefficients should be minor when DS2002 is used.

H. D. Royal, MD

Cancer Mortality Risk Among Workers at the Mayak Nuclear Complex

Shilnikova NS, Preston DL, Ron E, et al (Southern Urals Biophysics Inst, Ozyorsk, Russia; Radiation Effects Research Found, Hiroshima, Japan; Natl Cancer Inst, Bethesda, Md; et al)

Radiat Res 159:787-798, 2003 3–8

Background.—Workers at the Mayak Production Association received cumulative radiation doses far higher than those received by nuclear workers in other countries. Leukemia and solid cancer risks for these Russian workers were described.

Methods.—The cohort studied included about 18,800 people who worked in Mayak's nuclear reactor complex, radiochemical plant, or plutonium production plant and about 2700 people who worked only in auxiliary plants (water treatment facility, mechanical repair plant). Workers were hired from 1948 to 1972, and the 24% of women workers had the same exposures as men. Workers in the 3 main facilities had high exposure to external whole-body γ rays (average cumulative dose, 0.8 Gy, with some doses more than 10 Gy).

Workers in the radiochemical and plutonium plants also had potentially high internal exposure from inhaled plutonium (average plutonium body burden, 2.1 kBq). Workers at the auxiliary plants had lower exposure levels (average cumulative whole-body external γ-ray dose, 0.17 Gy) than other Mayak workers, but their levels are much higher than in similar workers in other countries. The excess relative risks of death due to solid cancers or leukemia that were associated with external γ radiation dose (after adjustment for effects of plutonium exposure) were calculated.

Results.—As of December 31, 1997, there have been 1730 deaths due to solid cancer, 77 deaths due to leukemia, and 213 deaths due to unknown causes. Among the solid cancer deaths, 569 were caused by lung cancer, 67 by liver cancer, 32 by skeletal cancer (ie, the sites of primary plutonium deposition), and 1062 by other solid organ cancers. Mortality rates for both solid cancer and leukemia increased significantly as the external γ-ray dose increased.

Assuming a linear dose-response model, the excess relative risk for lung, liver, and skeletal cancers combined (after adjustment for plutonium exposure) was 0.30 per gray. The excess relative risk for all other solid organ cancers was 0.08 per gray. The solid cancer excess risk estimates at doses <3 Gy were about two times higher than those predicted by a linear model, which suggests the dose-response relationship is nonlinear.

Internal exposure to plutonium also significantly increased the risk of lung, liver, and skeletal cancer combined, and the risk of other solid cancers as a group. Leukemia mortality rates increased significantly as the external γ-ray dose increased, but plutonium exposure did not appear to influence the leukemia death rate. The excess mortality risk associated with leukemia depended on how long ago the dose had been received. For doses received 3-5 years before death, the excess relative risk was about 7 per gray; however, for doses received 5-45 years before death, the excess relative risk was only about 0.45/Gy. None of the estimated relative risks for mortality differed significantly according to sex.

Conclusion.—External γ-ray exposure increased the risks of solid cancers and leukemia in the Mayak worker cohort; internal exposure to plutonium also increased the risk of solid organ cancers. Although it is difficult to determine precisely the risk associated with chronic radiation exposure, risks among Mayak workers who received 1 Gy or less appear to be slightly lower than those reported for A-bomb survivors with acute exposure.

► Studies of the workers at the Mayak Nuclear Complex are very interesting because the external radiation doses for this cohort are very high (average dose is 0.8 Gy and the highest doses exceeded 10 Gy). For a frame of reference, the average dose for the atomic bomb survivors is between 0.1 and 0.15 Gy. In addition, some of these workers have large radiation doses due to internal contamination with plutonium. Studies of these workers may allow us to better determine the cancer risk from protracted external radiation exposure as well as the risk from internal contamination with plutonium.

However, no one should underestimate the difficulties in studying chronically exposed populations. Accurately determining the radiation dose is very difficult. For the atomic bomb survivors, the dose could be reasonably estimated simply by knowing where survivors were in an instant in time. Calculating doses for chronic exposure is much more complicated. With this worker cohort, the doses will always be much less certain than the doses for the atomic bomb survivors. Uncertainty in dose will, in itself, tend to attenuate the dose-response relationship. How much the decreased risk from chronic exposure will be due to the increase uncertainty in dose and how much will be due to a real decrease in risk will be difficult to sort out.

H. D. Royal, MD

Thyroid Neoplasms After Therapeutic Radiation for Malignancies During Childhood or Adolescence

Acharya S, Sarafoglou K, LaQuaglia M, et al (New York Presbyterian Hosp and Cornell-Weil Med School; Mem Sloan-Kettering Cancer Ctr, New York; Univ of Washington, Seattle)

Cancer 97:2397-2403, 2003 3–9

Background.—Radiotherapy during childhood increases the risk of developing a thyroid neoplasm. The time course and outcomes of thyroid neoplasia developing after high-dose therapeutic radiation during childhood were examined.

Methods.—The medical records of 33 patients who developed a thyroid neoplasm after irradiation for childhood Hodgkin disease (18 patients), non-Hodgkin lymphoma (10 patients), or other malignancy (5 patients) were reviewed.

Results.—The patients (10 boys and 23 girls) ranged in age from 3.7 to 18.3 years (median age, 12.0 years) at the time the primary malignancy was diagnosed. Patients received 1000 to 4200 cGy to the thyroid gland (median, 2400 cGy), and it took between 6.2 and 30.1 years (median, 13.0 years) after radiation therapy for the thyroid neoplasm to be diagnosed. All lesions were diagnosed via physical examination.

Thirteen patients (39%) had malignant lesions, including 11 papillary carcinomas and 2 follicular carcinomas. Patients with malignant lesions were similar to patients with benign thyroid disease in terms of age at diagnosis, gender ratio, and time interval since radiotherapy. However, patients with malignant lesions received a significantly lower radiation dose to the thyroid gland (median, 2000 vs 2950 cGy). Eleven of the 13 patients with thyroid cancer were treated at the authors' institution with near total thyroidectomy plus radioactive iodine (8 patients) or with lobectomy (3 patients).

Disease was confined to the thyroid bed in 10 patients; 1 patient had regional lymph node involvement. None of these patients developed progressive or recurrent disease during up to 12 years of follow-up (median, 6.5 years), and there were no deaths related to thyroid cancer.

Conclusion.—About 40% of these clinically palpable thyroid neoplasms detected in patients with prior therapeutic radiation exposure were malignant. These cancers were not particularly aggressive, and patients have remained recurrence-free after curative excision. Nonetheless, these cancers developed up to 30 years after the radiation exposure, and thus patients who received radiotherapy as children should be followed up for the rest of their lives.

▶ Due to the Chernobyl accident, there has been renewed interest in the relationship between thyroid cancer and radiation exposure. It has become clear that children and adolescents are much more sensitive to external and internal radiation than are adults.

This article is not particularly helpful in answering many of the important questions that we still have about the relationship between thyroid cancer and radiation. The authors simply report on the subset of 33 patients who were identified as developing "thyroid neoplasm" after therapeutic radiation. Thirteen of these patients proved to have thyroid cancer.

One of the major problems with studying radiation and thyroid cancer is workup bias. Thyroid cancer has a low mortality so studies of mortality are usually uninformative because of the small numbers of patients and because most of the patients with thyroid cancer are excluded because they did not die. On the other hand, studying thyroid cancer incidence is difficult because the results are very dependent on how hard one looks for thyroid cancer (workup bias).

H. D. Royal, MD

Thyroid Cancer Risk After Thyroid Examination With ^{131}I: A Population-Based Cohort Study in Sweden

Dickman PW, Holm L-E, Lundell G, et al (Karolinska Institutet, Stockholm; Swedish Radiation Protection Board, Stockholm; Karolinska Univ, Stockholm; et al)

Int J Cancer 106:580-587, 2003 3–10

Background.—Ionizing radiation is the only established risk factor for thyroid cancer. The excess risks of thyroid cancer associated with a range of ^{131}I doses administered for diagnostic purposes were examined.

Methods.—A population-based cohort of all 36,792 people in Sweden who received ^{131}I for diagnostic purposes between 1952 and 1969, and who were alive and free of thyroid cancer 2 years after their exposure, was examined. Because tumors diagnosed within the first 2 years after exposure were unlikely to be due to ^{131}I, data regarding person-years at risk were calculated beginning 2 years after exposure and ending on December 31, 1998. Standardized incidence ratios (SIRs; ie, the ratio between the observed and the expected numbers of thyroid cancers) were estimated according to age at exposure, sex, previous exposure to external radiation therapy to the neck, indication for the scan, dose of ^{131}I, and time since exposure.

Results.—During 886,618 person-years of follow-up, there were 129 cases of thyroid cancer. The mean total absorbed ^{131}I dose to the thyroid was 1.07 Gy in the subjects without prior external radiation therapy to the neck, and 1.74 Gy in patients with prior exposure. No excess mortality was associated with age at exposure, sex, dose of ^{131}I, or time since exposure. Specifically, among the 2367 subjects (6.4%) with exposure before age 20 years, only 3 developed thyroid cancer (SIR, 1.01). However, patients with previous exposure to external radiation therapy to the neck (1767 patients) had a significantly increased mortality risk (SIR, 9.8), as did patients who were originally referred because of a suspected thyroid tumor (SIR, 3.5; 11,015 patients without previous external radiation therapy).

In all, 24,010 subjects (65.3%) did not have previous exposure to external radiation therapy to the neck and were referred for reasons other than a suspected thyroid tumor. In this cohort, the excess risk associated with ^{131}I exposure was actually less than that expected (SIR, 0.91).

Conclusion.—Exposure to ^{131}I during diagnostic procedures does not appear to increase the risk of thyroid cancer. However, almost 95% of these subjects were more than 20 years of age, and thus these results should not be extrapolated to children, in whom the thyroid gland may be particularly sensitive to the effects of ionizing radiation.

▶ Thyroid cancer risk after thyroid examination with ^{131}I is of considerable interest to nuclear medicine professionals. The article incorrectly states that the annual number of thyroid examinations using radioiodine is currently 5 per 1000 individuals worldwide. According to Table 38 on page 402 of the cited reference, the correct number would be less than 1 per 1000. According to this table, most studies are done with ^{99m}Tc-pertechnetate or ^{123}I.

One of the major problems with determining thyroid cancer risk after thyroid examination with ^{131}I has been that this examination has only been rarely done in children. The thyroids of children are much more sensitive to carcinogenic effects of radiation than are those of adults. Although this article does not find any dose-response relationship, few of the patients were under the age of 20 at the time of their exposure. Although it was commonly believed that ^{131}I would result in a lower risk than x-ray exposure, the dramatic increase in thyroid cancer in children following the Chernobyl accident has lead many to question this belief. The best summary for thyroid cancer risk following external radiation exposure is the pooled analysis that was published in 1995.[1] There is still considerable uncertainty about thyroid cancer risk following internal exposure.

H. D. Royal, MD

Reference

1. Ron E, Lubin JH, Shore RE, et al: Thyroid cancer after exposure to external radiation: A pooled analysis of seven studies. *Radiat Res* 141:259-277, 1995.

Depression and Anxiety During Isolation and Radionuclide Therapy

Brans B, van den Eynde F, Audenaert K, et al (Ghent Univ, Belgium)
Nucl Med Commun 24:881-886, 2003 3–11

Background.—A diagnosis of malignancy and hospitalization, isolation, and exposure to the radioactivity of a radionuclide therapy may have significant psychological effects on patients. Treatment acceptability and compliance may be compromised. The psychopathologic manifestations and underlying personality-related vulnerabilities of patients needing isolation for radionuclide therapy were investigated.

Methods.—Forty-eight patients, aged a mean of 57.8 years, were included in the study. Twenty-four were women. Twenty-six patients had a malignant condition and 22 had a nonmalignant condition necessitating isolation for radionuclide therapy. The patients completed a series of questionnaires to evaluate anxiety, depression, hopelessness, personality characteristics, and coping strategies.

Findings.—Compared with patients with low-state anxiety, those with a high level of state anxiety had greater levels of depression and hopelessness. The personalities of the latter group were characterized by significantly higher scores on harm avoidance as well as lower scores on self-directedness. This group's coping strategies were more passive and avoiding and less well aimed. The nature of the disease did not affect these results. Sex, age, years of education, being in or not in a relationship, and duration of hospitalization also did not influence results.

Conclusion.—Levels of anxiety are closely associated with individual personality traits and coping strategies inadequate for the experience of isolation for radionuclide therapy. Subgroup status such as that of women, the elderly, cancer patients, or people with less education does not correlate with a higher state anxiety level. Screening for trait anxiety before admission is easy to do and can help guide interventions to increase patient comfort and treatment acceptability.

► Unfortunately, this article did not answer what I thought was the most interesting question—that is, the difference between the depression and anxiety of patients treated as inpatients compared to those treated as outpatients. We now treat almost all patients as outpatients. When we first started doing this, we measured the radiation doses to family members.[1] The average administered activity was 116 mCi (4.3 GB) of ^{131}I, and the average radiation dose to family members was 0.24 mSv. Confining patients to hospitals based on the amount of activity within their body without any consideration of the biological half-life is irrational and wastes the limited resources that we have available to protect the public's health.

H. D. Royal, MD

Reference

1. Grigsby PW, Siegel BA, Baker S, et al: Radiation exposure from outpatient radioactive iodine (^{131}I) therapy for thyroid carcinoma. *JAMA* 283:2272-2274, 2000.

Large-Body Radiation Doses Following Radioiodine Therapy

Leslie WD, Havelock J, Palser R, et al (Univ of Manitoba, Winnipeg, Canada; Cancer Care Manitoba, Winnipeg, Canada)

Nucl Med Commun 23:1091-1097, 2002 3–12

Background.—The International Radiological Protection Commission has recommended reducing the maximum acceptable radiation dose limits for the public to 1 mSv in the United States, Canada, the United Kingdom and European Union nations. This recommendation has significantly affected radiation protection guidelines for contacts of patients treated with ^{131}I. Previously used models may overestimate dose rates at short distances. The current study measured ^{131}I dose rates using adult and infant phantoms, more accurately reflecting true geometry.

Methods and Findings.—Dose calculations and patient contact restrictions were derived from the direct dose measurements obtained by using the phantoms. Adult phantom doses were measured at 3 distances: contact, 1 m, and 2 m. Infant phantom doses were measured at contact in 2 orientations: adult cradling infant over the shoulder and cradling infant at the waist. The doses determined for the adult and infant phantoms were significantly lower than previously predicted. Doses received by the infant were markedly greater than those received by the adult because of the nature of the contact and the smaller size.

Conclusions.—Close contact between a patient receiving ^{131}I therapy and his or her small child is important and needs to be restricted. However, patient contact restrictions could be less stringent than those currently recommended.

► This is an important article for anyone who treats patients with radioactive iodine. The authors point out that the doses that were measured using phantoms are significantly lower than predicted because previous recommendations have relied on models that overestimate dose rates at short distances. Of particular importance are the conclusions that can be found in Tables 3 and 4 in the original journal article. As can be seen from these tables, the main restriction should be limited to close contact with an infant. The authors define close contact as being fifteen 35-minute periods of close contact for a total of 8.75 hours for every 24-hour period. Most caregivers would be able to considerably decrease the close contact time that they have with their infants and, at the same time, provide the necessary care.

In the United States, there is increasing concern for the inconvenience caused to patients due to the installation of radiation detectors. If a patient plans to travel following a nuclear medicine procedure, we give the patient a note identifying the radionuclide that has been administered. Most importantly, the note includes a hospital number that can be called 24 hours a day to verify the information in the note. The person at this number has access to the hospital information system, so the patient's procedure can be confirmed.

H. D. Royal, MD

Sister Chromatid Exchanges in Lymphocytes of Nuclear Medicine Physicians

Bozkurt G, Yuksel M, Karabogaz G, et al (Trakya Univ, Edirne, Turkey; Istanbul Univ, Turkey)

Mutat Res 535:205-213, 2003 3–13

Objective.—The aim of this study was to assess whether occupational exposure to chronic, low doses of Iodine 131 (I-131) and Technetium 99m (Tc-99m) may lead to genotoxicity. Medical personnel occupied in nuclear medicine departments are occupationally exposed to low doses of I-131 and Tc-99m. The determination of the frequency of sister chromatid exchanges (SCEs) and of cells with a high frequency of SCEs (HFC) is considered to be a sensitive indicator for detecting genotoxic potential of mutagenic and carcinogenic agents. Therefore, we examined peripheral lymphocytes from nuclear medicine physicians for the presence of both SCE and HFC.

Methods.—Sixteen exposed nuclear medicine physicians (non-smokers) were compared to 16 physicians (non-smokers) who had not been exposed to chemical or physical mutagens in their usual working environment at the same hospital.

Results.—A statistically significant difference was found between SCE frequencies and HFC percentages measured in lymphocytes from the exposed and control groups (Fig 1).

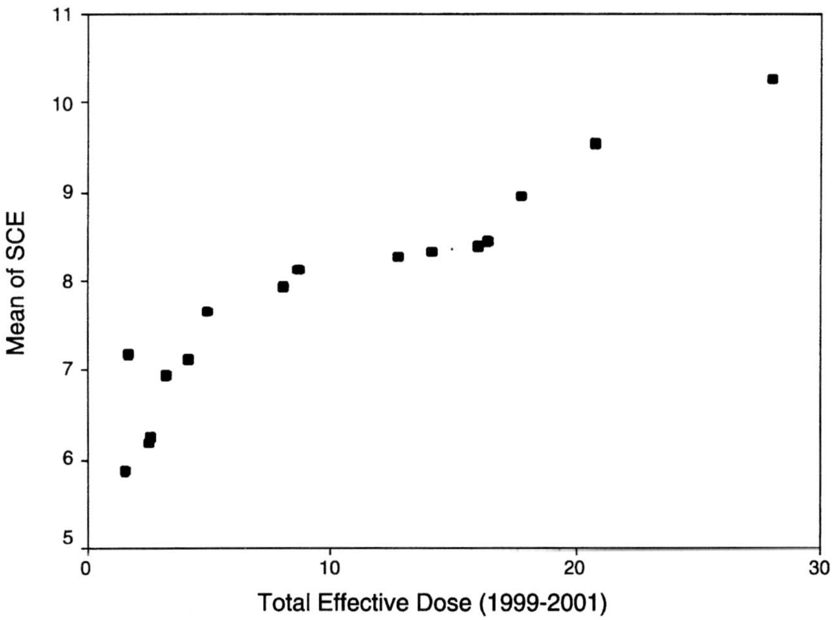

FIGURE 1.—Correlation plot of mean sister chromatid exchange (*SCE*) values and total effective dose. (Courtesy of Bozkurt G, Yuksel M, Karabogaz G, et al: Sister chromatid exchanges in lymphocytes of nuclear medicine physicians. *Mutat Res* 535:205-213. Copyright 2003 by Elsevier Science Inc.)

Conclusions.—The present observation on the effect of chronic low doses of I-131 and Tc-99m indicates the possibility of genotoxic implications of this type of occupational exposure. Hence, the personnel who work in nuclear medicine departments should carefully apply the radiation protection procedures and should minimize, as low as possible, radiation exposure to avoid possible genotoxic effects.

► The title of this article was intriguing. I am baffled by the data that are presented (see Fig 1). The units of dose in this graph are millisieverts so the average radiation dose is 3 or 4 mSv (300-400 mrem) per year. Despite these very low doses, the authors claim to get a very good correlation between the number of sister chromatid exchanges and the total effective dose. I know of no biodosimeter that gives these results at such low doses. I intend to wait until others reproduce these results before I use them.

H. D. Royal, MD

Second Neoplasms After Megavoltage Radiation for Pediatric Tumors

Gold DG, Neglia JP, Dusenbery KE (Univ of Minnesota, Minneapolis)

Cancer 97:2588-2596, 2003 3–14

Background.—Children exposed to therapeutic ionizing radiation require diligent long-term follow-up. The nature and risk of second neoplasms (SNs) in patients receiving megavoltage radiotherapy in childhood were further explored.

Methods.—Four hundred forty-six patients undergoing megavoltage radiotherapy for a primary malignancy between 1954 and 1980 were followed up. All patients survived for at least 5 years.

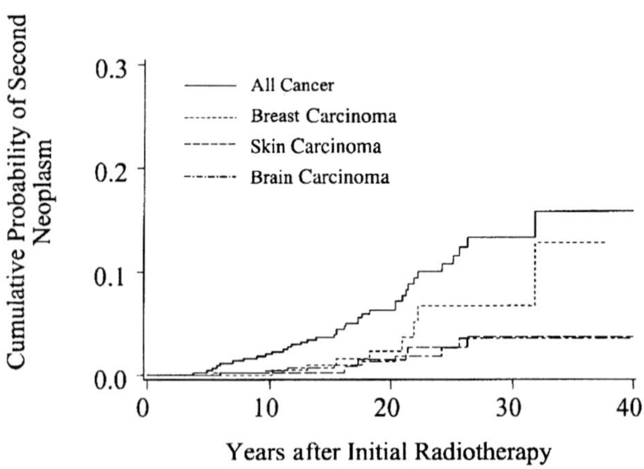

FIGURE 2.—The cumulative probabilities of second neoplasms as a function of time based on the study cohort. The *curve for breast carcinoma* is based only on the women in the cohort. (Courtesy of Gold DG, Neglia JP, Dusenbery KE: Second neoplasms after megavoltage radiation for pediatric tumors. *Cancer* 97(10):2588-2596. © 2003 American Cancer Society. Reprinted by permission of Wiley-Liss, Inc, a subsidiary of John Wiley & Sons, Inc.)

Findings.—At 30 years, the actuarial survival rate was 80% overall. SNs developed in 8.3% of the patients. Most occurred in the original radiation treatment field 3.8 to 31.8 years after radiotherapy. The cumulative risk of SN development was 13% at 30 years. The standardized incidence ratio for any SN development was 5.2. The most common SNs were breast carcinomas, occurring in 8 patients; skin carcinoma, including 5 basal cell carcinomas, 2 malignant melanomas, and 1 dermatosarcoma; and meningiomas, in 6 patients (Fig 2). All cases of breast carcinoma occurred in patients treated for childhood Hodgkin disease. Twelve of the 37 patients with SNs died from the second malignancy or from recurrent disease. The development of an SN was associated with initial diagnosis of Hodgkin disease, female sex, and initial diagnosis of acute lymphoblastic leukemia.

Conclusion.—This cohort of patients with childhood malignancies treated by radiotherapy had increased mortality, with an increased risk of developing an SN. Medical surveillance through adulthood is indicated for such patients.

▶ There is enormous literature about radiation effects. One way to confirm that the radiation effects predicted from studies of the atomic bomb survivors are reasonably accurate is by comparing the cancer incidence following other types of radiation exposure. There is ample scientific evidence to indicate that there is an increased incidence of SNs following radiation therapy for cancer. As Figure 2 shows, breast cancer is one of the most common secondary cancers.

The increased cancer risk following radiation therapy is not solely due to a genetic predisposition. Acknowledging the risk from radiation therapy provides the motivation for developing techniques that will prevent needless radiation of normal tissues. Clearly, the benefits of radiation therapy need to be balanced with the risks of radiation therapy.

H. D. Royal, MD

No Radiation Protection Reasons for Restrictions on ^{14}C Urea Breath Tests in Children

Gunnarsson M, Leide-Svegborn S, Stenström K, et al (Lund Univ, Malmö, Sweden; Malmö Univ, Sweden)

Br J Radiol 75:982-986, 2002 3–15

Background.—Because the radiation exposure involved is not known, traditional ^{14}C urea breath tests are usually not used in younger children. High-sensitivity accelerator mass spectrometry and an ultra-low amount of ^{14}C urea were used to diagnose *Helicobacter pylori* (HP) infection in young children. Radiation dose estimates in this setting were also established.

Methods.—Seven children aged 3 to 6 years were included. The activity applied was 250 times lower than that used for adults and 125 times lower than that used for older children; the amount of ^{14}C urea used was 440 Bq.

Findings were compared with previously published biokinetic and dosimetric data on adults and 7- to 14-year-old children.

Findings.—^{14}C activity levels in urine and exhaled air per unit of activity delivered to the young children corresponded well to that for 7- to 14-year-olds. In an HP-negative child aged 3 to 6 years, the urinary bladder wall received the highest absorbed dose, at 0.3 mGy/Mbq. Effective doses for a 3-year-old and for a 6-year-old were 0.1 and 0.07 mSv/Mbq, respectively. In 2 children, the 10- and 20-minute post–^{14}C administration samples of exhaled air were found to have a significantly greater amount of ^{14}C activity than in the other young children.

These values were 6% and 19%, respectively, of administered activity exhaled per hour, compared with 0.3% to 0.9% in the other children, indicating HP positivity in the former 2 children. A 3-year-old HP-positive child had an absorbed dose to the urinary bladder wall of 0.3 mGy/MBq. The effective dose per unit of administered activity was 0.4 mSv/MBq.

Conclusion.—Normal ^{14}C urea breath tests can be performed safely, even in young children. Using 55 kBq, the effective dose for a 3-year-old HP-negative child is about 6 μSv, and for a 3-year-old HP-positive child, it is 20 μSv.

► Another more expensive, less available technique (accelerated mass spectrometry) was being considered in order to avoid radiation doses of 6 to 20 μSv (0.6 to 2 mrems). Although I do not believe that we should have a cavalier attitude about exposing individuals to radiation, I continue to be amazed by the level of concern about radiation exposure expressed by our European colleagues.

I strongly believe that there are limited resources available to protect the public's health. Given that scenario, it is important that we spend these limited resources wisely. When we spend these resources to avoid very small risks, they are no longer available to prevent much larger risks and in the end, that causes society to be less healthy.

One of my favorite articles discusses the cost-benefit of various life-prolonging interventions.[1] Protecting members of the public from the risks of radiation is one of the more expensive things we do. The authors of this article divided life-prolonging interventions into 3 categories: medical, injury reduction, and toxin control. The median costs (in 1995 dollars) per quality-adjusted life-year were $19,000, $48,000, and $2,800,000, respectively.

H. D. Royal, MD

Reference

1. Tengs TO, Adams ME, Pliskin JS, et al: Five-hundred life-saving interventions and their cost-effectiveness. *Risk Anal* 15:369-390, 1995.

Introduction, Audit and Review of Guidelines for Delegated Authorization of Nuclear Medicine Investigations in Compliance With the Ionising Radiation (Medical Exposure) Regulations 2000

Harris AM, Greaves CD, Taylor CM, et al (Sheffield Teaching Hosps, England)
Nucl Med Commun 24:939-942, 2003 3–16

Background.—In Great Britain, the Ionising Radiation Regulations 2000 require that every nuclear medicine examination be justified by a practitioner with an appropriate certificate from the Administration of Radioactive Substances Committee. The practitioner may authorize the radiation exposure directly or delegate it to a trained operator using written, practitioner-approved guidelines. The process of implementation, audit, and review of a set of Delegated Authorization Guidelines (DAGs) was elucidated.

Methods.—After the DAGs were introduced, nuclear medicine referrals were audited at 2 sites for 3 months. Referrals were compared with the DAGs. If a referral was not consistent with the DAG criteria, it was categorized as insufficient referral information or clinical indication not included in the DAGs. The practitioner reviewed all inconsistent requests.

Findings.—Sixty-nine percent of 632 referrals were consistent with the DAGs. Twelve percent required clarification from the referrer before meeting criteria. Nineteen percent were authorized directly by the practitioner. Among directly authorized referrals, additional indications were identified, and the DAGs were subsequently revised.

Conclusion.—These data suggest that delegating authorization for nuclear medicine examinations can be successful. This procedure must be audited regularly.

▶ I hope the practice of nuclear medicine in the United States does not follow the example set by our British colleagues. Recent legislation requires that a practitioner formally document the justification for any study that exposes a patient to radiation. Generally, the most important reason for avoiding unnecessary studies is the harm caused by wasting limited resources rather than the harm caused by the radiation. Ironically, no formal justification is required when a practitioner exposes a patient to the risk of a new medication.

H. D. Royal, MD

Evidence for a Lack of DNA Double-Strand Break Repair in Human Cells Exposed to Very Low X-ray Doses

Rothkamm K, Löbrich M (Universität des Saarlandes, Homburg, Germany)
Proc Natl Acad Sci U S A 100:5057-5062, 2003 3–17

Background.—The most biologically significant lesion by which ionizing radiation produces cancer and hereditary disease is DNA double-strand breaks (DSBs). The induction and processing of DSBs after physiologically relevant radiation doses are not understood. Many techniques for measur-

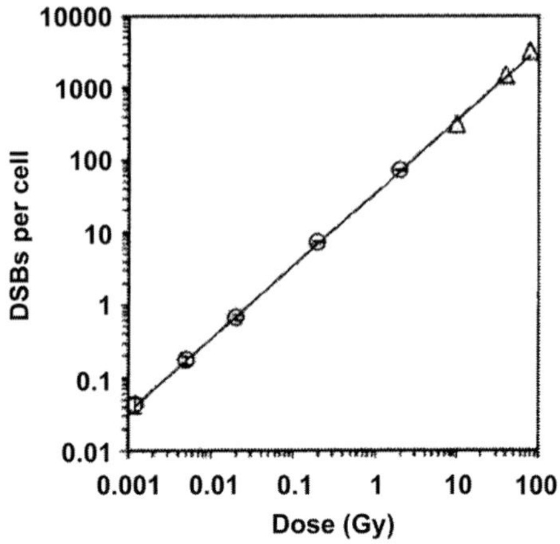

FIGURE 2.—Double-strand break (*DSB*) induction in MRC-5 cells. γ-H2AX foci were counted 3 minutes after irradiation, and the mean values of foci per cell are shown (*circles*). *Triangle* represent DSB induction data obtained from pulsed-field gel electrophoresis analysis. The *line* is a linear fit to the data points with a slope of 35 DSBs/cell/Gy. (Courtesy of Rothkamm K, Löbrich M: Evidence for a lack of DNA double-strand break repair in human cells exposed to very low x-ray doses. *Proc Natl Acad Sci U S A* 100:5057-5062. Copyright 2003 National Academy of Sciences, U. S. A.)

ing DSB repair inadvertently introduce this damage. Evidence for a lack of DSB repair in human cells exposed to very low x-ray doses was reported.

Methods and Findings.—Foci of γ-H2AX, a phosphorylated histone, were detected by immunofluorescence (Fig 2). These foci were quantitatively the same as DSBs. This finding enabled examination of DSB repair after radiation doses as low as 1 mGy, a marked improvement over current methods. DSBs induced in cultures of nondividing primary human fibroblasts by radiation doses of about 1 mGy remained unrepaired for many days, whereas DSB repair at higher doses is very efficient. However, DSB levels in irradiated cultures declined to that of nonirradiated cell cultures when the cells were allowed to proliferate after irradiation, an effect that may result from elimination of the cells carrying unrepaired DSBs.

Conclusion.—These data provide strong evidence that a γ-H2AX focus represents a DSB. These foci formations can be used to measure repair of individual DSBs in human cells. The findings contrast with current models of risk assessment that assume that cellular responses are equally efficient at low and high doses.

► The effects of radiation exposure at very low doses (less than a 5-10 rad) are so small that we will be unable to detect them by using epidemiologic studies. The linearity of DSBs is quite remarkable, even down to doses as low as 100 mrem (0.001 Gy) (see Fig 2). Some argue that the additional DNA breaks caused by radiation are very small compared to the number of DNA breaks caused by oxidative processes. What they don't acknowledge is that the DNA breaks caused by radiation are qualitatively different than the DNA breaks by oxidative process. The former are much more likely to be DSBs and the latter to be single stranded breaks. DSBs are much more difficult to repair.

Whether the linear no threshold hypothesis (LNT) is "true" at low doses seems to be a great controversy to many. The complex biological events that must occur for a cell to develop into a cancer is unlikely to be a linear process; however, for radiation protection purposes, use of the LNT is attractive because of its simplicity and because of the lack of good data to support an alternative model.

Further delineation of the dose-response curve for low doses of radiation exposure will only be possible using various biological models. This article is of interest since the authors use a technique that is able to detect DNA DSBs due to radiation at doses as low as 1 mGy. Using this technique, the authors found that DNA repair was less efficient at lower doses rather than higher doses. The long-term biological consequences of the existence of such a mechanism are difficult to predict.

H. D. Royal, MD

4 Pulmonary

Introduction

What an interesting time to highlight literature relevant to pulmonary radionuclide imaging! Dramatic changes are occurring in the workup of patients with suspected pulmonary embolism. The use of spiral CT has become firmly entrenched. Despite all odds, VQ imaging in patients suspected of pulmonary embolism remains a common procedure. Unfortunately, changes in the workup of patients with suspected pulmonary embolism are driven by diagnostic accuracy studies rather than patient outcome studies. Will we ever get the diagnosis and treatment of PE right? Correct management of patients depends on balancing the benefits and harms of true positives, false negatives, true negatives, and false positives. This balancing act requires the use of probabilities (apologies to the "Yes/No" boys) and risk stratification for PE, as well as for anticoagulation.

Major advances are also occurring in our understanding of the use of FDG-PET and FDG-PET/CT in the workup of and in the monitoring of therapy for pulmonary malignancies. Hope springs eternal for a clinically useful thrombus-imaging agent. I certainly have my fingers crossed.

Henry D. Royal, MD

V/Q Imaging

Is a Lung Perfusion Scan Obtained by Using Single Photon Emission Computed Tomography Able to Improve the Radionuclide Diagnosis of Pulmonary Embolism?

Collart J-P, Roelants V, Vanpee D, et al (Université Catholique de Louvain, Yvoir, Belgium)

Nucl Med Commun 23:1107-1113, 2002 4–1

Background.—The desire to increase the specificity of testing for pulmonary embolism (PE) and thereby avoiding the problems that attend the unneeded use of anticoagulation therapy prompted the development of the radionuclide ventilation study. The ventilation/perfusion (V/Q) scan has been used, but recently spiral CT was proposed as an appropriate initial diagnostic test in most patients suspected of having PE. With the emergence of multiple head cameras and SPECT, the diagnostic potential has been further improved. The ability of perfusion SPECT to enhance the radionuclide diagnosis of PE was investigated.

Methods.—Planar and SPECT lung perfusion scans plus planar ventilation scans were performed in 114 consecutive patients suspected of having PE. An algorithm that included D-dimer measurement, leg US, a V/Q scan, and chest spiral CT along with patient outcome formed the basis for the final diagnosis. If 1 or more wedge-shaped defects were present on a planar perfusion scan, it was considered positive for PE; if 1 or more wedge-shaped defects with sharp borders or 3-lane visualization with any photopenia were found on SPECT, it was considered positive.

Results.—PE was found in 40 women and 30 men; of these, D-dimers were obtained in 92.9%, venous US of the leg in 68.6%, and spiral CT in 52.9%. The PE prevalence was 23%. SPECT showed higher intraobserver and interobserver reproducibility values than did planar studies and had a greater specificity than planar imaging. False positive results were obtained in 4% of the SPECT studies; the false negative rate was 20%. Eight of 9 intermediate and 31 of 32 low probability scans were identified as negative on SPECT.

Conclusion.—While SPECT did not improve the sensitivity of the planar images, it significantly increased the specificity in diagnosing PE with the use of pulmonary perfusion studies. Most of the low probability and intermediate V/Q scans were also resolved by SPECT, and the reproducibility of the results was better than for planar studies. Finding a negative result on SPECT could be used to rule out PE among patients who had planar perfusion defects.

▶ We continue to do planar V/Q studies in our division. Numerous colleagues, particularly those in Australia, give convincing testimonials to the value of SPECT V/Q imaging for the diagnosis of PE. One of the major obstacles to exploring this technique in the United States is the lack of availability of pertechnegas. Table 4 in the original journal article indicates that SPECT V/Q imaging significantly improves the specificity of V/Q imaging for the diagnosis of PE. Observer variability is also decreased.

H. D. Royal, MD

Comparision of Observer Variability and Accuracy of Different Criteria for Lung Scan Interpretation

Hoekstra OS, for the ANTELOPE Study Group (Vrije Universiteit, Amsterdam; et al)

J Nucl Med 44:739-744, 2003 4–2

Background.—Ventilation/perfusion (V/Q) lung scanning is the test used to diagnose most cases of pulmonary embolism (PE), since the gold standard, pulmonary angiography, is invasive and of limited availability. The interpretation of a V/Q scan can be based on several different diagnostic classification schemes, with physicians often using an integration of the various criteria along with personal experience to make the diagnosis. This is termed the Gestalt interpretation. Interobserver variability and accuracy of the Hull criteria, the Prospective Investigation of Pulmonary Embolism Diagnosis (PIOPED) criteria, and the Gestalt interpretation were investigated.

Methods.—The 3 different diagnostic schemes were used by 2 experienced observers on the V/Q scans of 328 patients. The results were analyzed with respect to the presence or absence of PE as determined by pulmonary angiography or spiral CT angiography in each case.

Results.—A definitive result concerning the presence or absence of PE was obtained in 316 of the 328 patients. A normal perfusion lung scan was present for 117 patients, subsegmental perfusion defects were found for 54 patients, and at least 1 segmental perfusion defect, requiring ventilation scintigraphy, was found for 145 patients. A disagreement between the PIOPED criteria in at least 2 categories occurred in 2 cases (0.6%). The calculated κ values of the PIOPED criteria, Hull criteria, and Gestalt interpretation were 0.70, 0.79, and 0.65, respectively.

Statistically significant differences were found between the Hull and PIOPED criteria and between the Hull criteria and the Gestalt interpretation. The low probability PIOPED result obtained in 16 patients with a normal lung scan by the Hull criteria would have prompted additional tests, with 14 of the 16 patients eventually found not to have PE. An intermediate result was found by the PIOPED criteria in 21 of 73 patients who had a high probability V/Q lung scan result by the Hull criteria; 12 of these had PE and 5 had none.

The areas under the receiver-operating characteristic curve were 0.90 for the PIOPED criteria, 0.89 for the Hull criteria, and 0.89 for the Gestalt interpretation for observer 1, with similar values for observer 2.

Conclusion.—The interobserver variation was good for each of the 3 schemes but was best when V/Q lung scans were interpreted according to the Hull criteria. Using the PIOPED criteria would have increased the number of additional investigations undertaken to obtain a final diagnosis among these patients suspected of having PE.

► The search for the Holy Grail—the correct interpretation criteria! There are a variety of interpretation and revised interpretation criteria that have been published. I regard these schemes as educational tools to teach residents and others how to begin to interpret V/Q imaging studies. I don't take any of these interpretation criteria too seriously because they are such oversimplifications of a complex task. For experienced readers, the Gestalt method of interpretation works as well as any of the formal explicit methods. Diagnostic accuracy studies are flawed because the reference standard used to determine truth is also imperfect. A much better reference standard for imaging tests is patient outcome. When this standard is used, V/Q imaging does quite well.[1]

H. D. Royal, MD

Reference

1. Wells PS, et al: Use of a clinical model for safe management of patients with suspected pulmonary embolism. *Ann Intern Med* 129:997-1005, 1998.

Comparison of Two Clinical Prediction Rules and Implicit Assessment Among Patients With Suspected Pulmonary Embolism

Chagnon I, Bounameaux H, Aujesky D, et al (Univ Hosp, Lausanne, Switzerland; Centre Hospitalier d'Angers, France)

Am J Med 113:269-275, 2002 4–3

Purpose.—Two prediction rules for pulmonary embolism have been described recently: the Wells' rule, which was derived from both outpatients and inpatients, and which includes a subjective element; and the Geneva rule, which is entirely standardized and is suitable only for emergency department patients. We compared the predictive accuracy and the concordance of the two methods, as well as the Geneva score overridden by implicit clinical judgment.

Subjects and methods.—We studied 277 consecutive patients admitted to the emergency departments of three teaching hospitals. Clinical probability was assessed prospectively with the Geneva score and the Geneva score overridden by implicit clinical judgment in case of a disagreement. The Wells' score was calculated retrospectively.

Results.—The three methods classified similar proportions of patients as having a low (53% to 58% of patients), intermediate (37% to 41% of patients), or high (4% to 10% of patients) probability of pulmonary embolism (Table 4). The actual frequencies of pulmonary embolism in each category were also similar (5% to 13% in the low, 38% to 40% in the intermediate,

TABLE 4.—Proportions of Patients and Frequency of Pulmonary Embolism in the Three Clinical Probability Categories According to Each Scoring Method*

Clinical Probability Category	Geneva Score (n = 277)	Wells' Score (n = 277)	Geneva Score Overridden by Implicit Evaluation (n = 277)
	Number (%, 95% Confidence Interval)		
Proportion of patients in category			
Low	152 (55, 49-61)	162 (58, 53-64)	146 (53, 47-59)
Intermediate	113 (41, 35-47)	104 (38, 32-43)	103 (37, 32-43)
High	12 (4, 2-7)	11 (4, 2-7)	28 (10, 6-14)
Frequency of pulmonary embolism†			
Low	20 (13, 8-18)	19 (12, 7-17)	8 (5, 2-10)
Intermediate	43 (38, 29-47)	42 (40, 31-50)	41 (40, 30-49)
High	8 (67, 35-90)	10 (91, 59-100)	22 (79, 59-91)

*There were no significant differences among the three scoring methods in the proportions of methods in the different categories.

†The denominators for the percentages can be found in the first three rows of the table.

(Courtesy of Chagnon I, Bounameaux H, Aujesky D, et al: Comparison of two clinical prediction rules and implicit assessment among patients with suspected pulmonary embolism. *Am J Med* 113:269-275. Copyright 2002, with permission from Excerpta Medica, Inc.)

and 67% to 91% in the high clinical probability categories). Receiver operating characteristic curve analysis showed no difference between the two prediction rules, but the Geneva score overridden by implicit evaluation had a marginally higher accuracy. Concordance between the two prediction rules was fair (κ coefficient = 0.43). Clinicians disagreed with the Geneva score in 21% of patients (n = 57).

Conclusion.—The two prediction rules had a similar predictive accuracy for pulmonary embolism among emergency department patients. The Geneva rule appears to be more accurate when combined with clinical judgment, although it does not apply to inpatients.

► One major shortcoming of the PIOPED study was that it implied that the posttest probability of pulmonary embolism was determined primarily by the VQ result. Today, many clinicians and some nuclear medicine physicians think that an intermediate result on a VQ study means that the posttest probability of pulmonary embolism is between 20% and 80%. If this is what you think, you are missing an extremely important point. Posttest probability of disease can only be estimated by combining the results of the test with an estimate of the pretest probability of disease.

In our hospital, we report the result of a VQ study as a likelihood ratio (which does depend solely on the result of the test) rather than a probability to make it clear that we are reporting the test result and not the posttest probability of disease. Initially, clinicians would ask why we were reporting likelihood ratios rather than probabilities. These questions gave us the opportunity to explain that one could only calculate the posttest probability of disease if they provided a pretest probability of disease.

Skeptics have always argued that if you ask 2 different clinicians what the pretest probability of disease is that you would get 2 different answers. In recent years, a number of simple clinical prediction rules have been developed and validated that allow the determination of pretest probability with simple objective criteria. Based solely on a clinical assessment, these simple predication rules are able to identify patients with a low (approximately 10%), intermediate (approximately 40%), and high (approximately 80%) pretest probability of PE.

H. D. Royal, MD

Comparison of Ventilation/Perfusion Scintigraphy and Helical CT for Diagnosis of Pulmonary Embolism; Strategy Using Clinical Data and Ancillary Findings

Bajc M, Albrechtsson U, Olsson C-G, et al (Univ Hosp, Lund, Sweden)

Clin Physiol 22:392-397, 2002 4–4

Background.—Advantages associated with the use of ventilation/perfusion scintigraphy (SCINT) in diagnosing pulmonary embolism (PE) include its noninvasive nature, ease of performance, high sensitivity, low radiation exposure, and minimal cost. Its value has been undermined by the high incidence of nondiagnostic findings, which led to the use of helical CT instead, even though this method also has drawbacks. A comparison of SCINT and helical CT was undertaken to determine which would be the best choice as the initial method for diagnosing PE.

Methods.—Over a period of 3 years, 128 patients suspected of having PE were examined with both methods. The SCINT and CT findings were evaluated by experts in each field who had no access to clinical or laboratory data. The categories used were no PE, PE, and nondiagnostic, with any findings other than PE also described. The patients' final diagnoses were based on CT, SCINT, and other data gleaned during a 6- to 24-month follow-up.

Results.—One hundred twenty-six patients received a final diagnosis, with 32 patients found to have PE. True-positive results were obtained by clinical SCINT in 29 patients, for a sensitivity of 91%; 3 patients had nondiagnostic results. The specificity of this method was 96%, with 3 false-positive results obtained; clinical SCINT was nondiagnostic in 10% of cases. With reviewed SCINT, 31 patients were found to have true-positive results, and none were nondiagnostic, for a sensitivity of 97%; the specificity was 100%, with no false-positive or false-negative results. The nondiagnostic report rate was 9%.

The sensitivity of clinical CT was 81%, with 26 true-positive results and 3 nondiagnostic findings. One false-positive case was identified, for a specificity of 99%; the rate of nondiagnostic reports was 8%. True-positives were found in 25 cases of reviewed CT, for a sensitivity of 78%; 1 patient had a nondiagnostic result, and the specificity was 100%. Twenty-three of the 32 patients had concordant clinical CT and clinical SCINT results.

The clinical and reviewed SCINT results differed in their detection of PE in 14 of the 126 patients, for a rate of 11%. The clinical and reviewed CT results differed in 10 patients, for a rate of 8%, with 1 report nondiagnostic in 8 of the 10 cases. Both CT and SCINT showed no embolism in 1 patient who had PE detected post mortem.

Conclusion.—The diagnostic rate of SCINT was higher than previously reported, and the usefulness of CT in diagnosing PE was supported. SCINT remains the initial method of choice for diagnosing PE because it is highly sensitive, is easy to perform, carries a low radiation burden, and has few nondiagnostic results. When SCINT is not available or produces nondiagnostic results, CT is helpful.

▶ I selected this paper for those of you who are looking for articles that continue to support the use of SCINT as the screening imaging test of choice for patients suspected of pulmonary embolism. Unfortunately, this article has a number of weaknesses.

Recently, the British Thoracic Society has recommended spiral CT as the diagnostic test of choice for the evaluation of patients with PE.[1] This recommendation was based on expert opinion rather than an explicit review of the published scientific literature. An evidence-based review of the spiral CT literature was published in 2000.[2] This review concluded that spiral CT needed further validation. I am unaware of any more recent recommendations that have been evidence-based.

In the United States, it is clear that spiral CT is being used routinely in the workup in patients suspected of PE. Spiral CT is ordered as the initial study in approximately 60% of patients being evaluated for PE. It is likely that this percentage will continue to get larger.

H. D. Royal, MD

References

1. British Thoracic Society guidelines for the management of suspected acute pulmonary embolism. *Thorax* 58:470-483, 2003.
2. Rathbun SW, Raskob, GE, et al: Sensitivity and specificity of helical computed tomography in the diagnosis of pulmonary embolism: A systematic review. *Ann Intern Med* 132: 227-232, 2000.

Heparin Plus Alteplase Compared With Heparin Alone in Patients With Submassive Pulmonary Embolism

Konstantinides S, for the Management Strategies and Prognosis of Pulmonary Embolism-3 Trial Investigators (Georg-August-Universität, Göttingen, Germany; et al)

N Engl J Med 347:1143-1150, 2002 4–5

Background.—Thrombolysis is an established treatment for patients with acute massive pulmonary embolism and hemodynamic instability or cardiogenic shock. In contrast, there has for several decades been an ongoing debate regarding the effect of thrombolytic agents on the outcome of hemodynamically stable patients who have submassive pulmonary embolism. Among the factors contributing to the ongoing controversy are the lack of a large, randomized study assessing clinical end points; the risk of serious hemorrhage associated with thrombolytic therapy; and the fact that patients' hemodynamic status may gradually improve with heparin therapy alone. This randomized placebo-controlled study compared the effects of treatment with heparin plus placebo with heparin plus alteplase on the outcome of patients with acute submassive pulmonary embolism.

Methods.—The study focused on 256 patients with acute pulmonary embolism and pulmonary hypertension or right ventricular dysfunction but without arterial hypotension or shock. Patients were assigned in double-blind fashion to either heparin plus 100 mg of alteplase (118 patients) or heparin plus placebo (138 patients). The primary end point was in-hospital death or clinical deterioration requiring an escalation of treatment. The treatment was catecholamine infusion, secondary thrombolysis, endotracheal intubation, cardiopulmonary resuscitation, or emergency surgical embolectomy or thrombus fragmentation by catheter.

Results.—The heparin-plus-placebo group had a significantly higher incidence of the primary end point than the heparin-plus-alteplase group, whereas the heparin-plus-alteplase group had a significantly higher probability of 30-day event-free survival (Fig 1). Mortality was low in both groups. However, treatment with heparin plus placebo was associated with

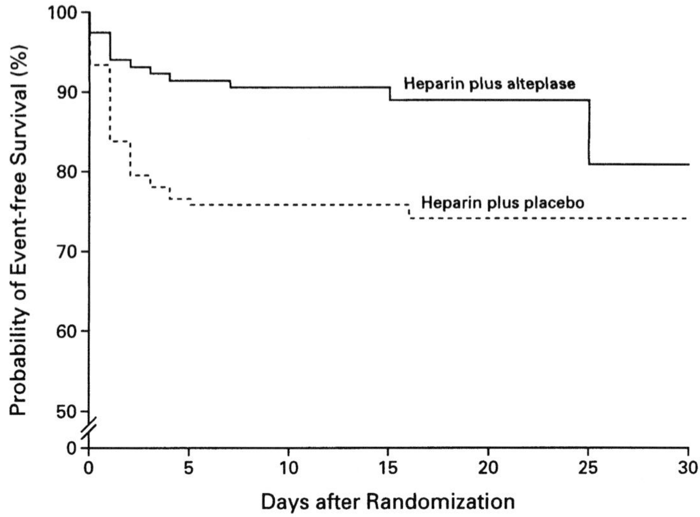

No. at Risk							
Heparin plus alteplase	118	107	96	57	26	11	6
Heparin plus placebo	137	105	87	53	24	3	2

FIGURE 1.—Kaplan-Meier estimates of the probability of event-free survival among patients with acute submissive pulmonary embolism, according to treatment with heparin plus alteplase or heparin plus placebo. An event was defined as in-hospital death or clinical deterioration requiring an escalation of treatment after termination of the infusion of the study drug. Escalation of treatment was defined as at least one of the following: infusion of a catecholamine because of arterial hypotension or shock (except for dopamine infused at a rate of no more than 5 µg/kg/min), secondary thrombolysis, endotracheal intubation, cardiopulmonary resuscitation, or emergency surgical embolectomy or thrombus fragmentation by catheter. $P = .005$ by the log-rank test for the overall comparison between the groups. (Reprinted by permission of Konstantinides S, for the Management Strategies and Prognosis of Pulmonary Embolism-3 Trial Investigators: Heparin plus alteplase compared with heparin alone in patients with submissive pulmonary embolism. *N Engl J Med* 347:1143-1150.)

nearly 3 times the risk of death or treatment escalation compared with heparin plus alteplase. There were no incidents of fatal bleeding or cerebral bleeding in patients receiving heparin plus alteplase.

Conclusion.—Alteplase administered in conjunction with heparin can improve the clinical course of stable patients who have acute submassive pulmonary embolism. Heparin plus alteplase also can prevent clinical deterioration requiring the escalation of treatment during the hospital stay.

► Why have I included an article about treatment of submassive pulmonary embolism in this review? There seem to be 2 very different schools of thought about the diagnosis and treatment of patients with pulmonary embolism. The first school of thought is that the diagnosis of pulmonary embolism is binary and that once you know that pulmonary embolism is present, those patients should be treated. The second school of thought views the management of patients with suspected pulmonary embolism as a delicate balance between the risk of not treating the patient who has pulmonary embolism and the risk of treatment itself. I fall into the latter camp.

Weighing the potential benefits and harms of treatment is complicated and requires an assessment of the risk of pulmonary embolism (risk stratification) and the risk of therapy. The importance of risk stratification is widely recognized with myocardial perfusion imaging. A great deal of useful information would be lost if myocardial perfusion imaging studies were only reported as positive or negative.

With pulmonary embolism, the prevailing (and wrong) view seems to be that risk stratification is unimportant. Why is this the wrong view? First, despite the fact that ventilation-perfusion (V/Q) imaging is often portrayed as a very imperfect diagnostic test for pulmonary embolism, I have always been impressed that patients who have low (and even intermediate) results on their V/Q studies do well when they are not treated. There are several articles in the literature that support this contention.[1-5] Yet we know that some of these patients who have not been treated would have been shown to have pulmonary embolism if they had had pulmonary arteriography or a CT pulmonary arteriogram. One unrecognized strength of V/Q imaging may be that patients who are a high risk for pulmonary embolism are readily identified by V/Q imaging.

Second, our technology for detecting pulmonary embolism continues to improve. Smaller emboli can be detected by spiral CT today than could be detected 5 years ago. At some point, we are going to have to ask ourselves the question, "When is pulmonary embolism clinically significant?" This article indicates that the addition of a thrombolytic agent in the treatment of patients with submassive pulmonary embolism results in better patient outcome (See Fig 1). More effective treatment tips the scales in favor of treatment.

H. D. Royal, MD

References

1. Lee ME, et al: Low-probability V-P scintigrams: Clinical outcomes in 99 patients. *Radiology* 156:497-500, 1985.
2. Smith R, et al: Clinical outcomes of patients with suspected pulmonary embolism and low probability aerosol-perfusion scintigrams. *Radiology* 164:781-788, 1987.
3. Kahn D, et al: Clinical outcomes of patients with a "low probability" of PE on V-P lung scans. *Arch Int Med* 149:377-379, 1989.
4. Hull RD, et al: Clinical validity of a normal perfusion lung scan in patients suspected of pulmonary embolism. *Chest* 97:22-26, 1990.
5. Wells PS, et al: Use of a clinical model for safe management of patients with suspected pulmonary embolism. *Ann Intern Med* 129:997-1005, 1998.

Diagnostic Strategies for Excluding Pulmonary Embolism in Clinical Outcome Studies: A Systematic Review

Kruip MJHA, Leclercq MGL, van der Heul C, et al (St Elisabeth Hosp, Tilburg, The Netherlands; Medisch Spectrum Twente, Enschede, The Netherlands; Univ of Maastricht, The Netherlands; et al)

Ann Intern Med 138:941-951, 2003 4–6

Background.—Pulmonary embolism is associated with high rates of morbidity and mortality if untreated. However, the diagnosis or exclusion of pulmonary embolism is difficult on the basis of clinical manifestations because such manifestations are nonspecific. Approximately 25% of patients with suspected pulmonary embolism have a diagnosis confirmed by objective testing. The goal of the first diagnostic strategies developed was to confirm, rather than exclude, the presence of pulmonary emboli. However, the most recently evaluated diagnostic approaches have focused on the identification of patients who do not have pulmonary embolism and therefore do not require anticoagulant therapy. Various diagnostic strategies for the exclusion of pulmonary embolism were evaluated.

Methods.—This retrospective study used the MEDLINE, EMBASE, and DARE databases; study investigators; and reference lists to identify prospective clinical outcome studies. Investigators recorded the frequency of symptomatic venous thromboembolism over a 3-month follow-up in patients in whom pulmonary embolism had been excluded according to various strategies. The strategies were divided into 3 categories according to the number of rounds of diagnostic tests needed to exclude pulmonary embolism.

Results.—Twenty-five studies involving more than 7000 patients were identified. In all the referred patients, normal results on pulmonary angiography or lung scintigraphy and normal D-dimer levels combined with low clinical probability safely excluded pulmonary embolism, with failure rates of 3% or less. In the second round of diagnostic tests, in patients with a nondiagnostic lung scan, pulmonary angiography and serial leg testing for venous thrombosis were accurate and safe (Table 5). When D-dimer testing

TABLE 5.—Summary Table of the Diagnostic Strategies for Excluding Pulmonary Embolism With an Upper 95% Confidence Limit of 3% or Less for 3-Month Thromboembolic Risk

Variable	3-Month Risk for VTE Complications (Upper 95% CL)
Diagnostic strategies for excluding pulmonary embolism in all referred patients	
Normal results on PA	0.8 (2.1)
Normal lung scan	0.9 (2.3)
Normal lung scan and normal leg testing results	0.6 (1.2)
Normal D-dimer level	0.0 (1.8)
Normal D-dimer level and low clinical probability	0.2 (0.8)
Diagnostic strategies for excluding pulmonary embolism after the first diagnostic round	
Abnormal lung scan plus normal results on PA	1.3 (2.8)
Nondiagnostic lung scan plus normal results on serial IPG	1.7 (2.8)
Nondiagnostic lung scan, normal results on serial CUS, and low to moderate clinical probability	0.5 (1.3)
Moderate to high clinical probability or elevated D-dimer level and low clinical probability plus normal lung scan	0.0 (1.1)
Moderate to high clinical probability or elevated D-dimer level and low clinical probability plus normal results on spiral CT and CUS	0.0 (1.3)

Abbreviations: CL, Confidence limit; *CUS*, compression US; *IPG*, impedance plethysmography; *PA*, pulmonary angiography; *VTE*, venous thromboembolism.

(Courtesy of Kruip MJHA, Leclercq MGL, van der Heul C, et al: Diagnostic strategies for excluding pulmonary embolism in clinical outcome studies: A systematic review. *Ann Intern Med* 138:941-951, 2003.)

combined with clinical probability was inconclusive, a normal perfusion lung scan safely excluded pulmonary embolism. The evidence accumulated from these trials showed that normal results on spiral CT may also safely exclude pulmonary embolism.

Conclusion.—There is likely to be increasing interest in a fast, simple strategy for the exclusion of pulmonary embolism, starting with a normal perfusion lung scan or a combination of normal D-dimer levels and low clinical probability. This systematic review of the literature found that, after the initial round of testing, a reliable diagnostic method such as angiography or lung scintigraphy is warranted.

► In this systematic review, the authors examine the effectiveness of various diagnostic strategies to exclude pulmonary embolism in patients suspected of having pulmonary embolism. The authors identified 77 studies that would potentially be included in their review; however, only 25 studies met predefined criteria for inclusion.

The article lacks some focus in that so many different diagnostic strategies are included (pulmonary arteriography, CT, ventilation-perfusion imaging, serial compression US, serial impedance plethysmography, D-dimer testing, assessment of clinical probability, and MR angiography). However, the major strength of the review is that the reference standard used to assess diagnostic strategies was patient outcomes rather than diagnostic accuracy.

Table 5 in the original article summarizes the diagnostic strategies that resulted in a risk of subsequent thromboembolic events of less than 3% when these patients were not anticoagulated. Of particular note is that the 3-month thromboembolic event rate in a patient with a non-diagnostic (low or intermediate results) ventilation-perfusion scan, normal results on serial compression US, and a low to moderate clinical pretest probability, is only 0.5%. Note that the subsequent thromboembolic event rate using these criteria is less than the thromboembolic event rate in patients who have normal results on a pulmonary arteriogram.

H. D. Royal, MD

Spiral CT

Diagnostic Strategy for Patients With Suspected Pulmonary Embolism: A Prospective Multicentre Outcome Study

Simonneau G, for the Evaluation du Scanner Spiralé dans l'Embolie Pulmonaire Study Group (Hôpital Universitaire Antoine Béclère, Clamart, France; et al)

Lancet 360:1914-1920, 2002 4–7

Background.—We designed a prospective multicentre outcome study to evaluate a diagnostic strategy based on clinical probability, spiral CT, and venous compression ultrasonography of the legs in patients with suspected pulmonary embolism (PE). The main aim was to assess the safety of withholding anticoagulant treatment in patients with low or intermediate clini-

TABLE 3.—Venous Thromboembolic Events During 3-Month Follow-up in Untreated Patients With Low or Intermediate Clinical Probability and Negative Findings on Spiral CT and Leg Venous Compression Ultrasonography

	Untreated Inpatients (n=126)	Untreated Outpatients (n=381)	Total (n=507)
Symptomatic VTE	2 (2 DVT)	2 (1 PE, 1 DVT)	4 (1 PE, 3 DVT)
Death			
Certainly related to PE	0	0	0
Possibly related to PE	4	1	5
VTE events (95% CI)	4·8% (1·8-10·1)	0·8% (0·2-2·3)	1·8% (0·8-3·3)

Abbreviations: VTE, Venous thromboembolism; *PE*, pulmonary embolism; *DVT*, deep-vein thrombosis.

(Courtesy of Simonneau G, for the Evaluation du Scanner Spiralé dans l'Embolie Pulmonaire Study Group: Diagnostic strategy for patients with suspected pulmonary embolism: A prospective multicentre outcome study. *Lancet* 360:1914-1920, 2002. Reprinted with permission from Elsevier Science.)

cal probability of PE and negative findings on spiral CT and ultrasonography.

Methods.—1041 consecutive inpatients and outpatients with suspected PE were included. Patients with negative spiral CT and ultrasonography and clinically assessed as having a low or intermediate clinical probability were left untreated. Those with high clinical probability underwent lung scanning, pulmonary angiography, or both. All patients were followed up for 3 months.

Findings.—PE was diagnosed in 360 (34·6%) patients; 55 had positive ultrasonography despite negative spiral CT. Of 601 patients with negative spiral CT and ultrasonography, 76 were clinically assessed as having a high probability of PE; lung scanning or angiography showed PE in four (5·3% [95% CI 1·5-13·1]). The remaining 525 patients were assessed as having low or intermediate clinical probability, and 507 of them were not treated. Of these patients, nine experienced venous thromboembolism during follow-up (1·8% [0·8-3·3]). The diagnostic strategy proved inconclusive in 95 (9·1%) patients, and pulmonary angiography was done in 74 (7·1%) (Table 3).

Interpretation.—Withholding of anticoagulant therapy is safe when the clinical probability of PE is assessed as low or intermediate and spiral CT and ultrasonography are negative.

► The results of this multicenter study to assess diagnostic strategy consisting of the clinical probability of PE, spiral CT, and other sonography are more believable than many of the other studies on spiral CT. The fact that these authors recognize that they needed to assess the clinical probability of PE and that they also needed to determine the status of the lower extremities by using compression US is a step in the right direction. Notice that the subsequent venous thromboembolic event rate (Table 3) is higher (although not statistically different) than the 2 strategies (Perrier, Wells) that used VQ imaging in combination with other noninvasive test results.

H. D. Royal, MD

Single-Detector Helical Computed Tomography as the Primary Diagnostic Test in Suspected Pulmonary Embolism: A Multicenter Clinical Management Study of 510 Patients

van Strijen MJL, for the Advances in New Technologies Evaluating the Localisation of Pulmonary Embolism (ANTELOPE) Study Group (Leyenburg Ziekenhuis, The Hague; et al)

Ann Intern Med 138:307-314, 2003 4–8

Background.—The nonspecific nature of the symptoms of pulmonary embolism (PE) make its diagnosis difficult and require the use of objective diagnostic imaging modalities, with helical CT of the pulmonary arteries becoming more accepted as a diagnostic test for PE. The overall sensitivities for helical CT have been reported to be between 64% and 100%, with specificities in the range of 89% to 100%. Patients with suspected PE were evaluated according to a simple and relatively noninvasive diagnostic algorithm of single-detector helical CT followed by serial venous compression US of the lower limb veins. The focus of this investigation was the effectiveness and safety of helical CT of the pulmonary arteries as a primary diagnostic method of identifying PE.

Methods.—With the use of a multicenter, prospective clinical outcome design over a period of 3 months, 510 consecutive inpatients and outpatients with suspected PE were assessed by helical CT of the pulmonary arteries within 24 hours of exhibiting signs and symptoms of PE. For normal or inconclusive CT results, compression US was done on the same day, then repeated 4 and 7 days later if the initial findings were normal. Patients were to report any signs or symptoms of PE or deep venous thrombosis (DVT) over a follow-up of 3 months. Compression US or phlebography was done for suspected DVT; pulmonary angiography was performed if PE was suspected.

Results.—On CT, PE was found in 124 patients (24.3%); 130 patients had no PE on their CT results but were diagnosed with an alternative condition that related to the signs and symptoms reported (Table 3). Two hundred forty-eight patients (48.6% of the sample) had normal CT results; 3 developed clinical symptoms compatible with a diagnosis of DVT over the 3-month follow-up, of whom nonfatal PE was found in only 1 patient, yielding a false-negative rate of 0.4%. Of the 130 patients who were diagnosed with other conditions, 1 developed possible symptoms of venous thromboembolism and was diagnosed with DVT by compression US.

Of 129 patients given anticoagulant therapy, 124 had PE, 2 had DVT, and 3 had no definitive diagnosis. Symptoms were present in 7 of these patients, of whom 5 suffered a thromboembolic event. Indeterminate results were obtained in 8 patients (1.6%); 5 did not receive anticoagulant therapy and did

TABLE 3.—The 6 Main Categories of Alternative Diagnoses

Category	Patients, %
Pneumonia	51
Malignancy	17
Progression of pleural fluid (underestimated on conventional chest radiography)	8
Cardiac failure	8
Chronic obstructive pulmonary disease	5
Other (e.g., pneumothorax, aortic dissection)	11

(Courtesy of van Strijen MJL, for the Advances in New Technologies Evaluating the Localisation of Pulmonary Embolism (ANTELOPE) Study Group: Single-detector helical computed tomography as the primary diagnostic test in suspected pulmonary embolism: A multicenter clinical management study of 510 patients. *Ann Intern Med* 138:307-314, 2003.)

not develop symptoms of PE or hemorrhage. None of the patients who had normal results on helical CT died of PE.

Conclusion.—Helical CT proved to be safe as a principal diagnostic test in patients suspected of having PE. The use of serial compression US was of help in selected cases.

▶ This article provides data that support the use of spiral CT in patients suspected of PE. The authors found that the addition of serial compression US provided little value. I still think that examination of the lower extremities is important. The event that will potentially kill the patient is subsequent emboli. Certainly the risk of subsequent emboli is affected by the amount of thrombus that resides in the lower extremities.

In this article, the authors state that one of the reasons that spiral CT is valuable is that an alternative diagnosis was made in 130 patients (25.5%). Some of the alternative diagnoses are listed in Table 3. I have 2 problems with these alternative diagnoses. The first is that it is difficult to determine whether CT provided unique information about these alternative diagnoses. Certainly many of these diagnoses would have been evident from other clinical information. The second problem is the assertion that these alternative diagnoses somehow rule out the diagnosis of PE. PE and these alternative diagnoses are not mutually exclusive.

H. D. Royal, MD

Outcomes After Withholding Anticoagulation From Patients With Suspected Acute Pulmonary Embolism and Negative Computed Tomographic Findings: A Cohort Study

Swensen SJ, Sheedy PF II, Ryu JH, et al (Mayo Clinic, Rochester, Minn)

Mayo Clin Proc 77:130-138, 2002 4–9

Background.—The estimated annual incidence of acute pulmonary embolism in the United States is 69 per 100,000 persons. Observed survival after pulmonary embolism is worse than the expected survival, with a 7-day mortality rate of nearly 30%. However, even for patients living at least 7 days, survival is significantly reduced for the next 3 months, independent of other comorbid conditions. Anticoagulation with heparin or warfarin is effective therapy for pulmonary embolism, but it can have severe and even life-threatening complications. Thus, it is critical that a diagnosis of pulmonary embolism be sufficiently certain so that affected patients receive potentially lifesaving therapy, and unaffected patients are spared the unnecessary risk of complications. Clinical studies have shown that withholding anticoagulation in patients with suspected acute pulmonary embolism is safe if the results of perfusion lung scans are negative. The outcome of withholding anticoagulation from patients with suspected acute pulmonary embolism in whom CT findings are negative for pulmonary embolism was determined.

Methods.—A total of 1512 consecutive patients were included in this retrospective cohort study. All the patients were examined by electron beam CT, and findings were interpreted as either positive or negative. The main outcome measures were deep venous thrombosis, pulmonary embolism, and vital status within 3 months after the CT scan as well as the cause of death based on review of medical records, patient questionnaires, and telephone interviews.

Results.—CT scans were interpreted as negative for acute pulmonary embolism in 1010 patients (67%). Seventeen of these patients received anticoagulation and were excluded from the final analysis. Of the remaining 993 patients, deep venous thrombosis or pulmonary embolism developed in 8 patients; 118 patients died, 3 of pulmonary embolism. The 3-month cumulative incidence of overall deep venous thrombosis or pulmonary embolism was 0.5%. For fatal pulmonary embolism, the 3-month cumulative incidence was 0.3%.

Conclusions.—There is a low incidence of overall deep venous thrombosis or pulmonary embolism, or fatal pulmonary embolism among patients with suspected acute pulmonary embolism, negative CT results, and no other clinical evidence of venous thromboembolism. Thus, it would appear safe to withhold anticoagulation in these patients.

► I'm not sure what to make of this article. First, it is a retrospective review of the results using electron beam CT from August 1997 until November 1998 that is being reported in 2002. The technology is rapidly changing so that relevance of this article to conventional spiral CT is uncertain.

Two other issues caught my attention. First, it appears that these studies were read in a vacuum, without the use of clinical probability or the results of US of the lower extremities. Because all diagnostic tests are imperfect, use of pretest probability is important. Since pulmonary embolisms are a sequela of deep vein thrombosis, an assessment of the clot burden in the lower extremities is likely to be useful in risk stratification. Second, the apparent prevalence of acute pulmonary embolism was very high (33%). This is a very different population than the population that would routinely be referred for imaging to exclude pulmonary embolism.

H. D. Royal, MD

PET

^{18}F-FDG Accumulation With PET for Differentiation Between Benign and Malignant Lesions in the Thorax

Demura Y, Tsuchida T, Ishizaki T, et al (Fukui Med Univ, Japan)

J Nucl Med 44:540-548, 2003 4–10

Background.—Study of tumors using ^{18}F-FDG, combined with PET is both sensitive and specific in the diagnosis and staging of several types of malignancies, although some benign processes also show ^{18}F-FDG uptake, yielding false-positive results and misdiagnoses. Accumulations of ^{201}Tl on SPECT differ between benign and malignant tumors, and this method is more cost efficient and more generally available than ^{18}F-FDG PET.

It was hypothesized that measuring the uptake and metabolism of ^{18}F-FDG at 2 time points would be helpful in differentiating malignant from benign lesions, with this method being superior to the use of ^{201}Tl SPECT. The 2 methods were compared in patients who had thoracic abnormalities to determine whether ^{18}F-FDG PET delayed imaging was useful.

Methods.—Thoracic nodular lesions were found on the chest CT images of 80 patients. These were then evaluated using early and delayed ^{18}F-FDG PET and ^{201}Tl- SPECT within 1 week of each evaluation. The results were assessed and compared with documented findings on histopathologic evaluation.

Results.—Surgical resection confirmed that 50 lesions were malignant and 24 benign; 3 patients were diagnosed with organizing pneumonia and 3 with a mycobacterial infection. All of the malignant tumors had a higher standardized uptake value (SUV) at 3 hours than at 1 hour, while most benign lesions had significantly lower SUV levels at 3 hours than at 1 hour (Fig 1).

The mycobacterial infections and 1 case of nodular sarcoidosis had a higher SUV at 3 hours than at 1 hour. Well-differentiated adenocarcinoma and squamous cell carcinoma had significantly lower SUV levels at 1 and 3 hours than poorly differentiated adenocarcinoma and squamous cell carcinoma. A higher retention-index SUV (RI-SUV) was found for undifferentiated carcinoma than for low-grade malignant diseases.

While early and delayed images using ^{18}F-FDG PET and ^{201}Tl-SPECT were similar for thoracic lesions, the RI-SUV was significantly superior in accurately differentiating benign lesions from malignant ones. Thoracic CT was less accurate than ^{18}F-FDG PET and ^{201}Tl-SPECT in nodal staging, with excellent sensitivity in the use of ^{18}F-FDG PET. With delayed imaging, the specificity improved significantly, from 62.9% to 91.4%; ^{18}F-FDG PET delayed imaging proved to be significantly more accurate overall than the other modalities. The close correlation between the RI-SUV results of the primary lesion and lymph node metastasis was helpful in nodal staging.

Conclusion.—While no significant advantages were noted between ^{18}F-FDG PET early and delayed imaging and ^{201}Tl-SPECT imaging with respect to differentiating between malignant and benign diseases, ^{18}F-FDG PET RI

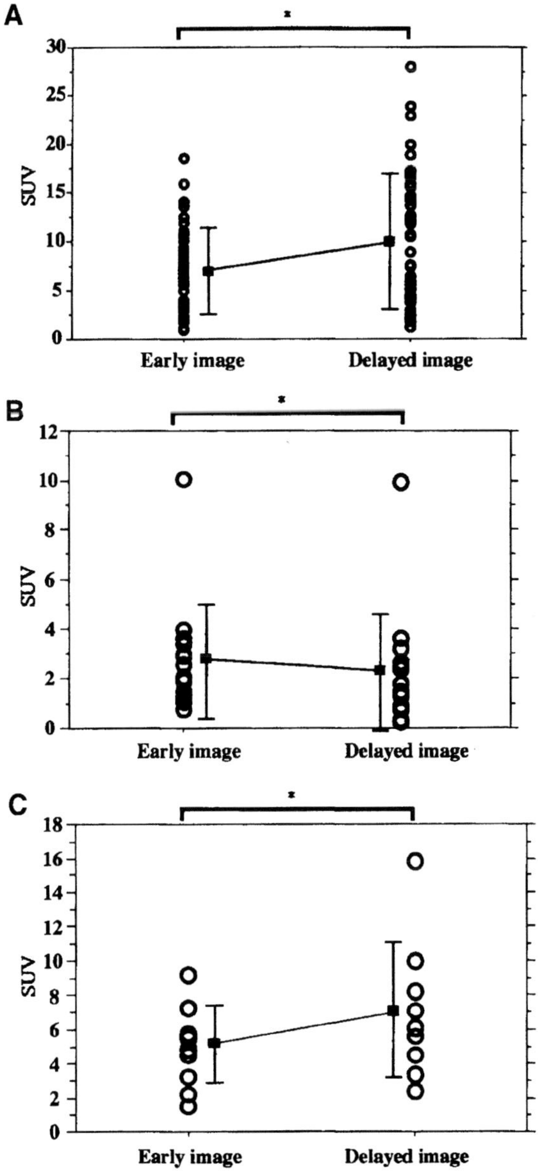

FIGURE 1.—Changes in ^{18}F-FDG accumulation (*SUV*) between early and delayed imaging in primary lesions of malignant lesion group (mostly lung cancer) (A), benign disease group (group 9) (B), and granulomatous disease group (group 10) (C). Significant increases of SUV in A and C and significant decrease of SUV in B were observed. *Bars* indicate mean ± standard deviation. *Asterisk* indicates $P < .05$. (Reprinted by permission of the Society of Nuclear Medicine from Demura Y, Tsuchida T, Ishizaki T, et al: ^{18}F-FDG accumulation with PET for differentiation between benign and malignant lesions in the thorax. *J Nucl Med* 44:540-548, 2003.)

(RI-SUV) was far superior to other scintigraphic methods for this application. Using ^{18}F-FDG PET at 2 points offered significant advantages in distinguishing between benign and malignant lesions.

► There are a number of ways that PET evaluation of solitary pulmonary nodules may be improved. One possible technique is to get additional delayed images. According to these authors, the SUV continues to increase in malignant lesions and decreases with benign lesions. Unfortunately, SUV also appears to increase in patients with granulomous disease (see Fig 1).

H. D. Royal, MD

Positron Emission Tomography in Non–Small-Cell Lung Cancer: Prediction of Response to Chemotherapy by Quantitative Assessment of Glucose Use

Weber WA, Petersen V, Schmidt B, et al (Technische Universität München, Germany)

J Clin Oncol 21:2651-2657, 2003 4–11

Background.—Patients with non–small-cell lung cancer (NSCLC) can be staged by PET, with the markedly accelerated glucose use producing high tumor uptake of the radiolabeled glucose analogue ^{18}F-FDG. PET imaging with FDG is significantly more sensitive and specific than conventional methods in detecting lymph nodes and distant metastases. Most patients

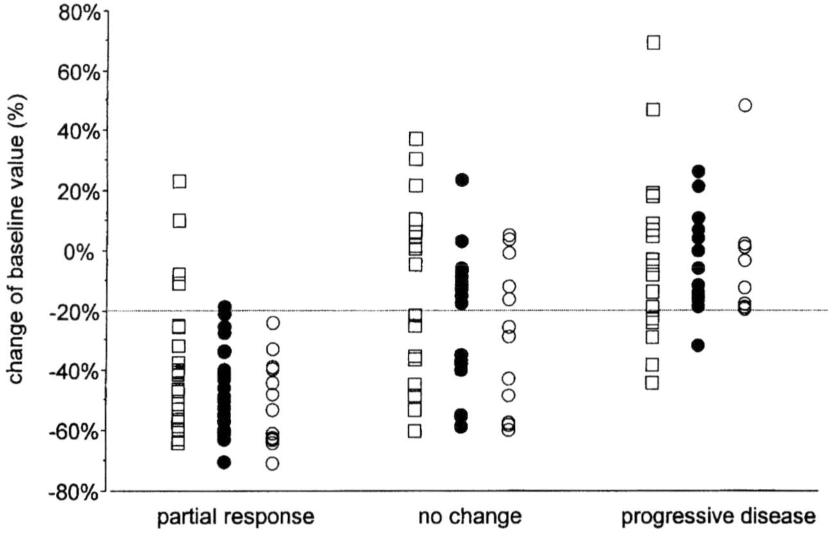

FIGURE 3.—Changes in tumor metabolic activity and best response to therapy. *Open boxes* indicates changes in tumor/muscle ratio; *black circles*, changes in standardized uptake values; *open circles*, changes in net-influx constants. (Courtesy of Weber WA, Petersen V, Schmidt B, et al: Positron emission tomography in non–small-cell lung cancer: Prediction of response to chemotherapy by quantitative assessment of glucose use. *J Clin Oncol* 21(14):2651-2657, 2003. Reprinted with permission from the American Society of Clinical Oncology.)

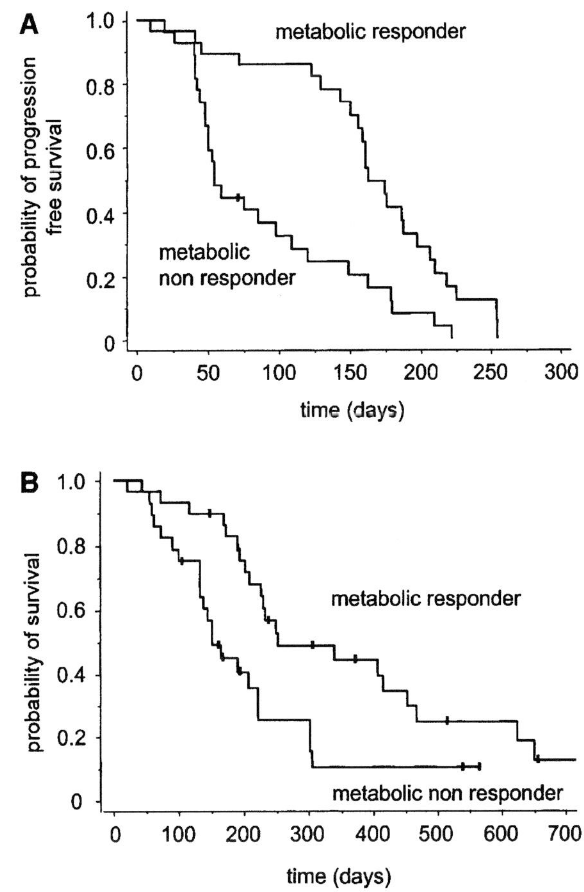

FIGURE 5.—Kaplan-Meier plots showing (**A**) progression-free and (**B**) overall survival. For both parameters, there is a significant difference between patients with and without a metabolic response in FDG-PET ($P = .0003$ and $P = .005$, respectively). (Courtesy of Weber WA, Petersen V, Schmidt B, et al: Positron emission tomography in non–small-cell lung cancer: Prediction of response to chemotherapy by quantitative assessment of glucose use. *J Clin Oncol* 21(14):2651-2657, 2003. Reprinted with permission from the American Society of Clinical Oncology.)

with NSCLC have unresectable disease and receive palliative therapy to improve quality of life and prolong median survival. One third of patients have tumor progression during first-line chemotherapy, and tyrosine kinase inhibitors have detected activity in patients who progress after platinum-based chemotherapy.

If the tumor response were predicted earlier, alternative therapies could be employed. Whether changes in tumor glucose use as determined by FDG-PET can predict tumor response and patient outcome after 1 cycle of platinum-based chemotherapy was studied by several techniques.

Methods.—Fifty-seven patients underwent FDG PET before and after their first cycle of platinum-based chemotherapy. A metabolic response was defined as reduced tumor FDG uptake by over 20% when using standardized uptake values (SUV); changes in tumor SUVs were compared with changes in the net-influx constants (Ki) and tumor/muscle (t/m) ratios of FDG.

Results.—Of 55 patients available for response assessment, the overall response rate was 38%. The metabolic response in FDG PET and the subsequent best overall response showed a highly significant correlation. Twenty of 28 patients with metabolic responses were also classified as responders by Response Evaluation Criteria in Solid Tumors (RECIST) criteria, while only 1 of 27 patients without a metabolic response had a partial response. The negative predictive value of a metabolic response for predicting the best response was thus 96%, sensitivity was 95%, and specificity was 76%.

Disease progression occurred after the first 2 chemotherapy cycles in only 1 patient who had a metabolic response. Tumor nonresponse based on the RECIST criteria was found in 8 patients with a metabolic response. The specificity was 84% and the sensitivity 96% for metabolic response predicting primary tumor response. Close correlation was found between relative changes in Ki and SUV; a higher scattering was found between the t/m ratio and SUV or Ki (Fig 3).

Follow-up ranged from 106 to 1404 days, during which time 44 patients died and 50 patients had diagnosed tumor progression. The survival rate at 1 year was 28%. Patients with a metabolic response had a median time to progression of 163 days, while for those with a less pronounced decline in SUV progression occurred in a median of 54 days (Fig 5). Patients with a metabolic response had a median overall survival of 252 days, while median survival for those lacking a metabolic response was 151 days. Survival rates at 1 year were 44% and 10%, respectively. While the results with Ki estimates of tumor glucose use were similar, considerable overlap was found for changes in the t/m ratio between responding and nonresponding lesions.

Conclusion.—Among patients with NSCLC, reduced metabolic activity after a single round of chemotherapy was closely related to the final outcome of therapy. Effective chemotherapy rapidly reduced tumor glucose use and yielded a response rate of 71%. In patients lacking a metabolic response, the response rate was only 4%.

► Another important article on the use of PET to predict response to therapy. More realistic expectations about how useful PET might be can be obtained by looking at Figures 3 and 5 of this article. Figure 3 demonstrates that there is considerable overlap in the change SUV among the 3 different patient groups (partial responders, no change, and progressive disease). Figure 5 indicates that, although there may be some improvement in life expectancy in those responders, the overall prognosis still is dismal.

H. D. Royal, MD

Staging of Non–Small-Cell Lung Cancer With Integrated Positron-Emission Tomography and Computed Tomography

Lardinois D, Weder W, Hany TF, et al (Univ Hosp of Zurich, Switzerland; Univ of Zurich, Switzerland)

N Engl J Med 348:2500-2507, 2003 4–12

Background.—Integrated PET-CT scanners have been recently introduced. The accuracy of integrated PET-CT and that of other imaging modalities in staging non–small-cell lung cancer (NSCLC) were compared in a prospective study.

Methods.—Fifty patients with proved or suspected NSCLC underwent integrated PET-CT scanning. In addition, CT alone, PET alone, and visually correlated PET and CT were undertaken. Tumor-node-metastasis (TNM) staging was assigned based on image analysis.

Findings.—In 41% of the patients, integrated PET-CT provided additional information beyond that available with visual correlation of PET and CT. The diagnostic accuracy of integrated PET-CT was greater than that of the other modalities (Tables 1, 2, and 3). In addition, tumor staging was significantly more accurate with integrated PET-CT than with CT alone, PET alone, or visual PET-CT correlation. Node staging was also significantly more accurate with integrated PET-CT than with PET alone. In 2 of 8 patients undergoing staging of metastasis, integrated PET-CT increased diagnostic certainty.

Conclusion.—When integrated PET-CT becomes more widely available, it will be the preferred modality for determining disease stage in patients with NSCLC. If further research verifies the current findings, integrated PET-CT may become the new standard for imaging lung cancer.

TABLE 1.—Comparison of the Diagnostic Accuracy of Integrated PET-CT With CT Alone, PET Alone, and Visual Correlation of PET and CT Images

Variable	*P* Value
Tumor stage (n=40)	
PET-CT vs. CT alone	0.001†
PET-CT vs. PET alone	<0.001†
PET-CT vs. visual correlation of PET and CT	0.013†
Node stage (n=37)	
PET-CT vs. CT alone	0.12
PET-CT vs. PET alone	0.013†
PET-CT vs. visual correlation of PET and CT	0.021

Note: The paired sign test was used to calculate *P* values. Stages assigned on the basis of CT alone, PET alone, and PET and CT were assessed by Review Board A, and stages assigned on the basis of integrated PET-CT were assessed by Review Board B.

*The *P* value was significant after Bonferroni's correction.

TABLE 2.—Diagnostic Accuracy of the Imaging Methods With Respect to Tumor Stage in 40 Patients

Imaging Method	Classification Correct (Score of 3)	Classification Correct But Equivocal (Score of 2)	Classification Incorrect (Score of 0 or 1)
		no. of patients (%)	
CT alone	23 (58)	8 (20)	9 (22)
PET alone	16 (40)	16 (40)	8 (20)
Visual correlation of PET and CT	26 (65)	5 (12)	9 (22)
Integrated PET-CT	35 (88)	4 (10)	1 (2)

(Reprinted by permission of Lardinois D, Weder W, Hany TF, et al: Staging of non–small-cell lung cancer with integrated positron-emission tomography and computed tomography. *N Engl J Med* 348:2500-2507.)

TABLE 3.—Diagnostic Accuracy of the Imaging Methods With Respect to Node Stage in 37 Patients

Imaging Method	Classification Correct (Score of 3)	Classification Correct But Equivocal (Score of 2)	Classification Incorrect (Score of 0 or 1)
		no. of patients (%)	
CT alone	22 (59)	2 (5)	13 (35)
PET alone	18 (49)	14 (38)	5 (14)
Visual correlation of PET and CT	22 (59)	4 (11)	11 (30)
Integrated PET-CT	30 (81)	1 (3)	6 (16)

(Reprinted by permission of Lardinois D, Weder W, Hany TF, et al: Staging of non–small-cell lung cancer with integrated positron-emission tomography and computed tomography. *N Engl J Med* 348:2500-2507.)

▶ PET/CT represents a major advance in imaging. The added accuracy of integrated PET and CT in the staging of non–small-cell lung cancer is documented by these authors. (See Tables 1, 2, and 3).

H. D. Royal, MD

In Vivo Assessment of Tumor Hypoxia in Lung Cancer With ^{60}Cu-ATSM

Dehdashti F, Mintun MA, Lewis JS, et al (Edward Mallinckrodt Inst of Radiology, St Louis; Washington Univ, St Louis)

Eur J Nucl Med Mol Imaging 30:844-850, 2003 4–13

Background.—When tumor hypoxia is detected, it signals an increased likelihood of local recurrence and distant metastasis, resistance to radiation therapy, and nonresponsiveness to certain types of chemotherapy. Methods of measuring tissue oxygen levels in tumors have been unsatisfying. ^{60}diacetyl-bis (N^4-methylthiosemicarbazone) (^{60}Cu-ATSM) has been shown to accumulate avidly in hypoxic cells and to wash out rapidly from normoxic cells. Whether ^{60}Cu-ATSM can be used to image hypoxic tissue with PET was evaluated in patients with non–small-cell lung cancer (NSCLC). The tumor uptake of ^{60}Cu-ATSM was compared with the tumor response to therapy.

Methods.—PET with ^{60}Cu-ATSM and with ^{18}F-FDG was used to study 19 patients with biopsy-proved NSCLC before therapy was initiated. The ^{60}Cu-ATSM uptake was assessed semiquantitatively by measuring the tumor-to-muscle activity ratio (T/M). PET results were then correlated with the outcome of therapy at 2 to 46 months.

Results.—FDG PET confirmed tumors in all patients before therapy was begun. Variable tumor uptake of ^{60}Cu-ATSM was found, with 17 patients having measurable uptake on PET of 2.3 for T/M and 3.2 for the tumor standardized uptake value (SUV). Response was determined in 14 patients, of

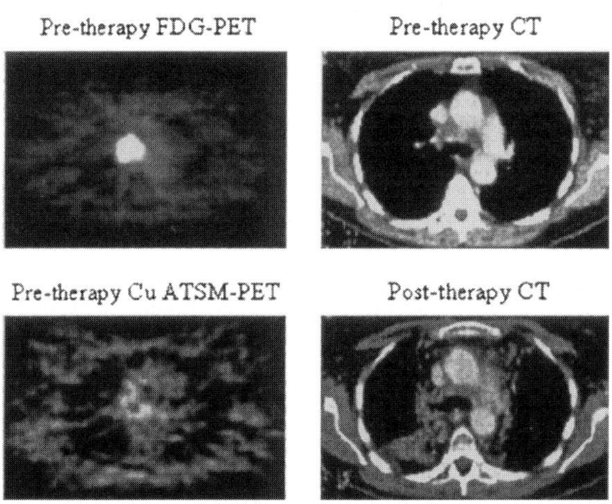

FIGURE 2.—Responder. Transaxial FDG PET image (**upper left**) of the chest shows moderately intense FDG uptake (standard uptake value, 4.9) in the known lung cancer. Transaxial ^{60}Cu-ATSM-PET image (**lower left**) at the same level demonstrates minimal uptake within the tumor (tumor-to-muscle activity ratio = 1.3). CT image prior to therapy (**upper right**) demonstrates increased soft tissue density in the precarinal space, consistent with patient's known cancer. CT image after radiotherapy (**lower right**) demonstrates postradiation changes but shows a good response of the tumor to the treatment. The patient was alive at last follow-up (46 months after the diagnosis of lung cancer) without evidence of tumor recurrence. (Courtesy of Dehdashti F, Mintun MA, Lewis JS, et al: In vivo assessment of tumor hypoxia in lung cancer with ^{60}Cu-ATSM. *Eur J Nucl Med Mol Imaging* 30:844-850, 2003.)

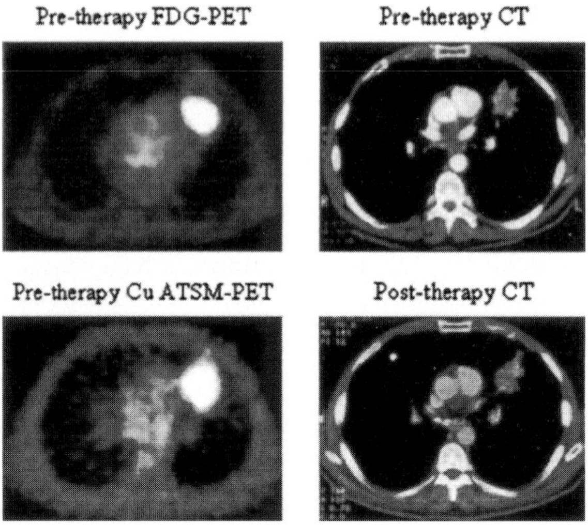

FIGURE 3.—Nonresponder. Transaxial FDG PET image (**upper left**) of the chest shows intense FDG uptake (standard uptake value, 17.3) in the known lung cancer in the lingula. Transaxial ^{60}Cu-ATSM-PET image (**lower left**) at the same level demonstrates intense uptake within the lingular cancer (tumor-to-muscle activity ratio = 3.0). CT image prior to therapy (**upper right**) demonstrates lingular mass, consistent with patient's known lung cancer. CT image (**lower right**) 3 months later, during chemotherapy, demonstrates an increase in the size of the tumor. The patient died with progressive disease 15 months after diagnosis. (Courtesy of Dehdashti F, Mintun MA, Lewis JS, et al: In vivo assessment of tumor hypoxia in lung cancer with ^{60}Cu-ATSM. *Eur J Nucl Med Mol Imaging* 30:844-850, 2003.)

whom 8 responded (5 complete and 3 partial) and 6 did not but had tumor progression. The 1 patient who had no discernible ^{60}Cu-ATSM uptake had a complete response to radiotherapy and no evidence of disease after 36 months.

Nonresponders had a significantly greater mean ^{60}Cu-ATSM T/M than responders (3.4 vs 1.5). In contrast, the mean tumor SUV did not differ significantly between responders and nonresponders. A threshold T/M of 3.0 served as an accurate cutoff value between responders and nonresponders, with the 8 responders having a T/M of less than 3.0 and the 6 nonresponders having a T/M of 3.0 or greater (Figs 2 and 3). No significant difference in mean tumor SUV for FDG was found between responders and nonresponders, nor was there a significant correlation between the tumor uptake of ^{60}Cu-ATSM and that of FDG.

Conclusion.—PET imaging with ^{60}Cu-ATSM proved to be feasible, with adequate imaging quality. The use of ^{60}Cu-ATSM in clinically assessing tumor hypoxia was shown to carry potential, possibly offering a reliable tool to monitor the effectiveness of various methods of overcoming hypoxia and improving cancer treatment.

► Hypoxia is a well-known determinant of the biological behavior of malignant solid tumors. Tumor hypoxia increases the chances of local recurrence and distant metastases. The results of this preliminary study of a tumor hypoxia marker in lung cancer are encouraging (see Figs 2 and 3).

H. D. Royal, MD

Miscellaneous

Imaging Characteristics of a Novel Technetium Tc 99m–Labeled Platelet Glycoprotein IIb/IIIa Receptor Antagonist in Patients With Acute Deep Vein Thrombosis or a History of Deep Vein Thrombosis

Bates SM, Lister-James J, Julian JA, et al (McMaster Univ, Hamilton, Ont, Canada; Berlex Labs Inc, Montville, NJ; Centre Hospitalier de l'Université de Montréal)

Arch Intern Med 163:452-456, 2003 4–14

Background.—To avoid missing a diagnosis of deep vein thrombosis (DVT), it is necessary to perform accurate objective testing. While there are several validated algorithms that address suspected first DVT, the diagnosis of recurrent DVT remains problematic. Venous compression US is widely used for the diagnosis of a first DVT, but persistent abnormalities occur in 80% of patients after 3 months and in 50% of patients after 1 year, so a noncompressible venous segment may represent a residual abnormality or new disease. Contrast venography can also be nondiagnostic, impedance plethysmography is obsolete, and radioactive fibrinogen uptake scanning is no longer done.

The use of scintigraphic imaging with radiolabeled peptides has been proposed for diagnosing recurrent DVT and has the potential to differentiate old from new thrombi. A pilot study was undertaken to determine the sensitivity of ^{99m}Tc-labeled synthetic arginine-glycine–asparatic acid (^{99m}Tc-apcitide) scintigraphy in patients with a first episode of acute DVT and to estimate the specificity of ^{99m}Tc-apcitide scintigraphy in patients who had a history of DVT, symptoms of postthrombotic syndrome, no acute DVT, and residual intraluminal abnormalities detected on compression US.

Methods.—The 78 patients ranged in age from 21 to 94 years (mean age, 63.1 years). Thirty-eight were newly diagnosed with a first DVT (group 1) and 40 had had previous DVT, symptoms of postthrombotic syndrome, and chronic intraluminal abnormalities (group 2). Two experts blinded to the clinical data and newly trained nuclear medicine physicians interpreted the images. The proportion of scans in group 1 patients read as positive for acute DVT and the proportion in group 2 patients read as negative for acute DVT were used to determine the sensitivity and specificity of ^{99m}Tc-apcitide scintigraphy.

Results.—With experts reading the scans, the sensitivity of ^{99m}Tc-apcitide was found to be 92% for both. The specificities according to the expert readers were 82% and 90%, respectively, and interreader agreement was excellent. For less experienced readers, both the accuracy and the interreader agreement were lower than for the experts.

Conclusion.—When expert readers are involved, the accuracy of the ^{99m}Tc-apcitide scintigraphy is high enough to qualify this test as an exclusionary method for initial and recurrent DVT. Most acute thrombi were detected and few false-positive results were obtained for patients with prior DVT. The training and experience of the interpreters proved to be a key factor in the accuracy of this method.

▶ Since the purpose of anticoagulation therapy is to prevent ongoing thrombosis, I have always thought that a radiopharmaceutical that detected ongoing thrombosis would be useful. Results so far have been disappointing, despite the fact that radioactive fibrinogen uptake scanning was the reference standard that was used to study postoperative lower extremity thrombosis many years ago. The radiopharmaceutical used in this study targets activated platelets and therefore may not be the best agent for venous thrombosis. Activated platelets are expressed in higher concentration in arterial thromboses.

H. D. Royal, MD

Pulmonary Activity on Labelled Leukocyte Images: Patterns of Uptake and Their Significance

Love C, Tomas MB, Palestro CJ (Long Island Jewish Med Ctr, New Hyde Park, NY)

Nucl Med Commun 23:559-563, 2002 4–15

Background.—Radiographs and sputum cultures are typically used to diagnose pulmonary infection, with labeled leukocyte imaging not generally employed. The pulmonary activity present on labeled leukocyte images was characterized and its significance determined.

Methods.—Within 7 days, 137 immunocompetent patients had ^{111}In-labeled autologous leukocyte chest imaging and chest x-ray studies. The pulmonary activity detected was deemed normal, focally increased, or diffusely increased, and an attempt was made to correlate the images with chest x-ray film results and final diagnoses.

Results.—Normal activity was identified in 112 patients and abnormal activity in 25 patients (18%), with focal abnormalities in 15 and diffuse abnormalities in 10. Normal chest x-ray results accompanied the normal leukocyte images in 68% of the cases; none of these patients were diagnosed with respiratory tract infection, for a negative predictive value of 100%. Various chest x-ray abnormalities were noted in the other 36 patients with normal activity, with pneumonia found in 1.

For 13 of the patients with focal abnormal pulmonary activity, the activity appeared segmental or lobar; 12 of these patients had pneumonia and 1 had cystic fibrosis. Abnormal chest x-ray results were also noted in 11 of the 12 patients with pneumonia and in the patient with cystic fibrosis. Of the 2 patients who had nonsegmental pulmonary activity, 1 chest x-ray showed pulmonary edema and the other was normal; neither had pulmonary infection.

The diffuse and bilateral abnormal pulmonary activity found in 10 patients was noted in the absence of any pulmonary infection, with 8 patients having normal chest x-ray results. One patient had pulmonary drug toxicity caused by methotrexate and 1 had persistent blood pool activity. The other 6 patients had various infections (none pulmonary) and sepsis. Two patients had an abnormal chest x-ray, with 1 having adult respiratory distress syndrome and 1 having pulmonary drug toxicity caused by paclitaxel.

Conclusion.—The 92% sensitivity of labeled leukocyte images was identical to that of the chest x-rays, meaning that a normal leukocyte study excluded pulmonary infection with a high level of certainty. Conditions other than pulmonary infection did not lead to an accumulation of labeled leukocytes. If the chest x-ray was abnormal, a negative leukocyte image could reliably exclude the presence of pyogenic infection. Thus, the use of leukocyte imaging was able to contribute useful information concerning pulmonary infection in these patients.

▶ This is a useful review of the various patterns of uptake of white blood cells in the lung. Make a mental note of this reference so you can find it the next time you have a scan with abnormal lung uptake with white blood cells.

H. D. Royal, MD

5 Gastrointestinal

Introduction

In the past year, several articles have been published on alternatives to the use of sincalide to induce gallbladder contraction in hepatobiliary imaging. Fortunately, sincalide is currently back on the market since few of the alternatives seemed to work as well. The remaining articles in this section cover a variety of topics including the usefulness of delayed GI bleeding images and the ability of GI bleeding studies to correctly determine the bleeding site. There continues to be interest in using nuclear techniques to monitor patients with inflammatory bowel disease. The remaining articles in this section cover a smorgasbord of topics. Bon appetite!

Henry D. Royal, MD

Comparison of Fatty Meal and Intravenous Cholecystokinin Infusion for Gallbladder Ejection Fraction

Krishnamurthy GT, Brown PH (Tuality Community Hospital, Hillsboro, Ore; Oregon Health and Science Univ, Portland)

J Nucl Med 43:1603-1610, 2002 5–1

Background.—The quantification of function is an essential component of hepatobiliary imaging in general and biliary dyskinesia specifically. The measurement of gallbladder ejection fraction (GBEF) with IV infusion of exogenous cholecystokinin (CCK) is an established technique for the diagnosis of biliary dyskinesia, including both chronic acalculous cholecystitis (CAC) and sphincter of Oddi spasm (SOS). Data collection for 30 minutes is usually adequate for generation of all the necessary parameters required for diagnosis. A fatty meal, which releases endogenous CCK, has also been used as a stimulant to empty the gallbladder. However, a direct comparison between CCK-8 and fatty meal has not been made in a sufficient number of healthy persons to facilitate a comparison of these 2 stimuli. This has become a more urgent need in the face of the current shortage and impending lack of availability of CCK-8. GBEF measured with a fatty meal was compared with GBEF measured with 2 equal IV infusions of CCK-8 in healthy subjects.

Methods.—GBEF was measured in technetium 99m-hepatic iminodiacetic acid cholescintigraphy in 13 healthy subjects. Each subject received 2 sequential doses of CCK-8 on day 1 and a 240-mL fatty meal (half-and-half milk) per 70 kg of body weight.

Results.—The mean ± SD GBEF with the fatty meal was 53.6% ± 20.2%, which was significantly lower than the mean of 75.8% ± 16.3% with the first dose of CCK-8 and 71.3% ± 17.4% with the second dose. There was a wide variation in the fatty meal GBEF, from 23.5% to 91.8% (Fig 3). The percentage rankings of the fatty meal GBEF were determined to be the preferred method for reporting results. In addition, latent and ejection periods were significantly longer with the fatty meal than with either dose of CCK-8.

Conclusions.—Gallbladder ejection fraction measured with a fatty meal can be an alternative to IV injection of CCK-8 when the hormone is no longer available for clinical use. However, careful attention to the details of

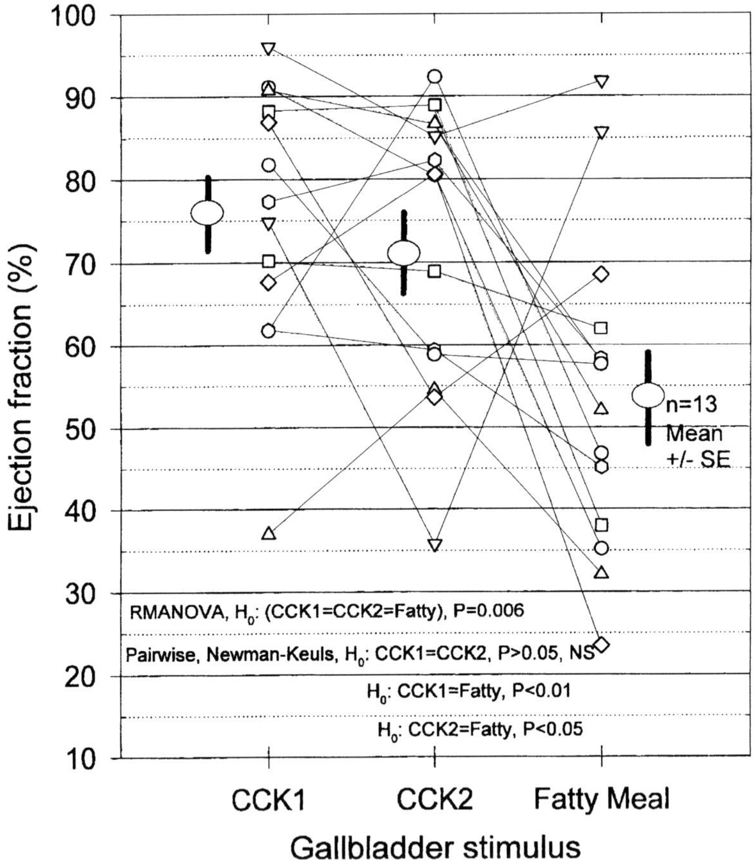

FIGURE 3.—GBEF obtained with CCK-1, CCK-2, and half-and-half milk fatty meal. Note that only 1 subject had GBEF >60% with CCK-1 and only 1 had <50% with CCK-2. GBEF values vary more with fatty meal. (Courtesy of Krishnamurthy GT, Brown PH: Comparison of fatty meal and intravenous cholecystokinin infusion for gallbladder ejection fraction. *J Nucl Med* 43:1603-1610, 2002. Reprinted by permission of The Society of Nuclear Medicine.)

the meal and time sequence is required for the measurement of GBEF with a fatty meal.

► During the shortage of CCK, nuclear medicine professionals were looking for alternative ways to stimulate gallbladder contraction. This study compares the results from sequential injections of CCK (CCK-1 and CCK-2) with the results obtained with half-and-half milk (fatty meal). In the past, I had thought that a fatty meal might be more physiologic and therefore might better differentiate normal from abnormal patients. However, the gallbladder ejection fraction measured with a fatty meal is lower and the ejection rate was slower than with CCK. Imaging needs to be extended to 60 minutes after the fatty meal because of the slower emptying rate.

During the CCK shortage, we used whole milk (not half-and-half milk) as the fatty meal. The results seemed less reliable than the results we obtained with infusion of CCK. For lactose-intolerant patients we used Ensure Plus as the fatty meal (see Abstract 5–2).

H. D. Royal, MD

Cholecystokinin Cholescintigraphy: Methodology and Normal Values Using a Lactose-Free Fatty-Meal Food Supplement

Ziessman HA, Jones DA, Muenz LR, et al (Georgetown Univ, Washington, DC)

J Nucl Med 44:1263-1266, 2003 5–2

Background.—Sincalide is used routinely for cholescintigraphy, including evaluation of gallbladder contraction and calculation of gallbladder ejection fraction for confirmation of exclusion of a preoperative diagnosis of chronic acalculous cholecystitis. However, there is a need for alternative methods for evaluating gallbladder contraction because sincalide was not in production or available from November 2001 to December 2002. Fatty meals have been used for evaluation of gallbladder contraction in oral cholecystography, ultrasonography, and cholescintigraphy. Milk has been well investigated, but one potential drawback is the prevalence of lactose intolerance in the general population. The use of a commercially available lactose-free fatty meal food supplement was investigated as an alternative to sincalide cholescintigraphy.

Methods.—The study group was composed of 20 healthy volunteers (7 men and 13 women) ranging in age from 21 to 47 years (mean ± SD, 33.2 ± 7.7 years) and weighing 59.8 to 94.5 kg (133 to 210 pounds) with a mean of 73.4 ± 13.5 kg (163 ± 30 pounds). All the volunteers had a negative medical history for hepatobiliary and gallbladder disease and no personal or family history of hepatobiliary disease and were not taking any medication known to affect gallbladder emptying. The study subjects were prescreened with a complete blood cell count, comprehensive metabolic profile, gallbladder and liver ultrasonography, and conventional cholescintigraphy. Three patients were not included in the final analysis because of abnormalities in one of these studies. After gallbladder filling on conventional cholescintigraphy, the subjects ingested the supplement and an additional 60-minute study was acquired.

Results.—Gallbladder ejection fractions ranged from 33% to 95% (mean, 62.6% ± 21.3%). On statistical analysis the lower range of normal was determined to be 32.6%. Maximal gallbladder emptying occurred between 55 and 60 minutes.

Conclusions.—This study established standard methods and normal gallbladder ejection fractions (≥33%) for cholescintigraphy by using a lactose-free fatty meal food supplement.

▶ The gallbladder ejection fraction and ejection rates obtained with Ensure Plus were similar to the results of the fatty meal. Now that CCK is available, our preferred method is a 30-minute infusion of CCK. The prolonged infusion period decreases the patient's symptoms and results in a higher, more reproducible ejection fraction in normal subjects.[1]

H. D. Royal, MD

Reference

1. Ziessman HA, Fahey FH, Hixson DJ: Calculation of a gallbladder ejection fraction: Advantage of continuous sincalide infusion over the three-minute infusion method. *J Nucl Med* 33:537-541, 1992.

Comparison of Gallbladder Function Obtained With Regular CCK-8 and Pharmacy-Compounded CCK-8

Krishnamurthy S, Cerulli-Switzer J, Chapman N, et al (Tuality Community Hosp, Hillsboro, Ore)
J Nucl Med 44:499-504, 2003 5–3

Background.—The measurement of gallbladder ejection fraction (GBEF) is a popular diagnostic technique for the evaluation of patients with a variety of hepatobiliary diseases, particularly those with biliary dyskinesia. Gallbladder emptying can be induced by a fatty meal or exogenous cholecystokinin (CCK). However, sincalide (CCK-8) is preferred because the fatty meal produces a significant degree of variability in the GBEF. CCK-8 is the only product approved for clinical use in the United States, but the nonavailability and subsequent shortage of CCK-8 has prompted stockpiling or a reluctant switch to fatty meal stimulation. Pharmacy-compounded CCK-8 has been made available, but there have been doubts expressed regarding its potency and reliability. Whether regular CCK-8 and pharmacy-compounded CCK-8 produce similar results in terms of gallbladder function was determined.

Methods.—The study group was composed of 20 patients with suspected gallbladder disease who were enrolled in quantitative cholescintigraphy. Each patient was infused for 10 minutes with 3 ng/kg per minute of regular CCK-8 and pharmacy-compounded CCK-8 sequentially, with 30 minutes between the beginning of the infusion. The GBEF, latent period, ejection period, and ejection rate were measured with both agents.

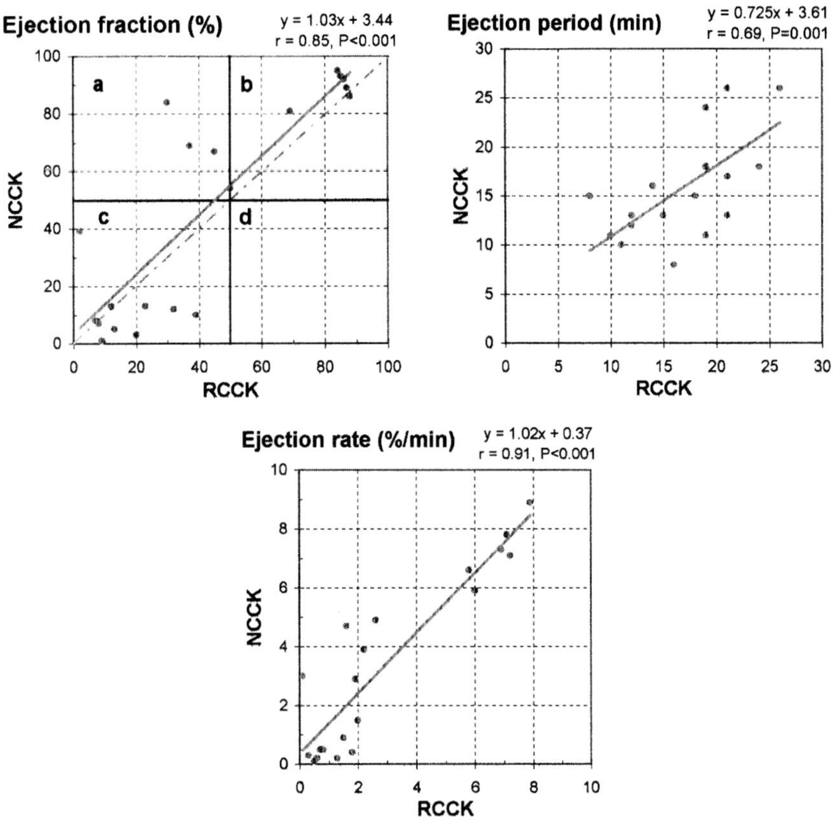

FIGURE 2.—Correlation of GBEF (r = 0.85), ejection period (*EP*) (r = 0.69), and ejection rate (*ER*) (r = 0.91) obtained with 10-min infusion of 3 ng/kg per minute of either sincalide (*RCCK-8*) or pharmacy-compounded CCK-8 (*NCCK-8*). Regression line (*solid line*) and line of identity (*broken line*) are shown. GBEF value of ≥50% is considered normal. In ejection fraction plot, lower left and upper right quadrants show concordant GBEF with both doses; in same plot, upper left quadrant shows 3 patients with discordant results, where GBEF value was >50% with NCCK-8 but <50% with RCCK-8. (Courtesy of Krishnamurthy S, Cerulli-Switzer J, Chapman N, et al: Comparison of gallbladder function obtained with regular CCK-8 and pharmacy compounded CCK-8. *J Nucl Med* 44:499-504, 2003. Reprinted by permission of The Society of Nuclear Medicine.)

Results.—Results were similar but not identical for regular and pharmacy-compounded CCK-8, with close correlation between the 2 agents in terms of all the main outcome measures (Fig 2). There was no evidence of either potentiation or inhibition of the first dose of pharmacy-compounded CCK-8 on the effects of the second dose of CCK-8.

Conclusions.—Pharmacy-compounded CCK-8 functions in a manner similar to that of regular CCK-8 as long as at least 30 minutes are allowed between doses.

► Sincalide (Kinavac, Bracco Diagnostics, Princeton, NJ) is the only product of its kind approved by the Food and Drug Administration (FDA) for clinical use. When FDA-approved CCK-8 became unavailable in September 2001, some state-based pharmacies compounded CCK-8 locally. The authors compared the results obtained with the FDA-approved CCK-8 with the pharmacy-compounded CCK-8 and found that the results were similar, although not identical.

Based on the results of these authors, the use of pharmacy-compounded CCK-8 seems to be the preferred alternative should FDA-approved CCK-8 become unavailable in the future.

H. D. Royal, MD

Quantitative Cholescintigraphy: Selection of Random Dose for CCK-33 and Reproducibility of Abnormal Results

Pons V, Sopena R, Hoyos M, et al (La Fe Univ Hosp, Valencia, Spain; Dr Peset Univ Hosp, Valencia, Spain)

J Nucl Med 44:446-450, 2003 5–4

Background.—Dynamic cholescintigraphy (DCG) has been shown to be a valid technique for the evaluation of gallbladder emptying. Several methodologic modifications have been incorporated since the first description of DCG in 1981, and there are much data on the role of DCG in the diagnosis of patients with clinically suspected gallbladder dysfunction. Cholecystokinin

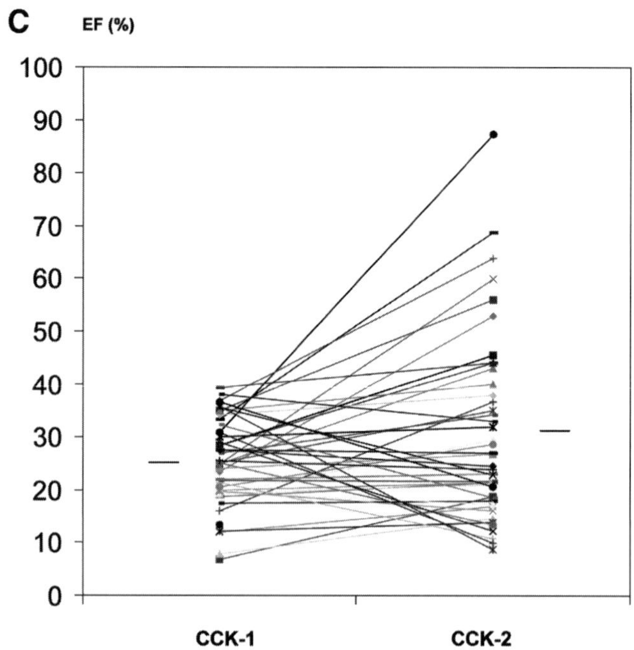

FIGURE 1.—Graphic representation of latency period (**A**), ejection period (**B**), and EF (**C**) for CCK-1 and CCK-2 doses. Only the data corresponding to those for patients with an abnormal EF (≤40%) in the first study are shown. *Horizontal bars* represent mean values. (Courtesy of Pons V, Sopena R, Hoyos M, et al: Quantitative cholescintigraphy: Selection of random dose for CCK-33 and reproducibility of abnormal results. *J Nucl Med* 44:446-450, 2003. Reprinted by permission of The Society of Nuclear Medicine.)

(CCK) as a slow infusion is recommended for stimulating contraction of the gallbladder. The normal ejection fraction (EF) has been shown to be reproducible, but the reproducibility of abnormal results has not been investigated. The CCK administration method was standardized, EF normality values were obtained, and the reproducibility of abnormal results was evaluated in patients with clinically suspected gallbladder dysfunction.

Methods.—The study was conducted in 3 phases. The first phase included 40 healthy volunteers divided into 4 groups and given IV CCK infusion according to 4 different regimens (0.25, 0.30, 0.40, and 0.60 Ivy dog units [IDU]/kg). In the second phase, 33 healthy volunteers were enrolled to determine DCG normality values; phase 3 evaluated the reproducibility of abnormal results in 44 patients having clinical manifestations compatible with gallbladder dysfunction and showing an abnormal EF in a previous study.

Results.—The most effective CCK infusion proved to be 0.40 IDU/kg over a 20-minute period because it afforded the least variability and a high EF (Fig 1). Application of this regimen to the healthy population provided an EF of 74.2% ± 17.1%; the inferior normality limit was estimated to be 40%. Abnormal results were recorded in 77% of the patients. Comparison of the 2 DCG studies demonstrated an EF correlation between them of 0.439.

Conclusions.—It would appear from these findings that slow CCK infusion is the best regimen for the stimulation of gallbladder contraction. It was estimated that an EF of less than 40% is representative of abnormality. This study also showed that the abnormal results for the EF in patients with clinically suspected gallbladder dysfunction are reproducible.

► These authors performed quantitative cholescintigraphy with CCK-33 (33-peptide molecular form of cholecystokinin) to standardize the technique for using this form of cholecystokinin. This form of cholecystokinin is not approved by the Food and Drug Administration for use in the United States; however, it is used in other countries.

In normal subjects, the highest EF was obtained with a slow, low-dose infusion. In the abnormal subjects, it is interesting to note that the second study done within 15 days of the first study was normal in 10 of 44 patients. This variability in EF may be due to the fact that the processes responsible for the abnormal ejection fraction wax and wane with time.

H. D. Royal, MD

Opioids Prolong Nuclear Hepatobiliary Imaging When Given Prior to Scanning

Barlas D, Margouleff D, Vignogna-Barlas L, Lesser ML (New York Univ, Manhasset)

J Emerg Med 23:231-236, 2002 5–5

Opioid-mediated contraction of the distal common bile duct (CBD) may delay tracer passage during nuclear hepatobiliary imaging (NHI), mimicking pathologic obstruction. We sought to determine if opioid administration

TABLE 2.—Summary of Imaging Results by Prior Opioid Administration* (95% Confidence Intervals Are Shown in Parentheses)

	No Opioid	Any Opioid	Meperidine	Morphine
Total subjects	142	56	40	14
Subjects with delayed CBD visualization at initial imaging	17	16	7	7
	12.0% (6.5-17.5%)	28.6% (16.5-40.7%)	17.5% (5.5-29.5%)	50.0% (23.3-76.7%)
Risk of delayed CBD visualization relative to patients not receiving opioids	—	2.39 (1.29-4.39)	1.46 (0.65-3.28)	4.18 (2.00-8.82)
Mean number of imaging sessions per subject	1.56 (1.47-1.66)	1.80 (1.67-1.91)	1.78 (1.64-1.91)	1.86 (1.55-2.17)
Proportion of subjects undergoing > 1 imaging session	53.5% (45.1-61.9%)	77.8% (66.7-88.9%)	77.5% (64.3-90.7%)	78.6% (56.7-100.5%)

*Two subjects received hydromorphone, too few for a meaningful analysis to be performed. Delayed visualization of the CBD was noted in both of these subjects.

Courtesy of Barias D, Margouleff D, Vignogna-Barias L, et al: Opiods prolong nuclear hepatobiliary imaging when given prior to scanning. *J Emerg Med* 23:231-236, 2002. Copyright Elsevier.)

before NHI delays CBD visualization and prolongs imaging. The records of 198 Emergency Department patients who underwent NHI were reviewed (after excluding those with evidence for pathologic CBD obstruction). Opioids were administered before NHI in 56 cases. Delayed CBD visualization occurred in 28.6% of subjects who had received opioids and in 12.0% of those who had not ($p < 0.01$). Delayed imaging was performed in 77.8% of those who had received opioids and in 53.5% of those who had not ($p < 0.01$). The relative risk of delayed CBD visualization was 1.46 [95%CI 0.65–3.28] for meperidine, 4.18 [95%CI 2.00–8.82] for morphine, and 2.38 [95%CI 1.29–4.39] for any opioid. We conclude that opioids given before NHI are associated with delayed CBD visualization and more imaging sessions.

► The authors defined delayed common bile duct visualization as incomplete visualization of the common bile duct and no activity in the small bowel at 1 hour. It is interesting to note that the relative risk for delayed visualization is 4.18 for morphine vs 1.46 for meperidine (Table 2 in the original journal article). The increased risk for meperidine was not statistically significant. These results confirm that morphine is more potent than meperidine in causing spasm of the sphincter of Oddi.

H. D. Royal, MD

Evidence of Impaired Gallbladder Function in Patients With Non-Insulin-Dependent Diabetes Mellitus by Quantitative Cholescintigraphy

Yang C-C, Sun S-S, Lin C-C, et al (China Medicine College Hosp, Taichung, Taiwan)

J Diabetes Complications 16:347-351, 2002 5–6

Non-insulin-dependent diabetes mellitus (NIDDM) is considered to predispose impaired gallbladder function and an increased prevalence of gallbladder disease. The aim of this study was to evaluate the gallbladder function of patients with NIDDM by quantitative technetium-99m-labeled imino-diacetic acid analogue (Tc-99m DISIDA) cholescintigraphy. One hundred and forty-five NIDDM patients (100 males, 45 females; age: 58.7 ± 9.5 years) with the absence of autonomic or peripheral neuropathy and without gallbladder or liver disorders were enrolled in this study. The patients were categorized by blood sugar control ($HbA_{1c} \geq 10\%$ as a poor blood sugar control group and $HbA_{1c} < 10\%$ as a good blood sugar control group) and disease duration (diabetic duration ≥ 10 years as a longer-duration group and diabetic duration < 10 years as a shorter-duration group). In addition, 60 normal controls (38 males, 22 females; age: 59.1 ± 10.2 years) were also studied for comparison. All NIDDM patients and normal controls underwent Tc-99m DISIDA cholescintigraphy, and the filling fraction (FF) and ejection fraction (EF) of gallbladder were calculated. The results showed significant difference between (1) NIDDM patients versus normal controls in FF and EF, (2) poor versus good blood sugar control of NIDDM patients in FF and EF, and (3) longer versus shorter disease duration of NIDDM patients in FF and EF. Our study, including a large number of subjects, showed that gallbladder function of patients with NIDDM is more impaired than the normal controls; and impaired gallbladder function in NIDDM patients is related to disease duration and blood sugar control.

► In this large study, the authors demonstrate that gallbladder ejection fractions are lower in non-insulin-dependent diabetes mellitus patients. Furthermore, they demonstrate that poor sugar control and a long duration of diabetes are also important factors to consider (Fig 2 in the original journal article). The fact that non-insulin-dependent diabetics have lower gallbladder ejection fractions should be kept in mind when interpreting hepatobiliary studies in this population.

H. D. Royal, MD

The Importance of Delayed Images in Gastrointestinal Bleeding Scintigraphy

Zettinig G, Staudenherz A, Leitha T (Univ of Vienna)
Nucl Med Commun 23:803-808, 2002 5–7

Background.—Radionuclide imaging methods for the detection of gastrointestinal (GI) bleeding have been available for more than 20 years. At first, most investigators obtained static images at 5- to 15-minute intervals. However, blood is a strong irritant in the bowel and causes rapid antegrade and retrograde movement; continuous computer imaging and review of dynamic images in a cinematic display will increase the accuracy of localizing the bleeding site. The standard protocol for GI bleeding scintigraphy mandates that dynamic anterior abdominal images be obtained at a frame rate of 10 to 60 seconds per frame over a 60- to 90-minute period. However, there is still controversy regarding the value of delayed images in GI bleeding scintigraphy, and they are recommended by some, but not all, investigators. The value of delayed images in GI bleeding scintigraphy was determined in patients with predominantly low-grade intermittent bleeding.

Methods.—A retrospective evaluation was conducted of 89 consecutive bleeding scintigraphic images of 75 patients. All the patients had been referred after other diagnostic methods had failed to identify the localization of GI bleeding. After the dynamic study, the delayed images were acquired for up to 24 hours until a bleeding site was identified. Data on clinical outcome were available in all but 5 patients.

Results.—There were no deaths from GI bleeding in any patient with a negative scan. Positive results were obtained in 41 patients (55%). In 11 of these patients (27%), the scans became positive during dynamic imaging. Immediate surgery was required in 4 patients, and 1 patient did not undergo surgery because of diffuse bleeding of the entire GI tract. One patient died without surgical intervention. In 33 scans of 30 (73%) of these 41 patients, findings were positive on delayed imaging only, resulting in surgery in 12 patients.

Conclusions.—The importance of delayed images in GI bleeding scintigraphy was demonstrated in these findings. In many cases patients who required surgery had scans that did not become positive for several hours.

▶ Until about 10 years ago, we used to routinely obtain delayed GI bleeding images up to 24 hours after injection unless signs of bleeding were identified on earlier images. Our purpose in obtaining delayed images were to determine which patients were likely to require emergent therapeutic interventions. As this study indicates, patients whose GI bleeding studies are negative at 24 hours are unlikely to require any emergent intervention. All patients with occult GI bleeding require a diagnostic work-up to determine the cause of their bleeding even if they don't require a therapeutic intervention to stop their bleeding.

We stopped doing delayed imaging because simply repeating the GI bleeding study if the patient continued to have evidence for active bleeding is a more efficient use of our resources. The problem with delayed imaging is that it is difficult to identify the site of bleeding with enough confidence to be able to localize the bleeding site for a therapeutic intervention. Blood within the GI tract can move antegrade or retrograde, so continuous imaging is required to localize the bleeding site most accurately. Occasionally, on delayed images one identifies the location of the bleeding site because the patient just happens to start bleeding again at the time of delayed imaging. Most of the time delayed images reveal activity within the colon and provide little information about the actual site of bleeding.

H. D. Royal, MD

The Clinical Utility of Nuclear Medicine Imaging for the Detection of Occult Gastrointestinal Haemorrhage

Howarth DM, Tang K, Lees W (Pacific Med Imaging, Newcastle, NSW, Australia; John Hunter Hosp, NSW, Australia; Goulburn Valley Imaging, Shepparton, Victoria, Australia)

Nucl Med Commun 23:591-594, 2002 5–8

Background.—Technetium 99m red blood cell (RBC) imaging has been shown to be an effective technique for the early detection of gastrointestinal bleeding. ^{99m}Tc RBC is often used in combination with angiography for more accurate localization of the bleeding site, but when angiography is not available a greater reliance is placed on ^{99m}Tc RBC imaging to localize the bleeding site. [^{99m}Tc]Pertechnetate imaging (Meckel's scan) may also be used to detect a Meckel's diverticulum to localize the source of intermittent and more occult bleeding. The clinical usefulness of ^{99m}Tc RBC imaging and Meckel's scan was evaluated for management of acute gastrointestinal bleeding.

Methods.—Over a 5-year period, ^{99m}Tc RBC imaging was used to investigate acute gastrointestinal bleeding in 137 patients ranging in age from 1 day to 95 years, with a median age of 66 years.

Results.—Of the 137 patients, 70 had positive ^{99m}Tc RBC imaging studies. Eleven of 24 patients whose imaging studies were performed beyond 3 hours had positive scans that would otherwise have been missed. Only 47 patients had a definite final diagnosis at the time of discharge from the hospital; 6 of these patients had negative findings on ^{99m}Tc RBC imaging. The correct site of bleeding was localized in 7 of 21 patients with foregut bleeding and in 15 of 20 patients with colonic bleeding. Endoscopy provided the diagnosis in 13 (28%) of 47 patients. Meckel's scans were performed in 11 patients, but all findings were negative. Angiography was diagnostic in 1 of 17 patients studied.

Conclusions.—The indication of these findings is that ^{99m}Tc RBC imaging is useful in the management of acute gastrointestinal bleeding. The bleeding detection rate may be further improved by imaging beyond 3 hours, but this test may be an unreliable method for the localization of bleeding, particularly in the foregut.

► The major role for gastrointestinal (GI) bleeding studies is to determine whether the patient is bleeding rapidly enough that an emergent arteriogram is likely to more precisely localize the bleeding site. In the appropriate patient population, arteriographic interventions can also be used to treat the site of bleeding. Occasionally the findings on GI bleeding scintigraphy are sufficient to precisely locate the GI bleeding site and thereby direct subsequent interventions.

These authors indicate that GI bleeding studies are less likely to correctly localize the bleeding site in patients with small bowel bleeding than in patients with colonic bleeding. I agree with this observation; however, further discussion of the words "correct localization" is warranted. I think correct localization should be determined by whether the results of the GI bleeding scintigraphy correctly guide the next steps in the patient's management. If the next step is angiography, the GI bleeding study provides useful information if it helps the arteriographer select the most likely major vessel that is the cause of bleeding. It also focuses the arteriographer's attention on the part of the abdomen where extravagation is most likely to be seen. If endoscopy is the next step, the bleeding site is correctly localized if it is correctly identified as being within the reach of a colonoscope. If surgery is the next step, the bleeding site is correctly localized if it correctly directs the surgeon to perform a right or left hemicolectomy. For surgery, it is unlikely that a GI bleeding study would be able to identify the site of bleeding in the small bowel well enough to help with the surgical intervention.

H. D. Royal, MD

Active Inflammatory Bowel Disease: Evaluation With ^{99m}Tc (V) DMSA Scintigraphy

Koutroubakis IE, Koukouraki SI, Dimoulios PD, et al (Univ Hosp Heraklion, Voutes, Crete, Greece)

Radiology 229:70-74, 2003 5–9

Background.—Agents used for radionuclide imaging of inflammatory bowel disease (IBD) include radiolabeled autologous leukocytes, polyclonal immunoglobulins, antigranulocyte monoclonal antibodies, and monoclonal antibodies that recognize activated endothelial adhesion molecules. The use of pentavalent (V) technetium 99m dimercaptosuccinic acid (DMSA) scintigraphy for assessing IBD activity was evaluated.

Methods.—Seventy-six patients underwent ^{99m}Tc (V) DMSA scintigraphy. Thirty-six had active IBD; 28 had inactive disease and 12 had miscellaneous bowel disease. For patients with active IBD, disease activity and laboratory indexes were also determined, along with endoscopic and histologic activity. These values were compared with the scanning activity index.

Findings.—The sensitivity and specificity of ^{99m}Tc (V) DMSA scintigraphy in detecting active IBD were 92% and 86%, respectively. Disease activity indexes correlated significantly with scintigraphy scores. The scanning activity score was also significantly associated with endoscopic and histologic activity. Of the patients with miscellaneous bowel disease, 3 with ischemic colitis had negative scintigraphic findings.

Conclusions.—Although ^{99m}Tc (V) DMSA scintigraphy cannot be used to diagnose IBD, it is useful for identifying patients with active disease and for assessing disease activity. It can also be used to evaluate response to various treatment schedules.

▶ ^{99m}Tc (V) DMSA is not available in the United States. We rarely do scintigraphy for active IBD since the presence or absence of active disease is usually determined noninvasively based on the patient's symptoms and the use of simple colitis activity scores. When we do perform studies in patients with active IBD, we use technetium-labeled white blood cells. These authors correctly state that DMSA is less expensive and easier to prepare. It is difficult to know the relative merits of the 2 radiopharmaceuticals without a direct comparison.

H. D. Royal, MD

^{99m}Tc-Interleukin-2 and ^{99m}Tc-HMPAO Granulocyte Scintigraphy in Patients With Inactive Crohn's Disease

Annovazzi A, Biancone L, Caviglia R, et al (Univ "La Sapienza," Rome; Univ "Tor Vergata," Rome; Univ "Campus Biomedico," Rome; et al)

Eur J Nucl Med 30:374-382, 2003 5–10

Background.—Crohn's disease (CD), a chronic inflammatory bowel disease, is characterized by marked intestinal T-cell and macrophage activa-

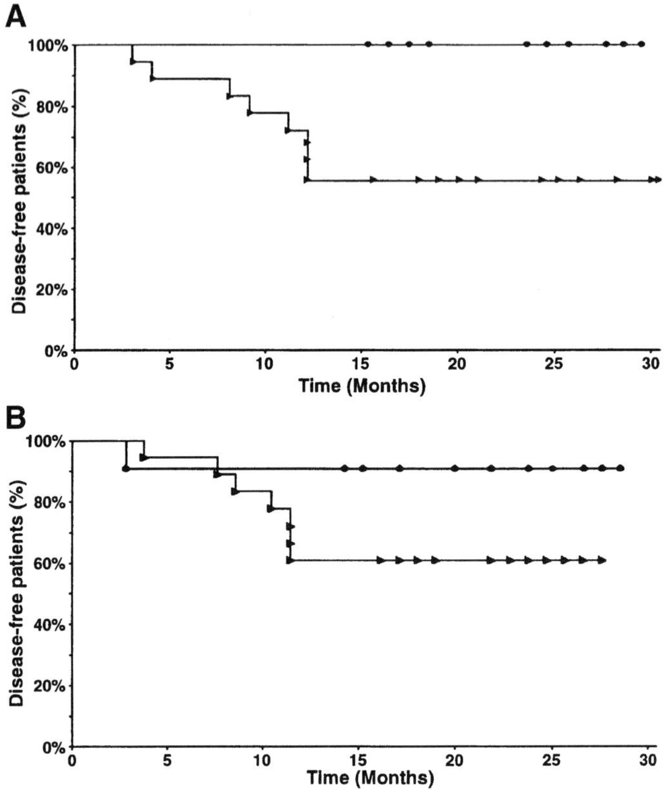

FIGURE 2.—Kaplan-Meier curves showing correlation between results of ^{99m}Tc-IL2 (**A**) and ^{99m}Tc-WBC (**B**) scintigraphy and percentage of patients free from disease relapse during follow-up. Curves with *circles* show the subgroups of patients who were negative on ^{99m}Tc-IL2 or ^{99m}Tc-WBC scan, whereas curves with *triangles* show those who were positive. (Courtesy of Annovazzi A, Biancone L, Caviglia R, et al: ^{99m}Tc-Interleukin-2 and ^{99m}Tc-HMPAO granulocyte scintigraphy in patients with inactive Crohn's disease. *Eur J Nucl Med* 30:374-382, 2003, copyright Springer-Verlag.)

tion. Polymorphonuclear cell infiltration also occurs, mostly during active inflammation. Scintigraphic detection of granulocytes and activated lymphocytes infiltrating the gut wall may help identify patients with clinically inactive CD undergoing early clinical relapse. The efficacy of scintigraphy was compared with that of technetium 99m/interleukin-2 (^{99m}Tc-IL2) and ^{99m}Tc/hexamethyl-propyleneamine oxine–labeled granulocytes (^{99m}Tc-WBC) in demonstrating the presence and extent of bowel inflammation in patients with CD inactive for more than 12 months. The accuracy of these methods for predicting future disease relapse was also determined.

Methods.—Twenty-nine patients with ileal or colonic CD in stable clinical remission underwent ^{99m}Tc-IL2 and ^{99m}Tc-WBC scintigraphy. In each patient, planar and single-photon emission CT images were obtained at 1 postinfusion. Quantitative analysis of ^{99m}Tc-IL2 uptake involved dividing the abdomen into 32 regions of interest.

Findings.—Although symptoms were absent, 62% of the patients had a positive ^{99m}Tc-IL2 and 62% had a positive ^{99m}Tc-WBC scan. Overall, 41.4% of the patients had positive findings on both scans. In most patients, the sites of IL2 and granulocyte bowel uptake were seen in different segments. As prognostic indicators, both modalities had a high negative predictive value but a low positive predictive value. Kaplan-Meier curves between scintigraphic findings and time free from disease relapse were significantly different only for ^{99m}Tc-IL2 scintigraphy (Fig 2).

Conclusions.—^{99m}Tc-IL2 scintigraphy appears to be useful for identifying patients with CD in clinical remission who may benefit from preventive treatment to avoid disease relapse. These data also show that in CD acute and chronic inflammation can occur at different sites.

► In this study, the authors compared the use of ^{99m}Tc-IL2 and ^{99m}Tc-WBC granulocyte scintigraphy to determine whether they could identify patients with clinically inactive Crohn's disease who are undergoing early clinical relapse. Kaplan-Meier curves were used to demonstrate that patients with positive ^{99m}Tc-IL2 studies or positive ^{99m}Tc-WBC granulocyte studies were more likely to relapse than patients with negative studies. The results were better for ^{99m}Tc-IL2. However, there is a large false-positive rate in that 50% to 60% of patients who have a positive study finding never had any clinical relapse. In this study, the management of patients was not changed based on the results of scintigraphy. An appropriate next study would be to randomize patients with positive ^{99m}Tc-IL2 studies to receive preventative treatment or to receive no treatment to see whether early treatment was effective.

H. D. Royal, MD

Effect of Altering Gastric Emptying on Postprandial Plasma Glucose Concentrations Following a Physiologic Meal in Type-II Diabetic Patients

Gonlachanvit S, Hsu C-W, Boden GH, et al (Temple Univ, Philadelphia)

Dig Dis Sci 48:488-497, 2003 5–11

Background.—Good glucose control is difficult to achieve in many patients with diabetes. An alternative to treating meal-induced hyperglycemia may be to delay glucose absorption. The effects of changing gastric emptying on postprandial plasma glucose levels after a physiologic meal in patients with type 2 diabetes mellitus were investigated.

Methods.—Nine diabetic patients were enrolled in the double-blind, randomized, 3-way crossover trial. Patients received erythromycin, 200 mg; morphine, 8 mg; or normal saline IV before eating a radiolabeled, dual-isotope, solid-liquid meal. At baseline and for 5 hours after meal ingestion, gastric emptying of solids and liquids was assessed along with serial plasma glucose, glucagons, and serum insulin concentrations.

Findings.—Compared with placebo, erythromycin accelerated solid- and liquid-phase gastric emptying, whereas morphine delayed emptying. During the first hour, postprandial plasma glucose levels were greater after erythro-

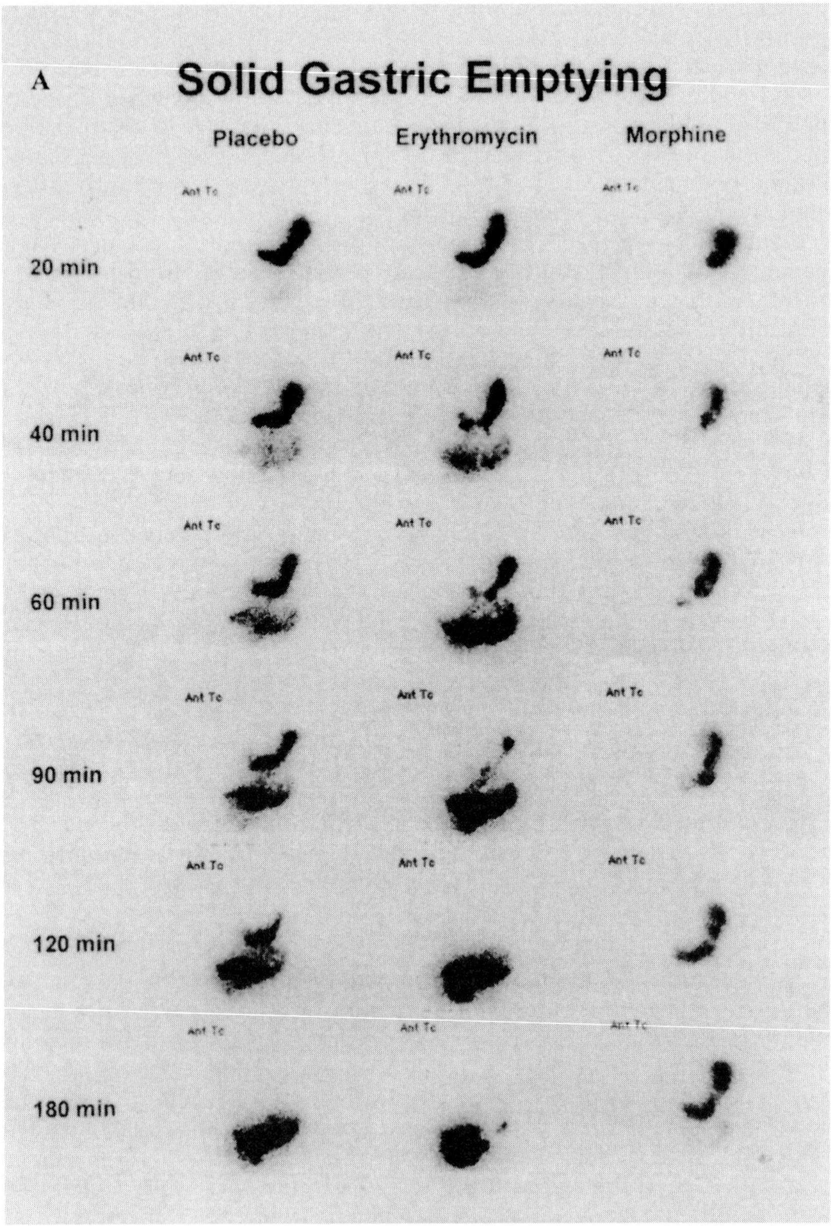

FIGURE 1.—Serial scintigraphic images of gastric emptying of solids over time in the same patient on the 3 different study days for placebo, erythromycin, and morphine. Solid gastric emptying with technetium 99m. After erythromycin infusion, at 2 hr, most of the radiolabeled solids had emptied from the stomach compared with placebo. In contrast, after the morphine infusion, most of the radiolabeled solids remained in the stomach. (Courtesy of Gonlachanvit S, Hsu C-W, Boden GH, et al: Effect of altering gastric emptying on postprandial plasma glucose concentrations following a physiologic meal in type-II diabetic patients. *Dig Dis Sci* 48:488-497, 2003, Plenum Publishing Corporation.)

mycin than after placebo. These levels were lower after morphine. In addition, peak postprandial plasma glucose levels were higher after erythromycin and lower after morphine than after placebo (Fig 1).

Conclusions.—Pharmacologic acceleration of gastric emptying appears to result in greater postprandial glucose levels after a physiologic meal in patients with type 2 diabetes mellitus. Delaying gastric emptying appears to lower postprandial glucose concentrations. Thus, administering opiate analgesics or prokinetic agents to such patients may affect glucose control. Modifying gastric emptying may help patients achieve glucose control.

► There is little doubt that gastric emptying can best be measured by using radionuclide techniques. The problem is controlling all the factors that may affect gastric emptying. This study nicely demonstrates that erythromycin increases gastric emptying and morphine decreases gastric emptying. In turn, the rate of gastric emptying affects the postprandial glucose concentrations. As the authors suggest, use of opiate analgesics or prokinetic agents in diabetic patients conceivably could be used to achieve better glucose control in type 2 diabetic patients.

H. D. Royal, MD

SPECT Imaging of the Stomach: Comparison With Barostat, and Effects of Sex, Age, Body Mass Index, and Fundoplication

Bouras EP, Delgado-Aros S, Camilleri M, et al (Mayo Clinic, Rochester, Minn)
Gut 51:781-786, 2002 5–12

Background.—Dyspeptic symptoms can result from impaired gastric accommodation. A noninvasive technique that uses SPECT for measuring gastric volumes has been developed. The accuracy of SPECT with 3-dimensional image analysis to determine balloon volumes in vitro was evaluated. In addition, gastric barostat balloon volumes measured after meal and after distension were compared with total gastric volumes measured simultaneously with SPECT.

Methods and Findings.—Healthy adult volunteers and postfundoplication patients were studied. Analysis showed that SPECT measures of in vitro balloon volumes were highly accurate. Postprandial/fasting ratios and postdistension volume ratios were very similar when determined simultaneously by gastric barostat and SPECT (Fig 3). Women had significant lower postprandial gastric volumes and gastric volume changes than men as measured by SPECT. Neither age nor body mass index affected the results. Compared with the healthy control subjects, patients who had fundoplication had lower postprandial/fasting gastric volume ratio on SPECT.

Conclusions.—These data show that SPECT can provide a noninvasive estimate of the effect of a meal on total gastric volume similar to balloon volume changes seen with the gastric barostat. The SPECT method may be useful in assessing gastric volumes and the effects of pharmacologic agents.

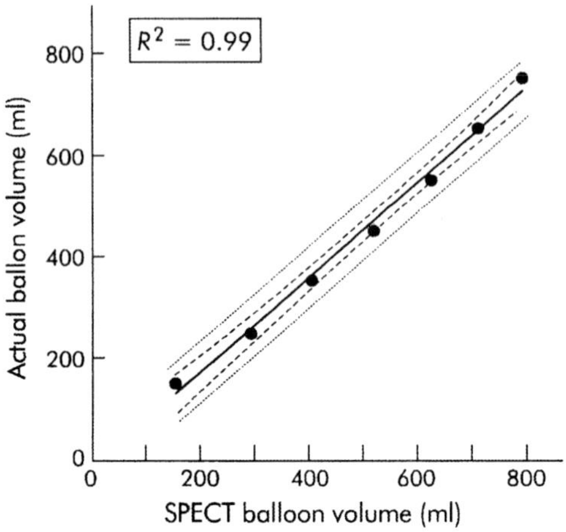

FIGURE 3.—Correlation of known balloon volumes with volumes measured in vitro by SPECT. (Courtesy of Bouras EP, Delgado-Aros S, Camilleri M, et al: SPECT imaging of the stomach: Comparison with barostat, and effects of sex, age, body mass index, and fundoplication. *Gut* 51:781-786, 2002, with permission of the BMJ Publishing Group.)

▶ These authors describe and validate the method for determining stomach volume in patients. It is likely that this technique will be applied in clinical research studies.

H. D. Royal, MD

Improved Detection of Splenosis in Patients With Haematological Disorders: The Role of Combined Transmission-Emission Tomography

Horger M, Eschmann SM, Lengerke C, et al (Eberhard-Karls Universität, Tübingen, Germany)

Eur J Nucl Med 30:316-319, 2003 5–13

Background.—Splenosis is common after traumatic rupture of the spleen or therapeutic splenectomy. Combined transmission and emission tomography (TET) consists of the fusion of single-photon ET and CT data acquired by using the same imaging device, enabling perfect overlap of anatomic and functional images. The use of TET for localizing heterotopic splenic tissue and differentiating splenosis from other masses was reported.

Methods.—The study included 7 patients with hematologic disorders and relapsing anemia, with thrombocytopenia after splenectomy, or who were immunosuppressed for various reasons. A total of 20 equivocal lesions were seen on CT or MRI. Splenic tissue was assessed by technetium-99m–labeled colloids or heat-damaged red blood cells.

Findings.—All patients had histologic confirmation by surgery or biopsy. TET correctly classified all 20 lesions as splenosis. In addition, 3 lesions not seen initially on CT or MRI were detected. The diagnostic relevance of TET was greatest for intrahepatic, intrapulmonary, and pleural splenic implants.

Conclusions.—Spleen scintigraphy combined with TET appears to be a reliable method for detecting or excluding splenosis in patients who have had splenectomy. Heterotopic splenic tissue can be localized precisely by using this technique.

► This technique is most likely to be helpful in patients who have relapses after a splenectomy for idiopathic thrombocytopenia purpura. In my experience it is usually possible to identify the location of splenic tissue by comparing the results of heat-damaged red blood cells to CT once you know where to look. However, the use of dedicated SPECT/CT systems will increase greatly in the future.

H. D. Royal, MD

The Role of Gallium-67 Scan in Defining the Extent of Disease in an Endemic Deep Mycosis, Paracoccidioidomycosis: A Predominantly Multifocal Disease

Yamaga LYI, Bernard G, Hironaka FH, et al (Sao Paulo Univ, Brazil)

Eur J Nucl Med Mol Imaging 30:888-894, 2003 5–14

Background.—Methods currently used to assess the extent of paracoccidioidomycosis (PCM) may not be useful for detecting subclinical lesions. The role of gallium 67 whole-body scanning in assessing disease extent in patients with active PCM was reported.

Methods.—Sixty-five patients were studied. Findings on ^{67}Ga scanning were compared with those of clinical evaluation, chest radiography, and/or high-resolution CT, abdominal US or CT, laryngoscopy, CT or MRI of the head, and technetium 99m methylene diphosphonate bone scanning before treatment.

Findings.—Imaging detected clinically unsuspected lesions in 32% of the patients. These were primarily in the lungs, adrenal glands, and superficial and deep lymph nodes. All cases with subclinical lung involvement were seen on ^{67}Ga scans. Scintigraphy was more effective than chest radiography in detecting lung disease. In addition, ^{67}Ga scanning demonstrated all suspected and nearly all unsuspected lymphatic lesions. In many of these cases, involvement was seen to be more extensive than clinically suspected. Agreement was good between ^{67}Ga scan findings and other imaging modalities for initially detecting thoracic and abdominal lymph nodes and bone involvement. Most cases of laryngopharyngeal disease with active inflammatory lesions seen on indirect laryngoscopy were also seen on ^{67}Ga images. However, ^{67}Ga scanning did not detect most adrenal and central nervous system lesions shown on abdominal US or CT and head CT or MRI.

Conclusions.—In patients with active PCM, ^{67}Ga imaging can demonstrate the location and extent of suspected and unsuspected lesions. This modality may be a useful screening tool before other diagnostic procedures are used.

► PCM is a deep mycosis endemic in Latin America. It is primarily a pulmonary disease but can affect other sites following hematogones spread. These authors demonstrate that the extent of the disease is better demonstrated with ^{67}Ga whole-body scintigraphy than with anatomic imaging studies such as chest radiography, CT, and abdominal US.

H. D. Royal, MD

6 Cardiovascular

Introduction

Nuclear cardiology continues to provide key information for medical decision making. It is often employed as a roadmap prior to coronary angiography, and as a major means of assessing outcome. Surveillance is performed with annual gated stress perfusion imaging, to determine if adjustments to doses of medical therapy are needed, or additional invasive procedures are necessary.

This year we have seen additional validation of the importance of radionuclide imaging for prognosis, validation of specific measurements (such as LV volumes and LVEF from gated SPECT), as well as enhancements of procedures (such as determination of perfusion reserve with SPECT, changes in the distribution of myocardial perfusion with inhalation of oxygen, and descriptions of apical hypertrophy with SPECT). Gated SPECT perfusion imaging remains the mainstay of nuclear cardiology practice. However, the recent Center for Medicare Studies approval of payment for routine PET perfusion studies suggests that the coming year will see further growth of PET as the preferred method of imaging patients with coronary disease. The routine application of PET will foster the development and clinical application of new radiopharmaceuticals to permit individualized therapy in patients with cardiomyopathy and coronary disease.

H. William Strauss, MD

Comparison of Late Outcome in Patients With Versus Without Angina Pectoris Having Reversible Perfusion Abnormalities During Dobutamine Stress Technetium-99m Sestamibi Single-Photon Emission Computed Tomography

Elhendy A, Schinkel AFL, van Domburg RT, et al (Thoraxcenter, Rotterdam, The Netherlands; Univ of Nebraska, Omaha)

Am J Cardiol 91:264-268, 2003 6–1

The aim of this study was to assess the prognostic significance of reversible perfusion abnormalities in patients without angina during dobutamine stress technetium-99m sestamibi single-photon emission computed tomography (SPECT). The study comprised 224 patients (age 60 ± 11 years, 144 men) with completely or partially reversible perfusion abnormalities during dobutamine stress sestamibi SPECT. Follow-up end points were hard cardiac events (cardiac death and nonfatal myocardial infarction). Angina occurred in 93 patients (42%) during the dobutamine stress test (symptomatic ischemia group). The 131 patients without dobutamine-induced angina represented the silent ischemia group. There was no significant difference between patients with and without angina with regard to summed stress perfusion score (5.3 ± 2.5 vs 5.2 ± 2.2, $p = 0.9$) or summed ischemic score (3.1 ± 1.7 vs 3.2 ± 1.4, $p = 0.7$). During a median follow-up of 7.2 years, cardiac death occurred in 14 patients (15%) with and in 21 patients (16%) without angina. Nonfatal myocardial infarction occurred in 8 patients (9%) with and in 13 patients (10%) without angina. In a multivariate analysis model of clinical and perfusion data, independent predictors of cardiac events were age (hazard ratio 1.02, confidence intervals [CI] 1.01 to 1.05 per year increment), diabetes mellitus (hazard ratio 1.9, CI 1.2 to 3.4), and ischemic perfusion score (hazard ratio 2.1, CI 1.3 to 3.8). Patients with silent ischemia defined as reversible perfusion abnormalities without associated angina during dobutamine stress sestamibi SPECT imaging had similar incidences of ischemia and similar cardiac event rates compared with patients with symptomatic ischemia. Therefore, the absence of angina in association with reversible perfusion abnormalities should not be interpreted as a sign of a more benign prognosis.

► The observations of this study are important because most of cardiac care is predicated on relieving symptoms. This study demonstrates that ischemia, whether silent or symptomatic, is equally serious.

H. W. Strauss, MD

The Effect of Nitroglycerin on Myocardial Blood Flow in Various Segments Characterized by Rest-Redistribution Thallium SPECT

Tadamura E, Mamede M, Kubo S, et al (Kyoto Univ, Japan; Natl Cardiovascular Ctr, Suita, Japan; Hokkaido Univ, Sapporo, Japan)
J Nucl Med 44:745-751, 2003 6–2

Introduction.—Several recent investigations have reported that the use of nitrates in perfusion imaging is effective in identifying viable myocardium and in prognostic evaluation. Few data are available regarding the absolute change in myocardial blood flow (MBF) after nitrates in the ischemic and nonischemic myocardium. The effect of nitroglycerin (NTG) on MBF and coronary vascular resistance (CVR) was examined in various segments characterized by rest-redistribution ^{201}Tl SPECT in patients with coronary artery disease.

Methods.—Twenty-three patients with coronary artery disease underwent both rest-redistribution ^{201}Tl SPECT and ^{15}O-labeled water PET at rest and after NTG spray (0.3 mg). Eleven healthy volunteers were evaluated with PET.

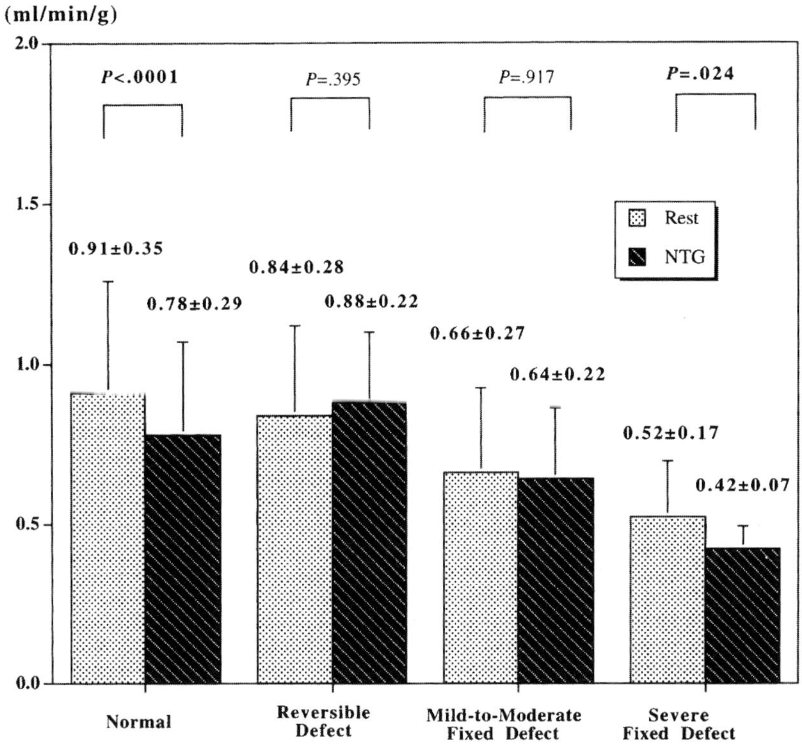

FIGURE 2.—Myocardial blood flow (MBF) at rest and after nitroglycerin (*NTG*), compared with rest-redistribution ^{201}Tl SPECT findings. (Reprinted by permission of the Society of Nuclear Medicine, from Tadamura E, Mamede M, Kubo S, et al: The effect of nitroglycerin on myocardial blood flow in various segments characterized by rest-redistribution thallium SPECT. *J Nucl Med* 44:745-751, 2003.)

Results.—Administration of NTG did not alter global MBF in volunteers or patients. In segments with normal ^{201}Tl uptake and in those with a severe, irreversible ^{201}Tl defect, the administration of NTG significantly decreased MBF without changing CVR. The administration of NTG decreased CVR in segments with a reversible ^{201}Tl defect (141 to 114 mm Hg/[mL/min/g]; P = .004) and in those with a mild-to-moderate irreversible ^{201}Tl defect (165 to 149 mm Hg/[mL/min/g]; P = .003), while maintaining MBF (Fig 2).

Conclusion.—NTG preferentially decreases CVR in the viable myocardium with ischemia. After NTG administration, tracer uptake in the ischemic myocardium will be relatively increased, compared with that in the nonviable and nonischemic myocardium, resulting in improvements in viability detection.

► NTG redistributes coronary flow to ischemic regions. This pharmacology helps identify viable ischemic myocardium.

H. W. Strauss, MD

Exercise Training Following Myocardial Infarction Improves Myocardial Perfusion Assessed by Thallium-201 Scintigraphy

Gunning MG, Walker J, Eastick S, et al (Univ College London; Royal Brompton Hosp, London)

Int J Cardiol 84:233-239, 2002 6–3

Aim.—We assessed the effects of a 6-week exercise programme on the thallium-201 myocardial perfusion characteristics of patients following myocardial infarction.

Methods.—Twenty-five patients presenting with a first acute myocardial infarction were randomised into two groups: (i) those undergoing a supervised exercise training programme over 6 weeks (n=15) and (ii) a control group who did not attend the exercise programme (n=10). All underwent three sequential stress thallium myocardial perfusion scans at 10 days, 6 weeks and 3 months after infarction. The stress conditions were identical on each occasion. The images were analysed using a polar plot with a computer assisted algorithm comparing stress and redistribution data. Values for extent, severity and percentage redistribution of the thallium images were generated.

Results.—A total of 29 perfusion defects were identified, 18 in the exercise group and 11 in the control group. Over 3 months in the exercise group the mean extent of the stress image defect fell from 109±64 to 95±51 pixels (P<0.05) while in the control group there was an increase from 133±57 to 144±57 pixels (P=ns). Stress defect severity fell in the exercise group from 581±417 to 494±346 S.D. (P<0.05) but increased in the control group from 765±494 to 877±543 S.D. (P=ns). On redistribution imaging in the exercise group a significant decrease was observed in both extent (94±56 to 76±43 pixels (P<0.05)) and severity (541±387 to 438±291 S.D. (P<0.05)) of the defects. However in the control group no significant change was observed for extent (125±54 to 125±52 pixels) or severity (745±485 to 820±503 S.D.) of the redistribution defects (P=ns). Reversibility of the defects increased slightly in both the exercise group (from 14.6±17 to 17.5±20%) and the control group (5.2±5 to 9.6±10%) (P=ns).

Conclusion.—Following myocardial infarction a 6-week exercise programme improves myocardial perfusion characteristics. An exercise programme should be integrated into cardiac rehabilitation protocols for patients after infarction.

► This is a preliminary study, involving small groups of patients, that suggests a favorable impact of exercise on myocardial perfusion following infarction, even in patients with limited work capacity (rate pressure product <16,000). This study should be repeated in larger groups of patients to determine the effectiveness of exercise training.

H. W. Strauss, MD

Long-term Prognostic Value of Dobutamine Stress ^{99m}Tc-Sestamibi SPECT: Single-Center Experience With 8-Year Follow-up

Schinkel AFL, Elhendy A, van Domburg RT, et al (Erasmus Med Ctr, Rotterdam, The Netherlands; Leiden Univ, The Netherlands)

Radiology 225:701-706, 2002 6–4

Background.—The purpose of risk stratification in patients with suspected or confirmed coronary arterial disease is to distinguish patients at high risk for disease who may benefit from further invasive strategies from low-risk patients who do not require further intensive evaluation. To overcome the problems of reduced exercise capacity and resultant insufficient testing, a variety of non–exercise-dependent pharmacologic stressors, such as dobutamine and adenosine, have been developed in conjunction with myocardial perfusion. This study is the first to report the long-term prognostic value of dobutamine stress ^{99m}Tc-labeled sestamibi SPECT in patients with limited exercise capacity.

Methods.—Clinical data and SPECT results were analyzed for 528 of 531 (99.4%) consecutive patients in whom follow-up was successful. Normal and abnormal findings were evaluated in the absence or presence of fixed or reversible perfusion defects. A summed stress score was calculated to determine the extent and severity of perfusion defects. Independent predictors of late cardiac events were identified with univariate and multivariate Cox proportional hazards regression models. The incremental value of myocardial perfusion scintigraphy compared with the value of clinical variables in predicting events was determined according to 2 models. Kaplan-Meier analysis was used to determine the probability of survival.

Results.—Of the 528 patients, findings were abnormal in 312 patients. In 8.0 ± 1.5 years of follow-up, 67 patients suffered cardiac death. Nonfatal myocardial infarction occurred in 34 patients, and late revascularization occurred in 49 patients. The annual rates for cardiac death, cardiac death or infarction, and all events were 0.9%, 1.2%, and 1.5%, respectively, after normal findings and 2.7%, 3.4%, and 4.4%, respectively, after abnormal findings. On multivariate Cox proportional hazards modeling, both an abnormal finding and the summed stress score provided incremental prognostic information in addition to clinical data. The hazard ratio for cardiac death was 1.09 per 1-unit increment of the summed stress score.

Conclusion.—This report on the long-term prognostic value of dobutamine ^{99m}Tc-sestamibi SPECT showed that this technique maintained its value over clinical data over an 8-year follow-up in patients with limited exercise capacity.

► The authors have excellent results addressing a very vexing question: How long are the data from a specific stress test meaningful? These results suggest that a single stress test carries prognostic value for 8 years. However, most events took place in the first 2 years. Since coronary disease progresses in steps, rather than continuously, it is important to retest patients periodically.

Retesting at 2- to 3-year intervals appears to detect significant disease progression prior to acute coronary events.

H. W. Strauss, MD

SPECT Imaging of Apical Hypertrophic Cardiomyopathy

Chu WW, Wallhaus TR, Bianco JA (Univ of Wisconsin, Madison)
Clin Nucl Med 27:785-787, 2002 6–5

Background.—Apical hypertrophic cardiomyopathy (HCMP) is common in Japan. In most patients with HCMP, the hypertrophy develops initially in the septum and extends to the free walls. This manifestation often gives the appearance of concentric hypertrophy. Apical hypertrophy is distinguished by hypertrophy in the apical segment of the left ventricular free wall, the ventricular septum, or both. Although the apical variant of HCMP accounts for only 1% to 2% of the non-Japanese population, apical HCMP accounts for 25% of cases of HCMP in Japan. Physical examination may show a displaced apical impulse and a prominent fourth heart sound. the echocardiograph often has symmetric, negative T waves.

The 2-dimensional echocardiograph often shows hypertrophy of the apex, while an apical view of the left ventricle shows hypertrophy of the apex with a spade-like configuration. A patient with the clinical, electrocardiographic, echocardiographic, and scintigraphic features of apical HCMP was presented.

> *Case Report.*—Man, 47, was examined after developing chest pressure and left arm discomfort with exercise during the preceding year. The patient had a history of dyslipidemia and a family history of coronary artery disease. He had no history of diabetes and denied using tobacco. The family history was negative for syncope and unexplained sudden death. Physical examination revealed a regular pulse, blood pressure of 120/95 mmHg, and a heart rate of 100 beats/min. Carotid upstrokes were brisk without delay. An electrocardiogram showed normal sinus rhythm, ST segment depressions in the anterolateral leads, and symmetric T-wave inversions in the anterior and lateral leads. The echocardiogram showed mildly increased left ventricular size with normal systolic wall motion and significant thickening of the apical wall segment. These findings were consistent with a diagnosis of apical HCMP. A rest-exercise SPECT myocardial perfusion study with ^{99m}Tc sestamibi showed no myocardial perfusion defects with significant apical tracer uptake and a spade-like deformity of the left ventricle consistent with apical HCMP (Fig 3).

Conclusion.—Although uncommon in other parts of the world, apical HCMP accounts for one fourth of the hypertrophic cardiomyopathy cases in Japan. This apical variant is characterized by giant negative T waves in the precordial echocardiographic leads, no intraventricular pressure gradient,

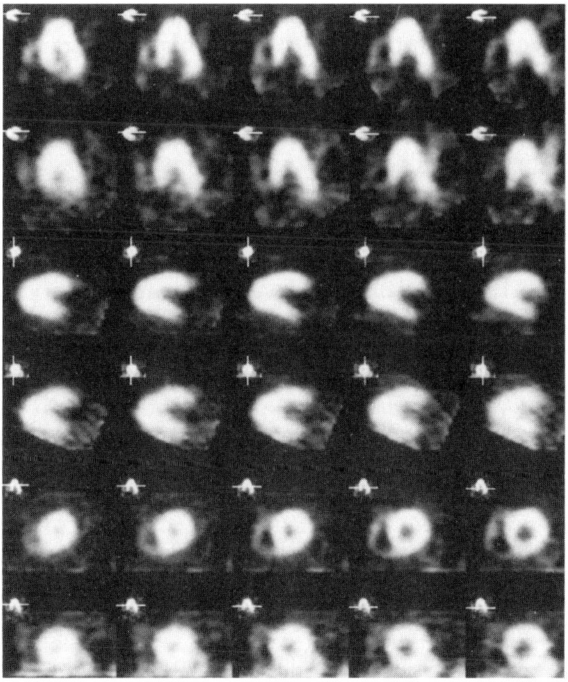

FIGURE 3.—Tomographic myocardial perfusion images show increased tracer uptake in the apex and a spade-like configuration of the left ventricular chamber. Representative stress perfusion images (**top**) and corresponding resting image (**bottom**) are shown for the horizontal long axis (anterior to inferior), the vertical long axis (septal to lateral), and the short axis (apex to base) planes, respectively. (Courtesy of Chu WW, Wallhaus TR, Bianco JA: SPECT imaging of apical hypertrophic cardiomyopathy. *Clin Nucl Med* 27(11): 785-787, 2002.)

and mild symptoms. SPECT imaging with ^{99}Tc agents allows direct determination of the relative thickness of the septum and the lateral wall in a patient with typical HCMP. Reversible myocardial perfusion defects are common in these patients in the absence of coronary artery disease.

► Although this entity is rare, it is important to recognize it when it occurs. In a very busy nuclear cardiology practice, there are probably several patients a year who have apical hypertrophy.

H. W. Strauss, MD

Effects of Abciximab on Microvascular Integrity and Left Ventricular Functional Recovery in Patients With Acute Infarction Treated by Primary Coronary Angioplasty

Petronio AS, Rovai D, Musumeci G, et al (Univ of Pisa, Italy; Clinical Physiology Inst, Pisa, Italy)

Eur Heart J 24:67-76, 2003 6–6

Aim.—To investigate the effect of abciximab on microvascular integrity and left ventricular (LV) functional recovery in patients with acute myocardial infarction (MI) treated by primary coronary angioplasty (PTCA).

Methods and results.—Thirty-one patients (27 males; age 39-76 years) with first, acute MI (<6 h after onset) were randomized to receive either abciximab + primary PTCA (n = 17) or primary PTCA alone (n = 14). Baseline characteristics of the two groups were similar. Myocardial reperfusion was studied shortly after PTCA by corrected TIMI frame count (cTFC) and intracoronary myocardial contrast echocardiography (MCE), after 48 h by intravenous MCE using intermittent, harmonic power Doppler, and after 1 month by intravenous MCE and 99 mTc-tetrofosmin SPECT. The patients treated with abciximab showed a shorter cTFC (23±4 vs 30±9 frames; $P<0.05$), a more preserved microvascular integrity shortly after PTCA (77% vs 55%; $P<0.01$), after 48 h (86% vs 50%; $P<0.005$) and at 1-month follow-up (86% vs 54% by MCE, $P<0.001$, and 68% vs 60% by SPECT, $P<0.005$) than patients treated with PTCA alone (Fig 2). Abciximab patients also showed a better recovery of LV function, as demonstrated by greater reduction in wall motion score index (1.4±0.3 vs 1.5±0.2; $P<0.05$) and increase in LV ejection fraction (53±7% vs 48±5%; $P<0.001$).

Conclusions.—Abciximab improves microvascular perfusion and LV functional recovery in primary PTCA.

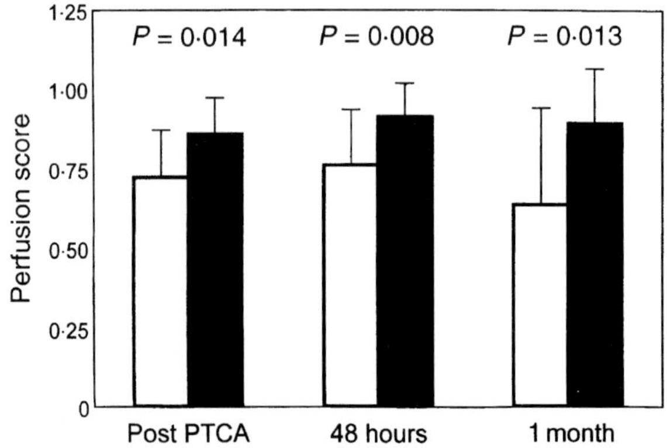

FIGURE 2.—Contrast perfusion scores in control (*open bars*) and abciximab patients (*solid bars*) after percutaneous transluminal coronary angioplasty (*PTCA*), at 48 h and at 1-month follow-up. (Courtesy of Petronio AS, Rovai D, Musumeci G, et al: Effects of abciximab on microvascular integrity and left ventricular functional recovery in patients with acute infarction treated by primary coronary angioplasty. *Eur Heart J* 24:67-76. Copyright 2003 The European Society of Cardiology with permission from the RCOG.)

► Controlling platelet thrombi appears to enhance distal flow—as judged by the angio TIMI frame count and both the acute and 1-month myocardial perfusion scans. Better flow results in more myocardial preservation, and a better outcome.

H. W. Strauss, MD

Single Photo Emission Computed Tomography Dual Isotope Myocardial Perfusion Imaging in Women With Systemic Lupus Erythematosus: II. Predictive Factors for Perfusion Abnormalities

Bruce IN, Gladman DD, Ibañez D, et al (Univ of Toronto; Toronto Western Hosp)

J Rheumatol 30:288-291, 2003 6–7

Introduction.—Subclinical coronary artery disease (CAD) in women with systemic lupus erythematosus (SLE) has been described with the use of several different modalities in up to 30% to 50% of patients. Factors associated with myocardial perfusion abnormalities in women with SLE without a known history of CAD were examined to determine the link between demographic characteristics, clinical and serologic features, therapy, and conventional CAD risk factors.

Methods.—Consecutive women with SLE being seen in a large lupus clinic underwent SPECT dual-isotope myocardial perfusion imaging (DIMPI) after undergoing pharmacologic stress with dipyridamole. All patients underwent a clinical and laboratory evaluation with a standard protocol. Traditional risk factors were compared, along with disease and therapy-associated factors, in patients with and without perfusion abnormalities.

Results.—The mean age of 129 patients was 44.8 years. The mean SLE Disease Activity Index was 4.2. Forty-nine patients (38%) had an abnormality of myocardial perfusion. Factors linked with an abnormal DIMPI included current hypertension (odds ratio [OR], 2.11; $P = .05$), elevated cholesterol ever (OR, 2.51; $P < .05$), and total cholesterol–to–high-density lipoprotein cholesterol ratio (OR, 1.96 for each increase of 1.0; $P < .008$).

Conclusion.—Myocardial perfusion abnormalities in women with SLE without known CAD are common, indicating a high burden of subclinical CAD. Several metabolic and therapy-associated factors seem to be linked with the process of atherogenesis in SLE. It may be that SLE is a predisposing factor for atherosclerosis.

► A very high prevalence of perfusion abnormalities in women in their mid 40s. The patients with perfusion abnormalities had slightly higher cholesterol, low-density lipoprotein (LDL), hypertension, and body mass index, but only the total cholesterol–to-LDL ratio was statistically significant.

H. W. Strauss, MD

Myocardial Sympathetic Denervation, Fatty Acid Metabolism, and Left Ventricular Wall Motion in Vasospastic Angina

Watanabe K, Takahashi T, Miyajima S, et al (Niigata Univ, Japan; Tsubame Rosai Hosp, Niigata, Japan; Daiichi Radioisotope Labs Ltd, Chiba, Japan)
J Nucl Med 43:1476-1481, 2002 6–8

Background.—Vasospastic angina is characterized by anginal attacks at rest, usually at night and in the early morning. A variety of noninvasive methods have been used to detect vasospasm, but none of these methods are sensitive enough for use in patients with sporadic attacks. Abnormal fatty acid metabolism and cardiac adrenergic neuronal damage are observed in ischemic myocardium, and so ^{123}I-15-(*p*-iodophenyl)-3-*R*,*S*-methyl pentadecanoic acid (BMIPP) and ^{123}I-metaiodobenzylguanidine (MIBG) have recently been proposed as useful tracers for detection of myocardial damage. The clinical implications of fatty acid metabolic imaging with BMIPP and of myocardial sympathetic nerve functional imaging with MIBG were clarified in patients with vasospastic angina.

Methods.—The study group included 50 patients with vasospastic angina (25 with clinically documented vasospasm and 25 with ergonovine-provoked vasospasm) and 25 control subjects with chest pain but with normal coronary arteries without ergonovine provocation of spasm. Sixteen patients with clinically documented vasospasm were reevaluated 6 months after medical treatment. The territorial regions of the vasospasm-induced coronary artery, wall motion determined by left ventriculography, and BMIPP and MIBG uptake were compared.

Results.—Regions manifesting a positive reaction to the ergonovine provocation were observed in the right coronary artery in 41 patients, in the left anterior descending artery in 33 patients, and in the left circumflex artery in 21 patients. Provocation occurred in multiple vessels in 29 patients (58%), and reduction of wall motion was observed in 19 patients (38%). Sensitivity and specificity for identification of vasospastic angina were 86% and 88%, respectively, for BMIPP scintigraphy and 100% and 56%, respectively, for MIBG scintigraphy. BMIPP or MIBG uptake was decreased in the region showing a reduction in left ventricular wall motion. The sensitivity and specificity of determination of vasospasm-induced coronary arteries were 71% and 95%, respectively, for BMIPP scintigraphy and 96% and 55%, respectively, for MIBG scintigraphy. At 6 months after medical treatment, vasospasm was reinduced by ergonovine provocation in 6 patients (group 1) and was not reinduced in 10 patients (group 2). Improvements in decreased BMIPP and MIBG uptake were lower in group 1 than in group 2, and the regions in which vasospasm was reinduced exhibited decreased BMIPP and MIBG uptake.

Conclusions.—In this group of patients with vasospastic angina, abnormal fatty acid metabolism and cardiac sympathetic denervation were observed more frequently than were wall motion abnormalities in the vasospastic region. BMIPP and MIBG scintigraphy are accurate, noninvasive techniques for determining the presence and location of vasospasm.

► This study demonstrates the influence of prolonged low-flow states (due to >90% stenosis of the involved vessel) on the reduction of sympathetic innervation and fatty acid catabolism. One hypothesis is that these patients are persistently ischemic, manifest at times with chest pain, at other times with no pain. The investigators also identify the importance of therapy that reduced myocardial oxygen requirements, as a means of improving fatty acid metabolism and sympathetic innervation.

H. W. Strauss, MD

Resting Echocardiography and Quantitative Dipyridamole Technetium-99m Sestamibi Tomography in the Identification of Cardiac Allograft Vasculopathy and the Prediction of Long-term Prognosis After Heart Transplantation

Ciliberto GR, Ruffini L, Mangiavacchi M, et al (CNR Clinical Physiology Inst of Pisa, Milan, Italy)

Eur Heart J 22:964-971, 2001 6–9

Background.—Cardiac allograft vasculopathy is the most significant limitation to long-term survival after heart transplantation. This process has been documented in 40% to 50% of transplant patients who survive to 5 years. In the absence of warning anginal symptoms, the clinical manifestations of coronary allograft vasculopathy are often severe and include life-threatening ventricular arrhythmias, congestive heart failure, silent myocardial infarction, and sudden death. Annual coronary arteriography had been introduced to monitor the development and progression of coronary allograft vasculopathy, but this invasive procedure has several significant limitations. The accuracy of echocardiography with quantitative high-dose dipyridamole ^{99m}Tc-sestamibi SPECT for the detection of coronary allograft vasculopathy was evaluated.

Methods.—A total of 78 consecutive heart transplant recipients underwent echocardiography at rest and high-dose dipyridamole SPECT within 48 hours of a yearly angiogram. Resting wall motion abnormalities were determined to be significant if they were present in 2 or more segments. SPECT findings were considered abnormal in the presence of reversible or fixed defects.

Results.—The coronary angiogram results were normal in 53 of 78 patients. Nonsignificant coronary allograft vasculopathy was present in 13 patients, and significant (50% or greater stenosis) coronary allograft vasculopathy was present in 12 patients. There were 9 patients with resting wall motion abnormalities and 20 patients with perfusion defects. Echocardiographic and SPECT findings were concordant in 59 patients (5 positive and 54 negative) (Table 1). Among these patients, accuracy was 100% for significant coronary allograft vasculopathy and 83% for any coronary allograft vasculopathy. Over a follow-up of 6.5 ± 2 years, 17 patients suffered coronary allograft vasculopathy–related events, including death in 6 patients and retransplantation in 3 patients. Statistical analysis showed that resting wall

TABLE 1.—Results of the Noninvasive Tests Versus Coronary Angiographic Findings

	n	ECHO Negative	ECHO Positive	SPECT Negative	SPECT Positive
No CAV	53	50	3	47	6
Non-significant CAV	13	13	0	10	3
Significant CAV	12	6	6	1	11
Total	78	69	9	58	20
		0·0001		0·0001	

Abbreviations: AV, Cardiac allograft vasculopathy; *ECHO*, resting echocardiography; *SPECT*, dipyridamole ^{99m}Tc-sestamibi tomography.

Reprinted from Ciliberto GR, Ruffini L, Mangiavacchi M, et al: Resting echocardiography and quantitative dipyridamole technetium-99m sestamibi tomography in the identification of cardiac allograft vasculopathy and the prediction of long-term prognosis after heart transplantation. *Eur Heart J* 22:964-971. Copyright 2001 The European Society of Cardiology, with permission from the RCOG.)

motion abnormalities, SPECT perfusion defects, and angiographic coronary allograft vasculopathy were significant predictors of cardiac events.

Conclusion.—In many heart transplant patients, the presence of normal resting wall motion at echocardiography in conjunction with normal stress myocardial perfusion will exclude the presence of significant coronary allograft vasculopathy. However, resting wall abnormalities and perfusion defects are strongly predictive of cardiac events. Thus, a safe and cost-effective strategy would be one that reserves angiography for patients with resting wall abnormalities or perfusion defects.

► After rejection, transplant vasculopathy is probably the second major problem for heart transplant patients. Many of these patients are catheterized and have intravascular US to evaluate their coronaries on a regularly scheduled basis. This study suggests that stress myocardial perfusion imaging can be used to identify the patients in need of catheterization, thereby reducing the complexity of managing these patients.

H. W. Strauss, MD

Total and Partial Cardiac Sympathetic Denervation After Surgical Repair of Ascending Aortic Aneurysm

Momose M, Kobayashi H, Ikegami H, et al (Tokyo Women's Med Univ)
J Nucl Med 42:1346-1350, 2001 6–10

Background.—The proximity of the sympathetic cardiopulmonary nerves to the great arteries creates a risk for cardiac sympathetic denervation in patients who have just undergone surgery for the repair of an ascending aortic aneurysm. A newly available norepinephrine analogue, ^{123}I-metaiodobenzylguanidine (MIBG), accumulates in the endings of sympathetic nerves through an uptake-1 mechanism and reflects cardiac sympathetic nervous function. In theory, the mechanical interruption of the cardiac sympathetic nerves can be expected to reduce the accumulation of ^{123}I-MIBG in the

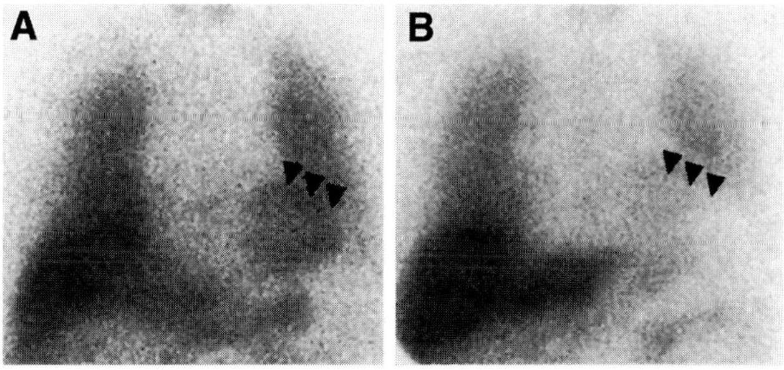

FIGURE 1.—A 66-year-old man with thoracic aortic aneurysm from ascending aorta to total aortic arch. Ascending and total arch graft replacement was performed. **A**, ^{123}I-MIBG early image shows normal accumulation (*arrowheads*) in whole heart (heart-to-mediastinum ratio, 1.83) before operation. **B**, One month after operation, MIBG accumulation is markedly decreased (heart-to-mediastinum ratio, 1.33). (Reprinted by permission of the Society of Nuclear Medicine from Momose M, Kobayashi H, Ikegami H, et al: Total and partial cardiac sympathetic denervation after surgical repair of ascending aortic aneurysm. *J Nucl Med* 42:1346-1350, 2001.)

heart. Previous studies have shown that ^{123}I-MIBG uptake is absent from transplanted human heart early after transplantation (less than 1 year). Cardiac sympathetic nervous function early after surgical correction of an ascending aortic aneurysm was evaluated.

Methods.—Cardiac ^{123}I-MIBG imaging was performed on 12 patients with a mean age of 47 ± 17 years before and after the surgical repair of an aneurysm. A control group consisting of 7 patients scheduled for coronary artery bypass grafting also underwent ^{123}I-MIBG. Heart rate variability was assessed with Holter 24-hour electrocardiography before and after the operation to produce a time-domain index of heart rate variability, which was used as an index of autonomic balance.

Results.—Both early and delayed heart-to-mediastinum ratios (H/Ms) were significantly decreased after surgery (early H/M, 1.84 ±0.16 before vs 1.40 ± 0.16 after; delayed H/M, 1.79 ± 0.38 before vs 1.37 ± 0.18 after). Visual analysis of ^{123}I-MIBG accumulation in early images showed absence of ^{123}I-MIBG accumulation in 3 of 12 patients, a score of 1 in 7 patients, and a score of 2 in 2 patients (Fig 1). However, there were no significant differences evident between H/M before surgery and H/M after surgery in patients who underwent coronary artery bypass graft. The time-domain index of heart rate variability was significantly lower after surgery than before surgery.

Conclusion.—Total or partial denervation of the cardiac sympathetic nerves occurs after the surgical repair of an ascending aortic aneurysm.

► Yet another condition affecting cardiac sympathetic innervation.

H. W. Strauss, MD

Acute Myocardial Infarction: Myocardial Viability Assessment in Patients Early Thereafter—Comparison of Contrast-Enhanced MR Imaging With Resting ^{201}T1 SPECT

Kitagawa K, Sakuma H, Hirano T, et al (Matsusaka Central Hosp, Mie, Japan; Mie Univ, Japan)

Radiology 226:138-144, 2003 6–11

Background.—Myocardial stunning may cause reversible left ventricular dysfunction in the early course of patients who suffer acute myocardial infarction. As a result, regional left ventricular wall motion at rest cannot be used for the evaluation of myocardial viability because both necrotic and viable myocardium may show impaired contractile function in the acute stage. The differentiation of viable from nonviable myocardial segments is an important clinical challenge in these patients. This study compared contrast-enhanced MRI with resting ^{201}Tl SPECT for the prediction of myocardial viability in patients early after acute myocardial infarction.

Methods.—The study group comprised 22 patients with acute myocardial infarction. ^{201}T1 SPECT images were obtained 4.3 ± 0.2 days after acute infarction, and inversion-recovery contrast-enhanced MR images were obtained 7.9 ± 1.6 days after the ^{201}T1 SPECT imaging. The transmural extent of hyperenhancement on the contrast-enhanced MR images and regional

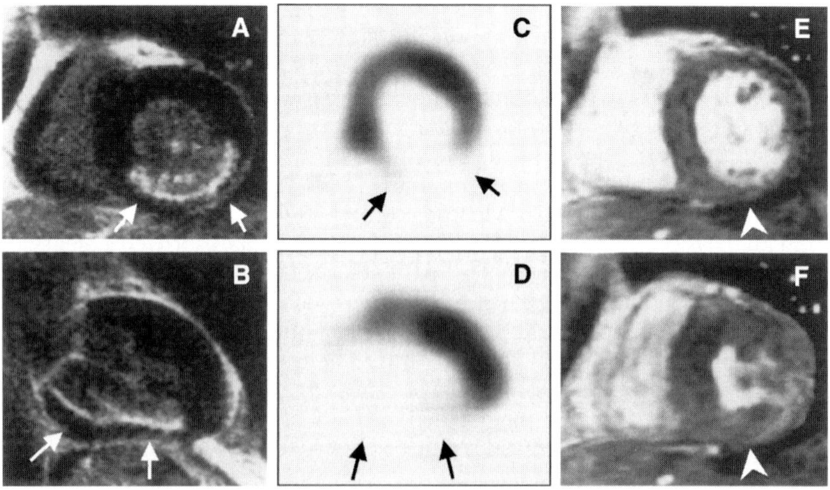

FIGURE 3.—Contrast-enhanced MR images obtained with a segmented inversion-recovery fast low-angle shot sequence (6.0/3.4/200) in **A**, short-axis and **B**, long-axis imaging planes and resting ^{201}T1 SPECT images obtained in **C**, short-axis and **D**, long-axis imaging planes in a 59-year-old man with inferior myocardial infarction. Transmural extent of hyperenhancement in the inferior wall (*white arrows*) was less than 50% of wall thickness, which indicates preserved regional viability. The ^{201}T1 SPECT images show reduced uptake of less than 60% of peak, which indicates nonviable myocardium (*black arrows*). Follow-up short-axis cine MR images obtained with a segmented fast low-angle shot sequence (50/4.8) at **E**, the end of diastole and **F**, the end of systole demonstrate preserved regional contractile function in the inferior wall (*arrowheads*). (Courtesy of Kitagawa K, Sakuma H, Hirano T, et al: Acute myocardial infarction: Myocardial viability assessment in patients early thereafter—Comparison of contrast-enhanced MR imaging with Resting ^{201}T1 SPECT. *Radiology* 226(1):138-144, 2003. Radiological Society of North America.)

^{201}T1 activity were quantitatively analyzed with a 12-segment model. Follow-up cine MR images were obtained at 67 ± 17 days after the contrast-enhanced MR images, and regional wall thickening visualized on these follow-up images was used as an index for myocardial viability. Statistical analyses included the χ^2 and 2-tailed Student *t* tests.

Results.—Both resting ^{201}T1 SPECT images and contrast-enhanced MR images showed significant correlation with regional wall thickening on follow-up MR images (Fig 3). The sensitivity, specificity, and accuracy of contrast-enhanced MRI for the prediction of viable myocardium were significantly higher than those values for resting ^{201}T1 SPECT (98% vs 93%, 75% vs 54.4%, and 92% vs 81.1%, respectively).

Conclusion.—These findings show that delayed contrast-enhanced MRI can aid in the prediction of myocardial viability as demonstrated on follow-up cine MR images in patients who have suffered acute myocardial infarction. Contrast-enhanced MRI demonstrated significantly improved sensitivity, specificity, and accuracy in this comparison with resting ^{201}T1 SPECT.

► The kinetics of thallium in the myocardium are much slower than those of gadopentetate dimeglumine. This may explain why the investigators found a lower sensitivity for thallium, because only immediate thallium images were recorded.

H. W. Strauss, MD

Effect of O_2-Enriched Breathing on Myocardial Uptake of ^{99m}Tc-Sestamibi

Basoglu T, Yapici O, Aksakal E, et al (Ondokuz Mayis Univ, Samsun, Turkey)

Eur J Nucl Med 29:1496-1501, 2002 6–12

Background.—Sestamibi (MIBI) has become the most frequently used radiopharmaceutical in the initial diagnosis of coronary artery disease in many centers. In addition to its diagnostic capability, the favorable physical characteristics of technetium-99m and the 24-hour availability of MIBI are important advantages. It has been reported that MIBI is able to visualize viable tissue, but ^{201}Tl rest-redistribution imaging continues as the most widely performed method for detection of myocardial viability in the daily routine of many centers. Oxygen inhalation after acute myocardial ischemia is part of the standard therapy in cardiology. It has also been shown that therapeutic hyperoxia diminishes myocardial stunning. In a pilot study, it was determined whether the uptake kinetics of MIBI during oxygen-enriched breathing is modified in comparison with the kinetics observed under conventional rest imaging performed after injection during inhalation of room air.

Methods.—Nine patients scheduled for coronary intervention (CI) who had documented significant stenosis (≥50%) of at least one epicardial coronary vessel, and one patient with slow flow on coronary angiography were studied. Rest MIBI ECG-gated SPET (G-SPET) with 740 MBq was performed. The tracer was injected 2 days later after a 5-minute period of 100% oxygen-supported (nasal catheter) breathing at rest (6 L/min), and a second

G-SPET (oxygen plus MIBI G-SPET) acquisition was performed. Patients' medications were not withdrawn and were matched throughout the study.

Results.—The mean elevation of arterial oxygen saturation attained was 2.95%. There were no significant changes in arterial blood pressure or heart rate during the procedure. In comparison with the results of baseline G-SPET, on oxygen plus MIBI G-SPET, 5 patients scheduled for CI and the 1 patient with slow flow showed increased tracer uptake in initially ischemic regions with no alterations in other myocardial regions. Post-CI imaging was performed in 3 of these 5 patients and showed increased tracer uptake in all additional areas previously detected by oxygen plus MIBI imaging. In 3 patients, in addition to the improvement in ischemic regions, a mild reduction in tracer uptake was observed in myocardium that initially appeared normal. Thallium-201 redistribution SPET was performed in one of these patients and showed an uptake pattern with greater resemblance to the pattern seen on oxygen plus MIBI images than that on baseline MIBI G-SPET images. In one patient, there was no difference in tracer uptake in the pre- and post-CI studies. Seven of 10 patients showed improvement in the wall thickening images of the oxygen plus MIBI study, and 4 of these patients showed improvement in the same regions after CI.

Conclusions.—MIBI injection during oxygen-enriched breathing can be a useful technique for enhancing the detection of viable myocardial tissue.

► Amazing results! A major question is whether the data represent a real change in perfusion or a change in extraction.

H. W. Strauss, MD

Dipyridamole, Cold Pressor Test, and Demonstration of Endothelial Dysfunction: A PET Study of Myocardial Perfusion in Diabetes

Kjaer A, Meyer C, Nielsen FS, et al (Univ of Copenhagen; Steno Diabetes Ctr, Gentofte, Denmark)

J Nucl Med 44:19-23, 2003 6–13

Background.—There is an accumulation of evidence for the presence of endothelial dysfunction in diseases such as hypertension, hypercholesterolemia, and non–insulin-dependent diabetes mellitus (NIDDM), and of an important role for endothelial dysfunction in the development of myocardial ischemia. Correlation between changes in blood flow during intravascular acetylcholine infusion and during cold pressor testing (CPT) has supported the use of CPT as a noninvasive way to study coronary endothelial function with PET. The effect of CPT on coronary blood flow (CBF) measured by PET was compared with that of dipyridamole in patients with NIDDM and in healthy volunteers. In addition, the effect of acute angiotensin-converting enzyme (ACE) inhibition on the flow response was studied.

Methods.—Ten patients with NIDDM and 10 control subjects were studied. Myocardial perfusion was determined at baseline, during CPT, and after dipyridamole infusion by PET using IV ^{13}N-ammonia.

Results.—The patients and controls had similar resting CBF values. CPT increased CBF by 20% in the control group but did not increase CBF in the NIDDM patients. Infusion of dipyridamole increased CBF 2- to 3-fold in patients with NIDDM and 3- to 4-fold in control subjects. During ACE inhibitor infusion, which had no effect on resting CBF in patients or control subjects, CPT increased CBF by 14% in the NIDDM group. After infusion of dipyridamole, CBF increased 3- to 4-fold in both groups. During ACE-inhibitor infusion, the increase in CBF and maximal CBF in the 2 groups were not different.

Conclusions.—In these patients with NIDDM and no evidence of epicardial coronary disease, endothelial dysfunction is strongly suggested on the basis of an impaired increase in CBF both to dipyridamole and to CPT. Infusion of an ACE inhibitor reversed this dysfunction. ACE inhibition during CPT resulted in significant increases in CBF in the patients, but these changes were small in comparison with the response to dipyridamole. In addition, the absence of an increase in CBF during CPT in 3 of the 10 control subjects is a further limitation on the value of CPT for the study of coronary endothelial dysfunction.

► Although this is an interesting article addressing the important area of endothelial dysfunction, we need more data to understand how to use the information clinically. The study should be repeated with a larger group of patients, and the patients should be categorized by the duration and severity of diabetes.

H. W. Strauss, MD

Repetitive Supply–Demand Ischemia With Dobutamine Increases Glucose Uptake in Postischemic and Remote Myocardium

McFalls EO, Murad B, Her D, et al (Univ of Minnesota, Minneapolis)

J Nucl Med 44:85-91, 2003 6–14

Background.—Ischemic reperfused myocardium demonstrates a sustained increase in glucose uptake in comparison with remote tissue. In the absence of reperfusion, myocardium in the distribution of coronary artery disease also shows a transient increase in glucose uptake in relation to remote myocardium, either after exercise or after dipyridamole stress. It would be expected that dobutamine stress would induce the same response within postischemic myocardial tissues, but the sustained effects of adrenergic receptor stimulation may affect glucose metabolism in the remote myocardium independent of insulin-mediated changes in phosphoinositol 3-kinase. An understanding of the effects of dobutamine on glucose metabolism in remote tissues is important because it helps to define the utility of glucose metabolic imaging studies for discriminating postischemic from remote myocardial regions. Whether myocardial glucose uptake after repetitive ischemia differs in response to coronary occlusion–reperfusion versus supply-demand ischemia induced by dobutamine was determined.

Methods.—Repetitive ischemia was induced in 18 swine with a hydraulic occluder and flow probes on the circumflex artery. In the first group of 9 swine, the circumflex artery was occluded, whereas in the second group of 9 swine, the circumflex flow was decreased by 30% before dobutamine (40 µg/kg/min IV). Each pig underwent 15 minutes of ischemia twice daily for 5 days. Echocardiography and PET were performed after final ischemia to determine myocardial glucose (^{18}F-FDG) uptake, and tissue was then analyzed for activation of Akt, p38 mitogen-activated protein, and adenosine monophosphate (AMP) kinase.

Results.—Wall thickening in the circumflex region was lower than in remote regions in both groups. ^{18}F-FDG uptake was similar in both groups. In the remote region, ^{18}F-FDG uptake was lower than in the circumflex region in group 1 but was similar to that in the circumflex region in group 2. AMP kinase activity in the remote region was significantly lower than in the circumflex region in group 1 but was similar to that in the circumflex region in group 2.

Conclusions.—In contrast to repetitive coronary artery occlusion–reperfusion, repetitive supply–demand ischemia with dobutamine alters glucose uptake within the remote myocardium; this effect may be the result of AMP kinase activation. These findings suggest that ^{18}F-FDG studies have only a limited role in the discrimination of postischemic from remote myocardium after dobutamine stress.

▶ FDG uptake is increased for some time after the ischemic interval.

H. W. Strauss, MD

Quantitative Estimation of Myocardial Salvage After Primary Percutaneous Transluminal Coronary Angioplasty in Patients With Angiographic No Reflow

Nakamura S, Takehana K, Sugiura T, et al (Kansai Med Univ, Osaka, Japan; Kochi Med School, Japan; Takarazuka Hosp, Hyogo, Japan)

Eur J Nucl Med 30:383-389, 2003 6–15

Background.—In patients with acute myocardial infarction (MI), angiographic thrombolysis in myocardial infarction (TIMI) flow grade of 2 or less after primary percutaneous transluminal coronary angioplasty (PTCA), defined as angiographic no reflow, predicts poor left ventricular functional recovery and survival. The relationship between angiographic coronary flow and myocardial salvage in the acute phase of MI was determined.

Methods.—One hundred seventeen patients were studied. Serial ^{99m}Tc-tetrofosmin imaging was done before, immediately after, and 1 month after PTCA. Twenty percent of the patients (group 1) had angiographic no reflow, and 80% (group 2) did not.

Findings.—The 2 groups did not differ significantly in the defect score before PTCA. However, the defect score immediately after PTCA was significantly greater in group 1 than in group 2. Group 1 also had a significantly smaller change in the defect score after PTCA than did group 2. Eighty-seven percent of patients in group 1 had impaired myocardial reperfusion, compared with 36% in group 2. This difference was statistically significant. For estimating impaired myocardial reperfusion, angiographic no reflow had a 36% sensitivity, 95% specificity, and 67% accuracy.

Conclusions.—In patients with primary PTCA, angiographic no reflow is a very specific marker for predicting impaired myocardial reperfusion estimated by serial ^{99m}Tc-tetrofosmin imaging in the early phase of acute MI. However, it is not very sensitive.

► In patients with primary PTCA, no reflow is a bad outcome. There is increasing evidence that this phenomenon is caused by embolization of atheromatous debris into the distal vessel as a result of the angioplasty. Some fortunate patients will develop collateral flow into this territory that will provide sufficient oxygen delivery to keep a significant fraction of the jeopardized myocardium viable, but this flow will not offer the same degree of improvement in the risk area as a totally successful angioplasty.

H. W. Strauss, MD

Comparison of the Short-term Survival Benefit Associated With Revascularization Compared With Medical Therapy in Patients With No Prior Coronary Artery Disease Undergoing Stress Myocardial Perfusion Single Photon Emission Computed Tomography

Hachamovitch R, Hayes SW, Friedman JD, et al (Univ of California, Los Angeles)

Circulation 107:2900-2906, 2003 6–16

Background.—For patients with stable coronary artery disease, the choice of revascularization or medical therapy must be made, with the various clinical and angiographic findings supporting one or the other of these approaches. With the use of risk-adjusted techniques in an observational data series, the survival benefit of revascularization was compared with that accompanying medical therapy based on treatment assignment selected in the first 60 days after myocardial perfusion stress testing (MPS). Evidence concerning any relationship between the amount of inducible ischemia present on MPS and the presence of a short-term survival benefit was sought.

Methods.—Follow-up for a mean of 1.9 years was conducted for 10,627 consecutive patients having exercise or adenosine MPS and no previous myocardial infarction or revascularization.

Results.—A total of 146 cardiac deaths and 492 all-cause mortality deaths occurred; the revascularization cardiac death rate was 2.8%, and the medical therapy cardiac death rate was 1.3%. When there was no inducible ischemia, patients receiving medical therapy were at very low risk (Fig 2). When the amount of inducible ischemia was greater, mortality rose in patients receiving medical therapy but did not rise in patients receiving revascularization therapy. When patients had more than 20% of their myocardi-

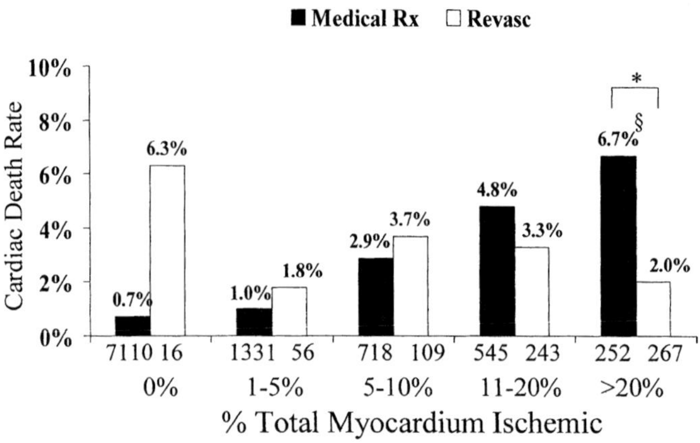

FIGURE 2.—Observed cardiac death rates over the follow-up period in patients undergoing revascularization (*Revasc*) versus medical therapy (*Medical Rx*) as a function of the amount of inducible ischemia. Increase in cardiac death frequency as a function of inducible ischemia, $P < .0001$. (Courtesy of Hachamovitch R, Hayes SW, Friedman JD, et al: Comparison of the short-term survival benefit associated with revascularization compared with medical therapy in patients with no prior coronary artery disease undergoing stress myocardial perfusion single photon emission computed tomography. *Circulation* 107:2900-2906, 2003.)

um ischemic, the cardiac mortality was lower with revascularization than with medical therapy.

The most accurate predictors of referral to revascularization were percentage of myocardium that was ischemic, anginal symptoms, percentage of myocardium fixed, ischemic ST-segment changes, elevated cholesterol levels, and previous catheterization. The most significant of these variables were percentage of myocardium that was ischemic and anginal symptoms. The increased likelihood of requiring revascularization was greatest in patients with typical angina pectoris and less in those with atypical angina or those who were asymptomatic.

An increased survival benefit for medical therapy was noted for patients who had no or only mild ischemia. An increased survival benefit for revascularization was found in patients when there was moderate to severe ischemia. Revascularization had an increased survival benefit over medical therapy for patients who were elderly, who were having adenosine stress, and were female, especially if they had diabetes.

Conclusion.—The absolute and relative risks of cardiac death were decreased by revascularization more than by medical therapy when patients had moderate to severe inducible ischemia on stress MPS, but medical therapy reduced the risk when lesser amounts of ischemia were present.

► This study provides substantial evidence to support the role of myocardial perfusion imaging as a guide to surgical or medical therapy. The study supports the contention that severe ischemia requires surgery, but mild ischemia is best treated medically.

H. W. Strauss, MD

Dobutamine-Induced Contractile Reserve in Stunned, Hibernating, and Scarred Myocardium in Patients With Ischemic Cardiomyopathy

Schinkel AFL, Bax JJ, van Domburg R, et al (Erasmus Med Ctr, Rotterdam, The Netherlands; Leiden Univ, The Netherlands)

J Nucl Med 44:127-133, 2003 6–17

Background.—Damage to cardiomyocytes and the contractile apparatus can result in less frequent observation of contractile reserve in hibernating myocardium than in stunned myocardium. The presence of contractile reserve in response to dobutamine infusion was investigated in a large group of patients with stunned and hibernating myocardium.

Methods.—One hundred ninety-eight consecutive patients with ischemic cardiomyopathy were studied. Resting 2-dimensional echocardiography was done to evaluate regional contractile dysfunction. Dysfunctional segments were categorized based on perfusion and glucose use. Dysfunctional segments showing normal perfusion were classified as stunned; those with a perfusion defect and a perfusion–^{18}F-FDG mismatch, as hibernating; and those with a perfusion defect and a perfusion–^{18}F-FDG match, as scar tissue. The latter segments were subgrouped into transmural and nontransmural

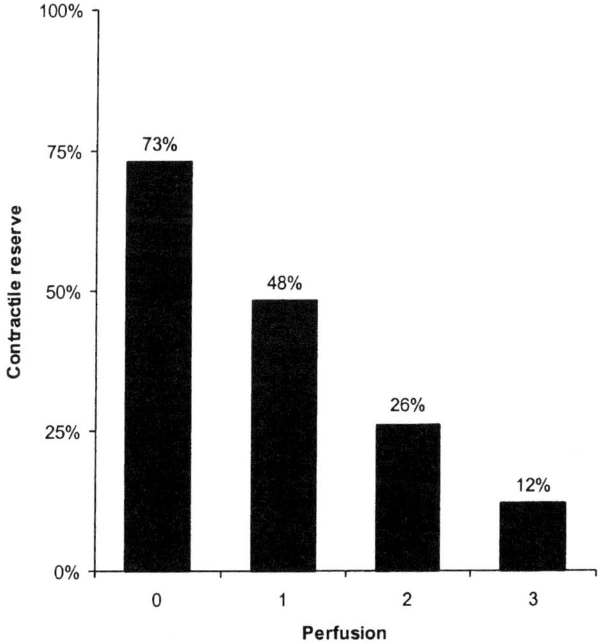

FIGURE 2.—Presence of contractile reserve according to resting ^{99m}Tc-tetrofosmin perfusion (0 = normal [100% ≥ uptake > 80%], 1 = mildly reduced [80% ≥ uptake > 50%], 2 = moderately reduced [50% ≥ uptake > 25%], 3 = severely reduced or absent [25% ≥ uptake ≥ 0%]). (Reprinted by permission of the Society of Nuclear Medicine, from Schinkel AFL, Bax JJ, van Domburg R, et al: Dobutamine-induced contractile reserve in stunned, hibernating, and scarred myocardium in patients with ischemic cardiomyopathy. *J Nucl Med* 44:127-133, 2003.)

scars. Dobutamine stress echocardiography was used to assess contractile reserve.

Findings.—Dobutamine-induced contractile reserve was documented in 61% of stunned myocardium and in 51% of hibernating myocardium (Fig 2). During dobutamine infusion, only 14% of the scarred segments improved in wall motion, which was significantly less than stunned or hibernating myocardium. Nontransmural scars demonstrated contractile reserve more often than did transmural scars.

Conclusions.—A progressive decrease in contractile reserve in stunned, hibernating, and scarred myocardium was documented. This supports the hypothesis that stunning, hibernation, and scarring are not circumscript pathophysiologic entities. Instead, they represent gradual ultrastructural damage on the myocyte level.

▶ This study supports the concept of a progressive loss of contractile function in hypoperfused areas. It suggests that patients with symptoms of cardiomyopathy should be studied early, and should undergo revascularization if ischemia is identified.

H. W. Strauss, MD

Prognostic Value of Normal Exercise and Adenosine ^{99m}Tc-Tetrofosmin SPECT Imaging: Results From the Multicenter Registry of 4,728 Patients

Shaw LJ, for the Myoview Multicenter Registry (Atlanta Cardiovascular Research Inst, Ga; et al)

J Nucl Med 44:134-139, 2003 6–18

Introduction.—Event rates correlated with normal or low-risk myocardial perfusion SPECT imaging have been shown by several trials to be linked with less than 1% per year of follow-up. This uniformly low event rate is important when applying myocardial perfusion imaging information to risk stratification. The prognostic value of a normal ^{99m}Tc-tetrofosmin study was examined in a geographically diverse registry of patients undergoing stress myocardial perfusion SPECT.

Methods.—A total of 4728 consecutively tested patients who underwent stress ^{99m}Tc-tetrofosmin SPECT at 5 US hospitals were included. Participants were monitored for the occurrence of major cardiac events and hospitalizations. Uniform methods for gathering data and standardized epidemiologic methods for follow-up were used at all 5 centers. Time to cardiac death was calculated by using a risk-adjusted Cox proportional hazards mode.

Results.—Of 4728 patients evaluated, one third underwent adenosine stress SPECT, and treadmill exercise was used in two thirds. The annualized survival rate for patients with a normal ^{99m}Tc-tetrofosmin study was 0.6%. Excellent survival rates were also seen in the male and female subsets of this patient population, for patients who could exercise, and for those who underwent pharmacologic stress testing. Compared with earlier published out-

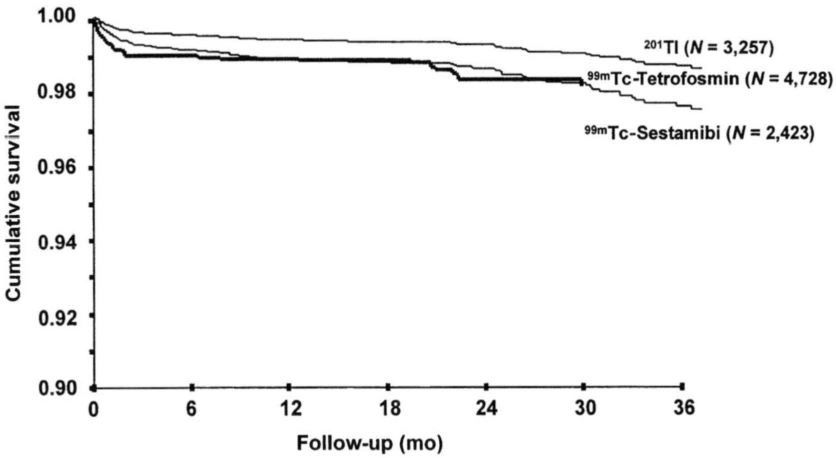

FIGURE 3.—Risk-adjusted (controlling for age, sex, and type of stress performed) Cox survival curve in patients with normal ^{201}Tl, ^{99m}Tc-sestamibi, and ^{99m}Tc-tetrofosmin SPECT. Similar survival rates were noted for all 3 isotopes—that is, at 3 y, ≥98% of patients with normal or low-risk perfusion scan were alive. (Reprinted by permission of the Society of Nuclear Medicine, from Shaw LJ, for the Myoview Multicenter Registry: Prognostic value of normal exercise and adenosine ^{99m}Tc-tetrofosmin SPECT imaging: Results from the multicenter registry of 4,728 patients. *J Nucl Med* 44:134-139, 2003.)

comes investigations on stress ^{201}Tl or ^{99m}Tc-sestamibi SPECT, the overall survival rates were similar and ranged between 99.3% and 99.7% (Fig 3).

Conclusion.—Data from this large multicenter registry provide further supportive evidence that the excellent prognosis linked with a normal SPECT scan is isotope independent.

▶ A normal tetrofosmin scan has similar prognostic value to that obtained with thallium and with sestamibi.

H. W. Strauss, MD

Exercise-Induced Electrocardiographic Changes in Patients With Chronic Respiratory Diseases: Differential Diagnosis by ^{99m}Tc-Tetrofosmin SPECT

Hirotani A, Maekura R, Okuda Y, et al (Toneyama Natl Hosp, Osaka, Japan; Osaka Univ, Japan)

J Nucl Med 44:325-330, 2003 6–19

Introduction.—The assessment of possible cardiac complications is crucial for safe and effective respiratory rehabilitation in patients with chronic respiratory diseases (CRDs). Myocardial perfusion SPECT was used to evaluate the pathophysiology of ECG changes during exercise and the prevalence of coronary artery disease in patients with CRD without any history of myocardial ischemia.

Methods.—Forty-two patients (16.9%) with exercise-induced ST depression by cardiopulmonary exercise testing were selected from 249 consecutive patients with CRD without any history of coronary artery disease. Car-

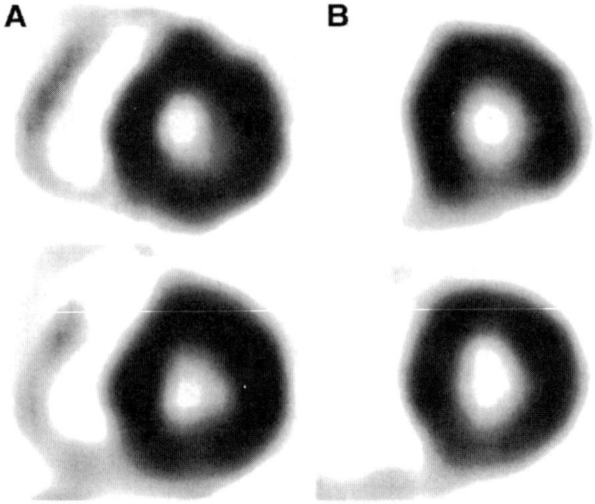

FIGURE 2.—Midventricular short-axis imaging of representative CRD patients with RV overload (**A**) and perfusion ischemia (**B**). **A**, Visualization and dilatation of RV both at rest (**bottom panel**) and during exercise (**top panel**). RV/LV ratio was greater during exercise than at rest (11.1% and 8.9%, respectively). **B**, Typical perfusion ischemia in inferior wall during exercise (**top panel**) and normal perfusion at rest (**bottom panel**). RV could not be visualized in either image. *Abbreviations: CRD*, Chronic respiratory disease; *RV*, right ventricular; *LV*, left ventricular. (Reprinted by permission of the Society of Nuclear Medicine, from Hirotani A, Maekura R, Okuda Y, et al: Exercise-induced electrocardiographic changes in patients with chronic respiratory diseases: Differential diagnosis by ^{99m}Tc-tetrofosmin SPECT. *J Nucl Med* 44:325-330, 2003.)

diopulmonary exercise testing was performed between January 1999 and December 2001. Thirty-three patients without respiratory diseases who had positive ST depression during exercise acted as controls. Exercise myocardial SPECT was performed to assess myocardial ischemia and right ventricular (RV) overload, as determined by increased RV uptake.

Results.—Only 2 of the 42 patients (4.8%) with exercise-induced ST depression had an ST depression other than in the II, III, or aVF leads. The rate of myocardial ischemia by perfusion SPECT was significantly lower in patients with CRD (26.2%), compared with controls (78.8%). The most frequently observed finding during exercise was RV overload without ischemia (26 cases; 61.9%). Ischemia was detected in 11 patients (26.2%), 10 of whom also had RV overload (Fig 2). Neither ischemia nor RV overload was identified in 5 patients (11.9%). These patients were considered normal.

Conclusion.—Perfusion SPECT revealed that the incidence of myocardial ischemia is low in patients with CRD with positive exercise-induced ECG changes. RV overload was observed in most of these patients. Cardiac perfusion SPECT is helpful in assessing cardiac ischemia and RV overload simultaneously. Before patients with CRD participate in respiratory rehabilitation, they should undergo cardiopulmonary exercise testing with 12-lead ECG monitoring. If positive ST depression is seen, further evaluation for ischemia is recommended.

► The RV should be reviewed in all myocardial perfusion studies. RV ischemia can be the cause of marked RV enlargement and should be considered in the differential diagnosis in these patients.

H. W. Strauss, MD

Dysregulation of Coronary Microvascular Reactivity in Asymptomatic Patients With Type 2 Diabetes Mellitus

Momose M, Abletshauser C, Neverve J, et al (Technischen Universität München, Munich; Novartis Pharma GmbH, Nürnberg, Germany; Institut für Diabetesforschung, Munich)

Eur J Nucl Med 29:1675-1679, 2002 6–20

Background.—Patients with diabetes mellitus are at increased risk for the development of microangiopathic and macroangiopathic cardiac disease. Impaired endothelial-dependent vasodilation in type 2 diabetes mellitus has been suggested by invasive coronary Doppler wire and by noninvasive methods. However, previous studies of vascular reactivity in diabetes mellitus have included either small and selected or relatively heterogeneous groups of diabetic patients. The pattern of dysregulation at the coronary microcirculatory level has not been clearly defined. Coronary microvascular function was characterized noninvasively in a homogeneous group of asymptomatic type 2 diabetic patients.

Methods.—A total of 46 patients with type 2 diabetes were studied. Myocardial blood flow (MBF) was quantified at baseline in response to cold pressor test (CPT) and during adenosine-mediated vasodilation by using PET and nitrogen-13 ammonia. None of the patients had been treated with insulin, and none had symptoms of cardiac disease.

Results.—Sixteen patients showed decreased MBF during CPT (CPT−), indicating microvascular dysregulation, and 30 patients showed increased MBF during CPT (CPT+). The response to CPT was mildly but significantly correlated with response to adenosine. However, there was no difference between the 2 groups in HbA1c, serum lipid levels, or serum endothelial markers. Microvascular dysregulation in the CPT− patients was associated with elevated baseline MBF, reduced baseline vascular resistance, and an abnormal increase in resistance during CPT.

Conclusions.—Coronary microvascular dysregulation is present in about one third of patients with asymptomatic, non–insulin-treated type 2 diabetes. This dysregulation is characterized by elevated baseline blood flow and reduced microvascular resistance at rest. These findings suggest that a state of activation of endothelial-dependent vasodilation exists at baseline, which appears to limit the flow response to conditions of stress.

► A controversial topic. This study does include a larger group of patients and better characterization of diabetes than the study of Kjaer et al (Abstract 6–13). It will take additional studies to determine which of these investigations is correct about the use of the CPT as an indication of the presence of endothelial dysfunction.

H. W. Strauss, MD

Myocardial Perfusion Imaging in Denmark: Activity From 1997 to 2001 and Current Practice

Petersen CL, Kjaer A (Univ of Copenhagen)

Eur J Nucl Med 30:137-140, 2003 6–21

Introduction.—National guidelines on clinical practice with myocardial perfusion imaging (MPI) were published in 1998 in an attempt to standardize referral and technique in Denmark. A survey was conducted to determine whether the activity is comparable with that of other European countries and the United States.

Methods.—A questionnaire was sent to all 20 departments of nuclear medicine in Denmark requesting details of MPI, including the number of patients examined each year from 1997 to 2001 and the current clinical and technical practice. All (100%) departments responded; all MPI studies performed in Denmark during the evaluation period were represented.

Results.—There were 2531 MPI studies in 1997 (0.47/1000/y) and 4961 (0.93 MPI/1000/y) in 2001; activity was doubled in 5 years. Nineteen departments (95%) performed MPI in 2001; 14 (74%) reported activity had increased during the past 5 years. MPI activity was unevenly distributed between hospitals and regions. In 2001, the university hospitals in the central Copenhagen region (capital) had the highest MPI activity (2.00/1000/y). The non-university hospitals, in general, had the lowest activity rate (0.73/1000/y). The most pronounced increment during that period was seen in the university hospitals outside Copenhagen, where activity increased by 300% (from 0.44/1000/y in 1997 to 1.33/1000/y in 2001). All departments with MPI used tomographic acquisition technique, and all departments used technetium tracers. The more sophisticated MPI procedures—gated acquisition, attenuation correction, and iterative reconstruction—were used in 74%, 32%, and 42% of departments, respectively. The stress mode in perfusion studies was dipyridamole/adenosine in 76%, exercise in 18%, and dobutamine in 6%. Despite these encouraging figures, MPI activity for 2001 remained below the recommendations set forth by other national and international societies. The anticipated further increase in nuclear cardiology is encouraging. The nuclear medicine community in Denmark needs to address the issues that prevent it from meeting demand. In general, the limited camera time and the limited number of appropriately educated personnel explain the excessive waiting lists in Denmark.

► It is interesting to see how a universal health care system works. Unfortunately, universal care results in a form of rationing, which leads to delays in getting important procedures, such as MPI. This often is detrimental to care.

H. W. Strauss, MD

Gated Myocardial Perfusion Tomography Versus Gated Blood Pool Tomography for the Calculation of Left Ventricular Volumes and Ejection Fraction

Vanhove C, Walgraeve N, De Geeter F, et al (Free Univ of Brussels, Belgium)

Eur J Nucl Med 29:735-741, 2002 6–22

Background.—Left ventricular (LV) volume and ejection fraction (EF) measurements are clinically important indications of the functional status of the heart and are predictors of prognosis in patients with cardiac disease. In nuclear cardiology, tomographic methods can be used to calculate LV function parameters from blood pool or from myocardial perfusion studies. The 3-dimensional nature of the ventricle is the rationale for the use of tomography rather than planar imaging. This study compared LV volumes and EF computed automatically from gated blood pool tomography (gBPT) using the new QUBE automatic algorithm with these same parameters obtained with gated myocardial perfusion tomography (gMPT) obtained with the QGS algorithm in patients with a known history of myocardial infarction.

Methods.—The effects of the extent and severity of myocardial perfusion defects were investigated in 37 patients. The patients were injected in a random sequence with 740 MBq of ^{99m}Tc human serum albumin and 925 MBq of ^{99m}Tc-tetrofosmin within an interval of 2 days. The gBPT and gMPT were obtained with the same triple-head gamma camera at the 360° step-and-shoot rotation, 32 stops (for 96 projections) at 30 seconds per stop, 64 × 64 matrix (at a pixel size of 5.8 mm) and 8 time bins. The projection data were reconstructed with filtered back-projection using a Butterworth filter.

Results.—The LV volumes calculated from gBPT were well correlated with those calculated on gMPT. However, LV volumes above 200 mL were significantly higher with gMPT than with gBPT. These discrepancies were related to the severity but not to the extent of the perfusion defects. In addition, there was good agreement between the 2 techniques for LVEF. No trend was identified on the Bland-Altman plot, but a systematic error of 5.57% and a random error of 6.85% were noted. For LVEF, the differences between these 2 techniques were not related to either the extent or the severity of the perfusion defects.

Conclusion.—LV volumes and EFs determined on gMPT were well correlated with these parameters measured on gBPT. Discrepancies were observed for large volumes, but these discrepancies are presumed to result from inaccuracies of gMPT in patients with severe perfusion defects.

► Additional proof that gMPT provides accurate data about ventricular function. The question to ask now is whether gMPT should be used in lieu of gBPT because of the additional data provided about perfusion.

H. W. Strauss, MD

Clinical Validation of Simultaneous Dual-Isotope Myocardial Scintigraphy

Weinmann P, Faraggi M, Moretti JL, et al (Paris XIII Univ, Cedex, France; Centre d'Imagerie Nucléaire, Annecy, France)

Eur J Nucl Med 30:25-31, 2003 6–23

Introduction.—The routine use of simultaneous dual-isotope (rest thallium-201/stress technetium-99m sestamibi) myocardial single-photon emission tomography (SPET) is limited by ^{99m}Tc cross-talk on the ^{201}T1 window. Photon energy recovery (PER) is a spectral deconvolution method validated for scatter and cross-talk removal in phantom imaging and a limited series of

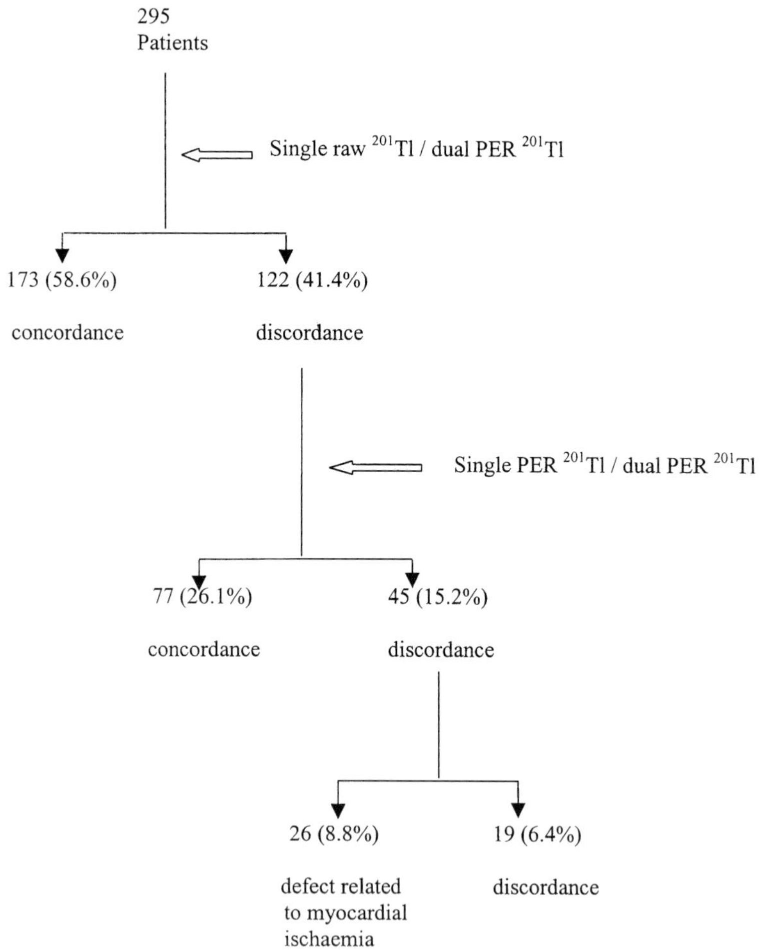

FIGURE 1.—Steps involved in the comparison between separate and simultaneous ^{201}Tl data sets and their results. (Courtesy of Weinmann P, Faraggi M, Moretti JL, et al: Clinical validation of simultaneous dual-isotope myocardial scintigraphy. *Eur J Nucl Med* 30:25-31, 2003. Copyright Springer-Verlag.)

patients. The validation of this technique was examined in 295 patients within the context of routine clinical practice.

Methods.—Of 295 patients evaluated, 64 had a history of past myocardial infarction, 102 had significant ST depression, and 69 had angina during stress testing. All patients underwent 2 SPET acquisitions: 1 during rest and 1 after a stress test. Visual analysis was performed by 2 qualified independent observers. Conventional separate rest ^{201}Tl myocardial SPET data sets were visually examined and compared with simultaneous dual-isotope data sets corrected by PER.

Results.—Conventional separate rest ^{201}Tl data sets were identical to dual PER-corrected ^{201}Tl data sets in 173 participants (58.6%). As dual PER ^{201}T1 data sets were corrected for ^{99m}Tc cross-talk and for ^{201}Tl scatter, they were compared with separate rest ^{201}T1 data sets corrected by PER in 122 discordant patients. No difference was seen in 77 patients (26.1%). In 26 patients (8.8%), the difference involved the presence of a defect on dual PER ^{201}Tl data sets only, mirroring an ischemic defect on ^{99m}Tc-sestamibi data sets (Fig 1). This difference may be attributed to the impact of stress on the kinetics of ^{201}Tl injected at rest. In the remaining 19 patients (6.4%), the difference between separate and simultaneous PER-corrected data sets was rated as mild in 11 and moderate in 8, and appeared to be associated with multiple methodological factors.

Conclusion.—PER correctly eliminates ^{99m}Tc cross-talk. With the addition of an appropriate attenuation correction, the PER method may soon allow the routine use of simultaneous dual-isotope myocardial scintigraphy.

► Although the proposed technique of simultaneous imaging of thallium and technetium look attractive, sufficient cross-talk remains to result in difficulty interpreting the thallium images in 15% of patients. This fraction is substantial enough to urge caution in adopting this methodology.

H. W. Strauss, MD

Left Ventricular Mass Measured by Myocardial Perfusion Gated SPECT: Relation to Three-Dimensional Echocardiography

Akinboboye O, Germano G, Idris O, et al (St Francis Hosp, Roslyn, NY; Cedars-Sinai Med Ctr, Los Angeles; Columbia Univ, New York)

Clin Nucl Med 28:392-397, 2003 6–24

Introduction.—Since gamma cameras cannot identify actual myocardial thickness, myocardial perfusion gated SPECT (GSPECT) techniques have used different assumptions for the definition of myocardial wall boundaries to calculate myocardial mass. Left ventricular mass (LVM) calculated from GSPECT data was examined to determine whether it corresponds with echocardiographic estimates, and whether mass accuracy diminishes as relative myocardial wall thickness increases.

Methods.—Of 37 patients referred for clinically indicated perfusion scintigraphy, 18 had Tl-201 and 19 had Tc-99m sestamibi GSPECT poststress

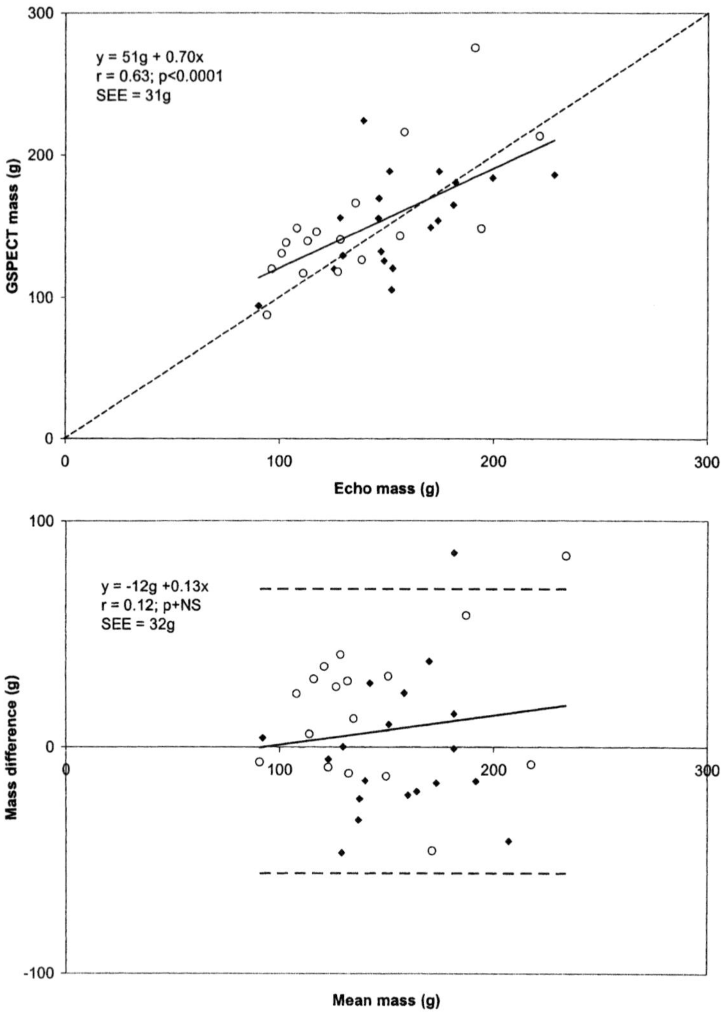

FIGURE 3.—Linear regression results for all patients. **Top**, Gated SPECT values for mass are plotted versus echocardiographic mass values. The *dashed line* is the line of identity, and the *solid line* is the least-squares fitted line. **Bottom**, Differences between gated SPECT and echocardiographic values are plotted versus the means of these values. The *dashed lines* are the 95% confidence limits, and the *solid line* is the least-squares fitted line. For both graphs, *solid circles* represent values derived from Tc-99m data, whereas *open circles* represent measures derived from Tl-201 data. *Abbreviations: SEE*, Standard error of estimate; *GSPECT*, gated SPECT. (Courtesy of Akinboboye O, Germano G, Idris O, et al: Left ventricular mass measured by myocardial perfusion gated SPECT: Relation to three-dimensional echocardiography. *Clin Nucl Med* 28(5): 392-397, 2003.)

data collections, which were subsequently processed with quantitative gated SPECT software. These patients also underwent clinically indicated echocardiograms for evaluation of wall thickness and possible valvular involvement. In addition, LV internal diameter and posterior wall thickness were calculated at end-diastole with 2-dimensional guided M-mode echocardiography to evaluate relative myocardial wall thickness; LVM was determined with 3-dimensional echocardiography by using an acoustic spatial locator device.

Results.—The LVM values were not significantly different between GSPECT and 3-dimensional echocardiography (153 g vs 146 g, respectively). The GSPECT correlated significantly ($r = 0.63$, $P < .0001$) (Fig 3) with 3-dimensional echocardiography (mean difference, 7 g and a substantial root mean squared error of 31 g). The findings were similar for similar mass ranges when subgrouped by isotope and by the presence of significant myocardial perfusion defects. The findings were independent of relative myocardial wall thickness ascertained by 2-dimensional echocardiography. Both methods produced similar results in the highest mass range of 400 to 500 g.

Conclusion.—There was a significant correlation between GSPECT and 3-dimensional echo LVM. Given the wide spread of statistical errors, these 2 methods should not be considered interchangeable. Since gamma camera resolution is limited, GSPECT LVM should be considered an approximation.

▶ When high precision is needed, echo should be used. However, medicine has worked well with a 1 to 4+ system of quantitation for many diseases. This study confirms that gated perfusion SPECT can discern differences between normal, moderate, and severe hypertrophy.

H. W. Strauss, MD

Estimation of Myocardial Blood Flow and Myocardial Flow Reserve by ^{99m}Tc-Sestamibi Imaging: Comparison With the Results of [^{15}O]H_2O PET

Ito Y, Katoh C, Noriyasu K, et al (Hokkaido Univ, Sapporo, Japan)

Eur J Nucl Med 30:281-287, 2003 6–25

Introduction.—Myocardial perfusion imaging is widely used in the diagnosis and assessment of coronary artery disease (CAD). Perfusion imaging has limited utility, especially in patients with multivessel disease or diffuse CAD, since it documents relative myocardial perfusion. A noninvasive method for quantitatively estimating the myocardial blood flow (MBF) index and myocardial flow reserve (MFR) was developed by using dynamic and static data obtained with technetium-99m sestamibi. The results were compared with MBF and MFR measured by oxygen-15–labeled water ([^{15}O]H_2O) PET.

Methods.—Twenty patients with CAD and 9 normal controls underwent both ^{99m}Tc-sestamibi and PET imaging within a 2-week period. From the anterior view, dynamic data were acquired for 2 minutes immediately after injection of ^{99m}Tc-sestamibi. Planar static images were taken after 5 minutes at rest and during adenosine triphosphate (ATP) stress (0.16 mg kg^{-1} min^{-1} for 5 minutes) on another day. The area under the time-activity curve on the aortic arch (Aorta ACU), the myocardial weight with the SPET image (M), and the myocardial count on the planar image for 1 minute (C_m) were calculated. The following formula was used to determine the MBF index (MBFI): MBFI = C_m/Aorta ACU × 100/M. The MFR was calculated by dividing the MBFI at ATP stress by the MBFI at rest.

Results.—The MBFI determined by ^{99m}Tc-sestamibi was significantly associated with the MBF obtained with [^{15}O]H_2O PET (MBFI = 13.174 + 11.732 × MBF; $r = 0.821$; $P < .001$). The MFR determined by ^{99m}Tc-sestamibi was well correlated with that obtained by [^{15}O]H_2O PET, with some underestimation ($r = 0.845$; $P < .001$). In patients with CAD, the MFR measured with ^{99m}Tc-sestamibi was significantly lower than in normal subjects (CAD, 1.484 vs normal, 2.127; $P < .001$).

Conclusion.—The MBFI and MFR can be determined with ^{99m}Tc-sestamibi. This may be beneficial in the quantitative assessment of CAD, particularly in patients with diffuse coronary disease.

▶ The authors have done a marvelous job trying to make this measurement work. However, the change in myocardial extraction at high flow limits the dynamic range of measurements they obtained with MIBI. This creates overlap between the normal subjects and patients with CAD, reducing the value of measuring MFR with MIBI.

H. W. Strauss, MD

Attenuation and Scatter Correction in Myocardial SPET: Improved Diagnostic Accuracy in Patients With Suspected Coronary Artery Disease

Kjær A, Cortsen A, Rahbek B, et al (Univ of Copenhagen)

Eur J Nucl Med 29:1438-1442, 2002 6–26

Background.—Myocardial SPET has a high sensitivity for the detection of coronary artery disease and a high prognostic value. However, artifacts hamper the accuracy of this modality. Most commercially available camera systems provide the ability to compensate for attenuation and scatter, but there is some variation among vendors in both the hardware systems and the algorithms used to correct for attenuation and scatter. The performance of a commercially available system for attenuation and scatter correction was evaluated in everyday routine, with the use of coronary angiography as a reference.

Methods.—The study included 142 consecutive patients who were referred for myocardial SPET. Their studies were processed with and without scatter and attenuation correction (SCAC). Uncorrected and SCAC images were then scored by blinded, consensus readings. Coronary angiography was used when available as a reference if there were differences in the scoring of the images.

Results.—The readings differed in 37% of cases, of which SCAC caused disappearance of irreversible defects in 74% of cases, disappearance of reversible defects in 14% of cases, and change of irreversible to reversible defects in 9% of cases (Table 2). SCAC introduced 2 new defects. The defects

TABLE 2.—CAG Findings in Cases Where SCAC Differed From FBP Readings

Effect of SCAC (*n*)		Presumed Correct Angiographic Finding	No. With This Angiographic Finding
Disappearance of inferior defect	24	<70% narrowing of RCA or PDA in dominant LCX	20 (83%)
Disappearance of anterior defect	3	<70% narrowing of LAD	3 (100%)
Appearance of new anterior defect	1	>70% narrowing of LAD	1 (100%)
Irreversible inferior defect becoming reversible	2	Not possible to discriminate by CAG	—
Total (defects)	30	*Total in which CAG supported SCAC*	*Defects:* 24 (80%)
Total (cases)	29		*Cases:* 24 (83%)

Abbreviation: CAG, Coronary angiography; *SCAC*, scatter and attenuation correction; *RCA*, right coronary artery; *LCX*, left circumflex artery; *LAD*, left anterior descending artery; *PDA*, posterior descending artery.

(Courtesy of Kjær A, Cortsen A, Rahbek B, et al: Attenuation and scatter correction in myocardial SPET: Improved diagnostic accuracy in patients with suspected coronary artery disease. *Eur J Nucl Med* 29:1438-1442, 2002. Copyright 2002, Springer-Verlag.)

influenced were located inferiorly in 75% of cases, anteriorly in 14% of cases, septally in 7% of cases, laterally in 2% of cases, and apically in 2% of cases. Coronary angiography was available in 29 of the discrepant cases and supported SCAC image readings in 83% of cases and uncorrected image readings in 7% of cases.

Conclusions.—A commercial system for correction of attenuation and scatter in myocardial SPET was diagnostically helpful in a consecutive series of patients. With coronary angiography as a reference, the SCAC interpretation was confirmed in almost all cases.

► Attenuation correction of single-photon images with rod sources remains a controversial area. This study suggests that it really helps.

H. W. Strauss, MD

Comparison of Microsphere-Equivalent Blood Flow (^{15}O-Water PET) and Relative Perfusion (^{99m}Tc-Tetrofosmin SPECT) in Myocardium Showing Metabolism–Perfusion Mismatch

Schaefer WM, Nowak B, Kaiser H-J, et al (Aachen Univ of Technology, Germany)

J Nucl Med 44:33-39, 2003 6–27

Background.—Myocardial perfusion imaging with ^{99m}Tc-tetrofosmin is widely used for the diagnosis of coronary artery disease. This technique is based on the assumption that a linear correlation exists between myocardial blood flow (MBF) and tracer uptake. However, it is known that ^{99m}Tc-tetrofosmin uptake is directly related to energy-dependent transport processes, such as Na^+/H^+ ion channel activity, as well as cellular and mitochondrial membrane potentials. Thus, it would seem that cellular alterations that affect these energy-dependent transport processes would influence ^{99m}Tc-tetrofosmin uptake independently of blood flow. Because metabolism (^{18}F-

FDG)–perfusion (^{99m}Tc-tetrofosmin) mismatch myocardium (MPMM) is a reflection of impaired but viable myocardium showing cellular alterations, MPMM was selected to quantify the blood flow–independent effect of cellular alterations on ^{99m}Tc-tetrofosmin uptake. Microsphere-equivalent MBF (MBF_micr; ^{15}O-water PET) and ^{99m}Tc-tetrofosmin uptake were compared in MPMM and in "normal" myocardium.

Methods.—The study group comprised 42 patients with severe coronary artery disease who were referred for myocardial viability diagnostic evaluations. The patients were examined with ^{18}F-FDG PET and ^{99m}Tc-tetrofosmin perfusion SPECT. Relative uptake values for the 2 modalities were calculated by using 18 segments per patient. Normal myocardium and MPMM myocardium were classified with a previously validated ^{99m}Tc-tetrofosmin SPECT/^{18}F-FDG PET score. Other evaluations included ^{15}O-water PET for assessment of kinetic-modeled MBF (MBF_kin), the water-perfusable tissue fraction (PTF), and the resulting MBF_micr (MBF_kin·PTF), which is comparable to tracer uptake values. Values for ^{99m}Tc-tetrofosmin uptake and MBF_micr were calculated for all normal and MPMM segments and averaged within their respective classifications.

Results.—The mean relative ^{99m}Tc-tetrofosmin uptake was 86% ± 1% in normal myocardium and 56% ± 1% in MPMM, which demonstrated the significant difference that was expected from the classification (Fig 4). In contrast to these findings, mean MBF_micr in MPMM myocardium was 0.60 ± 0.03 mL·min^{-1}·mL^{-1}, a finding not significantly different from that for normal myocardium (0.64 ± 0.01 mL·min^{-1}·mL^{-1}).

Conclusions.—These findings suggest that the differences between reduced ^{99m}Tc-tetrofosmin uptake and the unchanged MBF_micr in MPMM

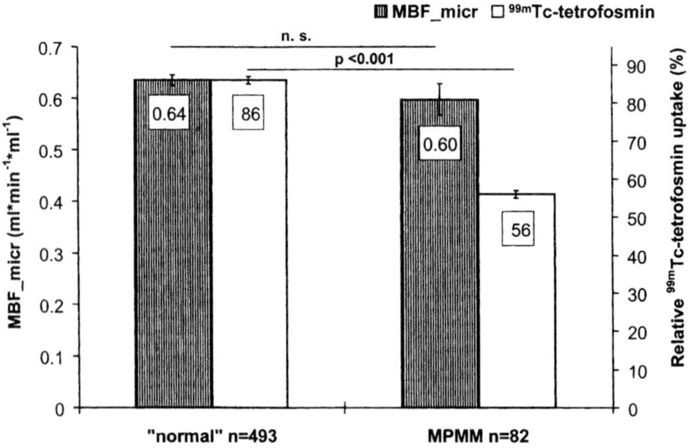

FIGURE 4.—Mean MBF_micr (mL·min^{-1}·mL^{-1}) and relative ^{99m}Tc-tetrofosmin uptake in normal myocardium and MPMM myocardium. ^{99m}Tc-tetrofosmin uptake values are normalized to respective patient's maximum uptake region, set as 100%. *Abbreviation: n.s.*, Not statistically significant. (Reprinted by permission of the Society of Nuclear Medicine, from Schaefer WM, Nowak B, Kaiser H-H, et al: Comparison of microsphere-equivalent blood flow (^{15}O-water PET) and relative perfusion (^{99m}Tc-tetrofosmin SPECT) in myocardium showing metabolism-perfusion mismatch. *J Nucl Med* 44:33-39, 2003.)

myocardium does not reflect reduced blood flow but rather cellular alterations that affect uptake and retention of ^{99m}Tc-tetrofosmin independently of blood flow. Thus, it would appear that perfusion deficits in MPMM myocardium are greatly overestimated by ^{99m}Tc-tetrofosmin, which has a tendency to provide false-positive findings.

► Fascinating and unexpected results. This study suggests that changes in extraction of the tracer, rather than a reduction in perfusion, are the cause of the mismatch. This study also lends credence to the observation that mismatch is probably caused by recurrent, episodic ischemia, rather than a persistent low-flow state.

H. W. Strauss, MD

A Comparison of Three Radionuclide Myocardial Perfusion Tracers in Clinical Practice: The ROBUST Study

Kapur A, Latus KA, Davies G, et al (Royal Brompton Hosp, London; Imperial College School of Medicine, London; Royal Free and Univ College Med School (UCL), London)

Eur J Nucl Med 29:1608-1616, 2002 6–28

Background.—Myocardial perfusion imaging is part of routine clinical cardiology, but there are no large studies available to guide the selection of thallium (Tl), methoxyisobutylisonitrile (MIBI), or tetrofosmin (Tf) for myocardial perfusion imaging. Most of the experience has been with Tl-201, whereas MIBI and tetrofosmin are newer agents and are used in an increasing number of studies. The technical and clinical performances of these 3 agents were compared in routine clinical practice.

Methods.—A total of 2560 patients were randomly assigned to receive Tl, MIBI, or Tf, with a 1-day stress/rest protocol used for MIBI and Tf. Tracer uptake was scored by means of a 17-segment model. Quanlity and artifact scores were assigned, and ratios of heart, liver, subdiaphragmatic, and lung activity were measured.

Results.—The mean quality scores (stress/rest) were 2.13/2.16 for Tl, 2.18/2.39 for MIBI, and 2.18/2.42 for Tf. For attenuation artifact, Tl > MIBI = Tf, and for low-count artifact, Tl > MIBI > Tf. For heart/subdiaphragmatic activity, Tl > MIBI = Tf; for heart/liver activity, Tl > MIBI = Tf; and for heart/lung activity, Tl < MIBI = Tf. Stress defects in patients with reversible or mixed perfusion defects were more severe for Tl than for the other tracers, but mean rest scores were more similar. In a subset of 137 patients undergoing diagnostic perfusion studies without prior infarction, angiography, or revascularization, the overall sensitivity for the detection of coronary disease defined by subsequent angiography was 91%, with a specificity of 87%. There were no significant differences between the tracers in sensitivity and specificity.

Conclusions.—Technical differences between the tracers exist. MIBI provides superior overall image quality with less low-count artifact and less attenuation. However, thallium showed slightly greater stress defect depth and extent, with no difference between MIBI and tetrofosmin. In clinical terms, all 3 of these tracers perform well, manifesting high sensitivity and specificity for angiographic stenosis and no differences in accuracy between the tracers.

► An important study. The conclusions differ from a previous study by Soman et al,[1] which found better contrast in studies done with MIBI than with tetrofosmin.

H. W. Strauss, MD

Reference

1. Soman P, Taillefer R, DePuey EG, et al: Enhanced detection of reversible perfusion defects by Tc-99m sestamibi compared to Tc-99m tetrofosmin during vasodilator stress SPECT imaging in mild-to-moderate coronary artery disease. *J Am Coll Cardiol* 37:458-462, 2001.

Simple and Accurate Assessment of Forward Cardiac Output by Use of 1-^{11}C-Acetate PET Verified in a Pig Model

Sörensen J, Ståhle E, Långström B, et al (Academic Hosp, Uppsala, Sweden; Uppsala Univ, Sweden)

J Nucl Med 44:1176-1183, 2003 6–29

Background.—PET with 1-^{11}C-acetate (AC-PET) provides a useful, noninvasive technique of measurement of myocardial oxidative metabolism. By means of first-pass analysis with the indicator-dilution method, it might be possible to measure cardiac output (CO) and stroke volume simultaneously with AC-PET. A pig model was used to assess the accuracy of AC-PET measurements of CO, and to evaluate the relationship between pulmonary acetate uptake and cardiac function measures.

Methods.—A series of experiments was performed in a validated model using invasively instrumented domestic pigs. The animals underwent AC-PET scanning at baseline and during infusion of dobutamine, high-dose metoprolol and morphine, or angiotensinamide. The CO by PET (CO_{PET}) was calculated by using regions of interest in the right and left ventricles, with calculation of time-activity curves and area under the curve. The values were compared with thermodilution measurements of CO. Pulmonary extravascular retention of tracer was measured and compared with left atrial filling pressures and ventricular function.

Results.—There was a significant linear relationship between CO_{PET} and CO measured by thermodilution (Fig 3). Slopes were close to 1 when CO_{PET} was measured with either right or left ventricular region of interest data; interobserver reproducibility was high. Pulmonary capillary wedge pressure ranged from 6 to 14 mm Hg, whereas pulmonary tracer uptake ranged from 2.7% to 8.5% of injected dose. Normalized to baseline volume, pulmonary tracer uptake was significantly correlated with pulmonary capillary wedge pressure and with left ventricular input resistance. A piecewise linear relationship was apparent on normalization of lung uptake and stroke volume to baseline.

Conclusions.—Findings in this animal model support the accuracy of AC-PET measurement of CO. With the use of right ventricular regions of interest, CO might be measured by any injected PET tracer. With further study,

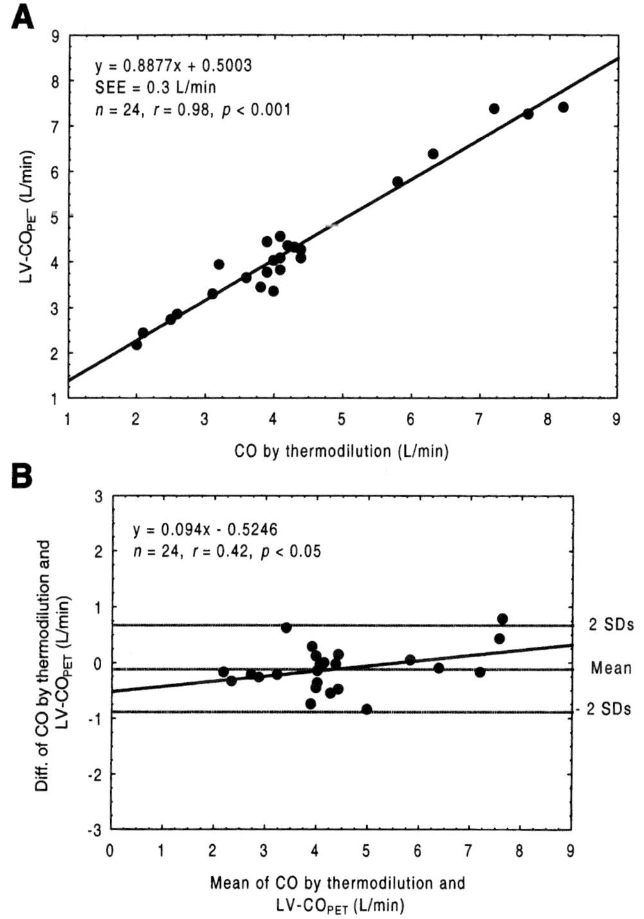

FIGURE 3.—A, Plot of estimates of CO_{PET} derived from LV ROI (LV-CO_{PET}) against standard thermodilution technique (CO_{thermo}). B, Bland-Altman plot shows difference (Diff.) between 2 methods plotted against mean values. Slope is significantly different from 0. *Abbreviations: CO_{PET}*, Cardiac output by PET; *LV*, left ventricular; *ROI*, regions of interest; *SEE*, standard error of estimate. (Reprinted by permission of the Society of Nuclear Medicine, courtesy of Sörenson J, Ståhle E, Långström B, et al: Simple and accurate assessment of forward cardiac output by use of 1-^{11}C-acetate PET verified in a pig model. *J Nucl Med* 44:1176-1183, 2003.)

assessment of pulmonary acetate uptake might be useful in the assessment of pulmonary congestion.

► Revalidating an old principle with a very high tech approach. It is helpful to know that PET data can be acquired with sufficient temporal and spatial resolution to provide these data.

H. W. Strauss, MD

Feasibility and Image Quality of Dual-Isotope SPECT Using ^{18}F-FDG amd ^{99m}Tc-Tetrofosmin After Acipimox Administration

Kam BLR, Valkema R, Poldermans D, et al (Erasmus MC, Rotterdam, The Netherlands; Leiden Univ, The Netherlands)

J Nucl Med 44:140-145, 2003 6–30

Introduction.—Coronary revascularization can improve function and long-term prognosis in patients with heart failure secondary to coronary artery disease. Studies of myocardial viability are required to guide treatment, and the most accurate method is that of metabolic imaging with ^{18}F-FDG and PET or SPECT. Because good image quality requires that ^{18}F-FDG stud-

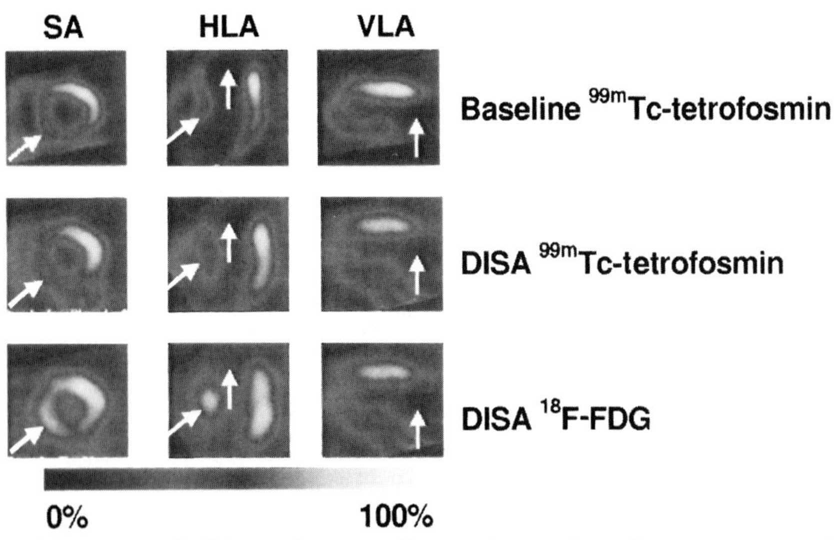

FIGURE 4.—Baseline ^{99m}Tc-tetrofosmin, DISA ^{99m}Tc-tetrofosmin, and DISA ^{18}F-FDG SPECT images of patients with known 2-vessel disease. **Top row**, Baseline ^{99m}Tc-tetrofosmin short-axis (*SA*), horizontal long-axis (*HLA*), and vertical long-axis (*VLA*) slices. **Center row**, Corresponding DISA ^{99m}Tc-tetrofosmin images. **Bottom row**, Corresponding ^{18}F-FDG slices. There is large severe defect in perfusion and glucose metabolism in area of apex (matched pattern, scar; *vertical arrows*). In septum, there is moderate perfusion defect with nearly normal glucose metabolism (mismatch pattern, viable; *oblique arrows*). Additionally, there is mild perfusion defect in basal posterior area with mismatch (best seen on HLA images, *no arrows*). DISA perfusion images are less sharp than baseline perfusion images, but diagnostic information is retained. *Abbreviation: DISA*, Dual-isotope simultaneous acquisition. (Reprinted by permission of the Society of Nuclear Medicine, from Kam BLR, Valkema R, Poldermans D, et al: Feasibility and image quality of dual-isotope SPECT using ^{18}F-FDG and ^{99m}Tc-tetrofosmin after acipimox administration. *J Nucl Med* 44:140-145, 2003.)

ies be performed during hyperinsulinemic euglycemic clamping, this approach is usually not feasible. Nicotinic acid derivatives such as acipimox may help to obtain better image quality in ^{18}F-FDG studies.

Methods.—The feasibility and image quality of ^{18}F-FDG SPECT (with dual-isotope simultaneous acquisition [DISA] using ^{99m}Tc-tetrofosmin to assess perfusion) after acipimox administration were studied in 50 nondiabetic patients. All patients had a history of coronary artery disease and of myocardial infarction. Image quality was evaluated visually and quantitatively by using myocardium-to–blood-pool ratios as a measure of target-to-background ratio. The image quality and diagnostic value of DISA ^{99m}Tc-tetrofosmin SPECT were compared with ^{99m}Tc-tetrofosmin SPECT at baseline (Fig 4).

Results.—After the injection of acipimox, plasma levels of free fatty acids were extremely low (mean, 68 nmol/L for the patient group). There were no severe side effects associated with acipimox administration, but paroxysmal flushing occurred in some patients. The ^{18}F-FDG image quality was considered good in 92% of patients, and moderate but interpretable in 8%. Clinical information of the baseline ^{99m}Tc-tetrofosmin SPECT was retained in the DISA ^{99m}Tc-tetrofosmin SPECT, and clinical judgment in patients was the same whether the baseline perfusion or the DISA image was used.

Conclusion.—Acipimox used with ^{18}F-FDG DISA SPECT was found to be safe in patients without diabetes mellitus or impaired glucose tolerance. This convenient method of metabolic cardiac imaging yielded good results in intrapatient comparison with standard resting perfusion SPECT.

► It may seem that the era of dual single photon approaches to FDG imaging are passé. However, it is likely that the era of SPECT CT will give new life to this approach. This study is interesting because of the influence of decreased fatty acid levels on enhanced FDG uptake.

H. W. Strauss, MD

Performance of OSEM and Depth-Dependent Resolution Recovery Algorithms for the Evaluation of Global Left Ventricular Function in ^{201}Tl Gated Myocardial Perfusion SPECT

Daou D, Pointurier I, Coaguila C, et al (Lariboisière Univ, Paris; Foch Hosp, Suresnes, France; Bichat Univ, Paris; et al)

J Nucl Med 44:155-162, 2003 6–31

Introduction.—ECG-gated SPECT (GSPECT) is an important nuclear cardiology study that provides valuable information on left ventricular function. The functional parameters are affected by the reconstruction method used, traditionally filtered backprojection (FBP). More accurate iterative reconstruction methods such as ordered-subsets expectation maximization (OSEM) have recently become available. The use of OSEM and depth-dependent resolution recovery (RR) was evaluated for evaluation of left ventricular function with GSPECT.

Methods.—The study included 56 patients undergoing rest thallium-201 GSPECT and planar equilibrium radionuclide angiography ($planar_{RNA}$) on the same day. Conventional angiography was also performed in 29 patients. The quantitative GSPECT software was used to calculate left ventricular functional parameters by using 4 different processing techniques: FBP alone, OSEM alone, RR plus FBP, and RR plus OSEM. The gold standards for comparison were $planar_{RNA}$ for left ventricular ejection fraction and conventional angiography for end-diastolic and end-systolic volume.

Results.—By all 4 calculation techniques, the GSPECT values for left ventricular ejection fraction were similar to and significantly correlated with the $planar_{RNA}$ value. The mean absolute difference in left ventricular ejection fraction was similar across the 4 GSPECT reconstruction methods, although limits of agreement were relatively large. The left ventricular volumes calculated by the GSPECT methods were lower than those calculated from conventional angiography, but were significantly correlated. Volumes calculated with FBP or OSEM alone were lower than those calculated with the addition of RR. Mean absolute differences in left ventricular volumes with the GSPECT methods versus conventional angiography were 56 mL for FBP, 57 mL for OSEM, 43 mL for RR plus FBP, and 46 mL for RR plus OSEM. For both left ventricular ejection fraction and volumes, variance of random effects was not significantly different between the 4 techniques.

Conclusions.—For GSPECT assessment of left ventricular function, the accuracy is similar when reconstruction is performed with OSEM or FBP. Combining either technique with depth-dependent RR improves the accuracy of left ventricular volume measurements, without affecting ejection fraction.

► Software improvements will be increasingly important as our instrumentation approaches the theoretical maximum resolution. We still have room for improvement in both areas. This study reaffirms the value of RR software.

H. W. Strauss, MD

---

^{125}I-BMIPP and ^{18}F-FDG Uptake in a Transgenic Mouse Model of Stunned Myocardium

Verberne HJ, Sloof GW, Beets AL, et al (Academic Med Ctr, Amsterdam; Oak Ridge Natl Lab, Tenn; Johns Hopkins Univ, Baltimore, Md)

Eur J Nucl Med 30:431-439, 2003 6–32

Background.—In previous research, metabolic patterns in myocardial stunning are not consistent. Relative myocardial perfusion, glucose, and fatty acid uptake were investigated by using a technetium-99 hexakis-2-methoxyisobutyl-isonitrile (MIBI), ^{18}F-FDG, and iodine-125 12-(*p*-iodophenyl)-3(*R,S*)-methylpentadecanoic acid (BMIPP) mixture.

Methods.—A recently developed transgenic mouse model that mimics stunned myocardium was used. Fourteen transgenic mice (TR group) and 13 age-matched wild type controls (C group) were divided into 4 groups and either fed or fasted. Two hours after injection, the mice were killed and examined using radiolabeled analogues.

Findings.—Pooled data demonstrated no differences in myocardial blood flow, glucose uptake, or fatty acid uptake. There were only minor differences in incorporation of ^{125}I-BMIPP into the myocardial triglyceride, diglyceride, free fatty acid, and phospholipid lipid pools. Myocardial FDG uptake was significantly reduced in a subgroup of fasted mice, including 4 of 10 TR mice and 3 of 9 C mice.

Conclusions.—This transgenic mouse model demonstrated normal myocardial perfusion and overall intact myocardial glucose and myocardial fatty acid uptake, determined by clinically applicable radiolabeled analogues. These findings are consistent with the hypothesis that the contractile inefficiency in stunned myocardium is unrelated to metabolic changes but is associated with an insufficient chemical to mechanical energy coupling.

► Additional support for the concept that stunning is not related to substrate uptake, but to the ability to convert the energy to contractile work.

H. W. Strauss, MD

Bicycle Exercise Stress in PET for Assessment of Coronary Flow Reserve: Repeatability and Comparison With Adenosine Stress

Wyss CA, Koepfli P, Mikolajczyk K, et al (Univ Hosp Zurich, Switzerland)

J Nucl Med 44:146-154, 2003 6–33

Background.—Absolute measures of myocardial blood flow (MBF) can be obtained with PET. The feasibility and repeatability of supine bicycle exercise stress in PET were compared with standard adenosine stress in PET.

Methods.—Eleven healthy volunteers were studied. MBF was assessed at rest, during adenosine-induced hyperemia, and immediately after supine bicycle exercise with the use of PET and $^{15}O\text{-}H_2O$. After 20 minutes, the assessment was repeated. Coronary flow reserve was determined as hyperemic/resting MBF for adenosine and exercise stress.

Findings.—The paired resting MBF and hyperemic MBF with adenosine or exercise stress did not differ significantly (Table 2). Coronary flow reserve with adenosine and exercise stress was reproducible. Repeatability coefficients for MBF were 0.26 at rest, 1.34 for adenosine stress, and 0.82 for exercise stress.

Conclusions.—Assessing coronary flow reserve with $^{15}O\text{-}H_2O$ and PET using bicycle exercise in the PET scanner is feasible. This method is at least as repeatable as with adenosine stress.

► These results are impressive. The perfusion measurement made immediately after bicycle exercise demonstrated a greater than 2-fold increase in myocardial flow, in keeping with the rate pressure product and the fact that perfusion decreases rapidly with cessation of exercise. Adenosine, however, was associated with a greater than 4-fold increase in perfusion. This marked

TABLE 2.—Myocardial Blood Flow

Parameter	Rest 1	Rest 2	Repeatability Coefficient		Adenosine 1	Adenosine 2	Repeatability Coefficient		Bicycle 1	Bicycle 2	Repeatability Coefficient	
			Abs.	% of Mean			Abs.	% of Mean			Abs.	% of Mean
Global												
Uncorrected	1.22 ± 0.16	1.26 ± 0.21	0.26	21	5.13 ± 0.74	4.97 ± 1.05	1.34	27	2.35 ± 0.66	2.25 ± 0.61	0.82	36
Corrected	1.75 ± 0.37	1.46 ± 0.29	0.58	37								
Regional												
Septal	1.14 ± 0.14	1.23 ± 0.50	0.66	55	4.75 ± 1.06	4.40 ± 0.90	2.68	59	2.53 ± 0.74	2.23 ± 0.73	1.64	68
Anterior	1.25 ± 0.27	1.35 ± 0.31	0.58	45	5.24 ± 0.99	5.37 ± 1.75	3.72	70	2.08 ± 0.63	2.14 ± 0.92	1.34	62
Lateral	1.14 ± 0.25	1.12 ± 0.14	0.52	46	4.94 ± 1.15	5.04 ± 1.46	3.44	69	2.36 ± 0.56	2.13 ± 0.63	1.06	46
Inferior	1.18 ± 0.26	1.21 ± 0.14	0.46	38	5.16 ± 1.15	5.13 ± 1.52	2.84	55	2.91 ± 0.84	2.48 ± 0.61	1.64	60

Values are given in mL/min/g.
Abbreviations: Abs., Absolute; *1*, initial test; *2*, repeated test.
(Reprinted by permission of the Society of Nuclear Medicine, from Wyss CA, Koepfli P, Mikolajczyk K, et al: Bicycle exercise stress in PET for assessment of coronary flow reserve: Repeatability and comparison with adenosine stress. *J Nucl Med* 44:146-154, 2003.)

increase is likely, in part, a reflection of the detailed approach the investigators used to make their measurement.

H. W. Strauss, MD

Factors Affecting Left Ventricular Ejection Fraction Using Automated Quantitative Gated SPECT

Gayed I, Cid E, Boccalandero F, et al (Univ of Texas, Houston)

Clin Nucl Med 28:290-295, 2003 6–34

Background.—Limited research is available on factors affecting the accuracy of left ventricular ejection fraction (LVEF) quantification using auto-

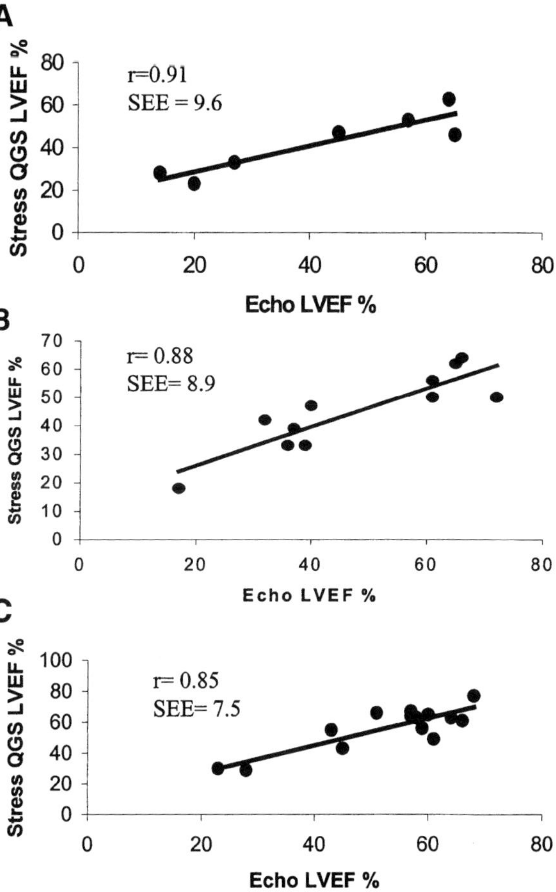

FIGURE 4.—Correlation of LVEF from stress QGS and echocardiography in patients with 3 or more segments of perfusion defect (**A**), 1 to 2 segments of perfusion defects (**B**), and normal perfusion (**C**). *Abbreviations: LVEF,* Left ventricular ejection fraction; *QGS,* quantitative gated SPECT; *SEE,* standard error of the estimate. (Courtesy of Gayed I, Cid E, Boccalandero F, et al: Factors affecting left ventricular ejection fraction using automated quantitative gated SPECT. *Clin Nucl Med* 28:290-295, 2003.)

mated quantitative gated SPECT (QGS) in clinical settings. The effect of defect size and ^{99m}Tc-tetrofosmin dose on the accuracy of LVEF calculation with the automated QGS program was determined.

Methods.—Thirty-two consecutive patients were studied. Gated rest and stress myocardial perfusion SPECT were performed after the administration of 8 and 27 mCi of ^{99m}Tc-tetrofosmin, respectively. The LVEF was acquired for the rest and stress studies with the use of the QGS program. Data were compared with LVEF data obtained from quantitative echocardiography performed within 2 weeks. In 12 left ventricular segments, myocardial perfusion defects were documented as scarring, ischemia, or mixed scarring and ischemia. The size of the defect was determined by adding the number of affected segments.

Findings.—The mean LVEF calculated with the use of high-dose stress QGS was 49.2%; with low-dose rest QGS, 46.2%; and with echocardiography, 48.7%. These differences were nonsignificant. The LVEF acquired with the use of high-dose stress QGS was more strongly associated with echocardiography than the LVEF obtained with low-dose rest QGS. Good correlation with echocardiography was observed when the high-dose stress LVEF in 14 patients with normal myocardial perfusion was compared with that in 11 patients with 1- or 2-segment perfusion defects as well as 7 patients with perfusion defects in 3 or more segments (Fig 4).

Conclusions.—Myocardial perfusion defects do not appear to affect the accuracy of LVEF calculation with automated QGS. High-dose gated myocardial SPECT correlated more strongly with quantitative echocardiographic LVEF data.

▶ The calculation of LVEF from myocardial perfusion SPECT is robust.

H. W. Strauss, MD

7 Oncology

Introduction

The role of nuclear medicine in diagnostic and therapeutic oncology continues to increase with the new indications for FDG-PET imaging and new radionuclide therapies. We are continuing to learn about the applications of PET in oncology as well as the limitations. FDG-PET is a tremendous modality that is useful in diagnosing and staging many cancers, but it is not a perfect test. Physicians interpreting PET scans must be aware of the causes of false-positive and false-negative images in patients with suspected and/or proven malignancy. PET-CT is having a major impact on the use of PET and is resulting in studies that are more accurate.

We continue to learn more about the use of somatostatin receptor scintigraphy and metaiodobenzylguanidine (MIBG) scintigraphy in neuroendocrine tumors. The therapeutic applications of these radiopharmaceuticals continue to be explored.

The use of lymphoscintigraphy for identification of sentinel lymph nodes continues to increase in its utilization. Refinement of the techniques and the evaluation of different radiopharmaceuticals are the topics covered by this review of the literature.

R. Edward Coleman, MD

Uptake in Supraclavicular Area Fat ("USA-Fat"): Description on ^{18}F-FDG PET/CT

Cohade C, Osman M, Pannu HK, et al (Johns Hopkins Hosp, Baltimore, Md)
J Nucl Med 44:170-176, 2003 7–1

Background.—Lymph node metastases is common in the supraclavicular region. On ^{18}F-FDG PET, malignancies in this region typically appear as a round focus of intense metabolic activity that may be single, multiple, or bilateral and is sometimes accompanied by other distant abnormal foci of uptake. Nonpathologic supraclavicular uptake is well known and is often attributed to muscle uptake, which is thought to result from muscle contraction in tense patients during the ^{18}F-FDG uptake phase. Muscle uptake of ^{18}F-FDG is a potential cause of false positive findings on imaging studies of patients with cancer.

Some authors have proposed the use of muscle relaxants and sedatives such as diazepam to reduce muscle uptake. However, in some patients imaged with PET/CT, it has been observed that ^{18}F-FDG activity in the supraclavicular area did not have a corresponding soft tissue mass or lymph node or muscle uptake on the CT scan. The potential for PET/CT scanners in the evaluation of how patterns of ^{18}F-FDG uptake in the supraclavicular region relate to CT findings was investigated.

Methods.—This retrospective review evaluated images for 359 consecutive clinical whole-body studies in 347 patients using ^{18}F-FDG and a PET/CT scanner. The supraclavicular region was evaluated for abnormal uptake on PET images, and the corresponding CT findings were assessed. Abnormal ^{18}F-FDG uptake was noted in 3 distinct patterns. Pattern A showed uptake localizing to supraclavicular area fat (USA-fat) without corresponding lymph node or muscle uptake. Pattern B showed uptake localizing to muscle

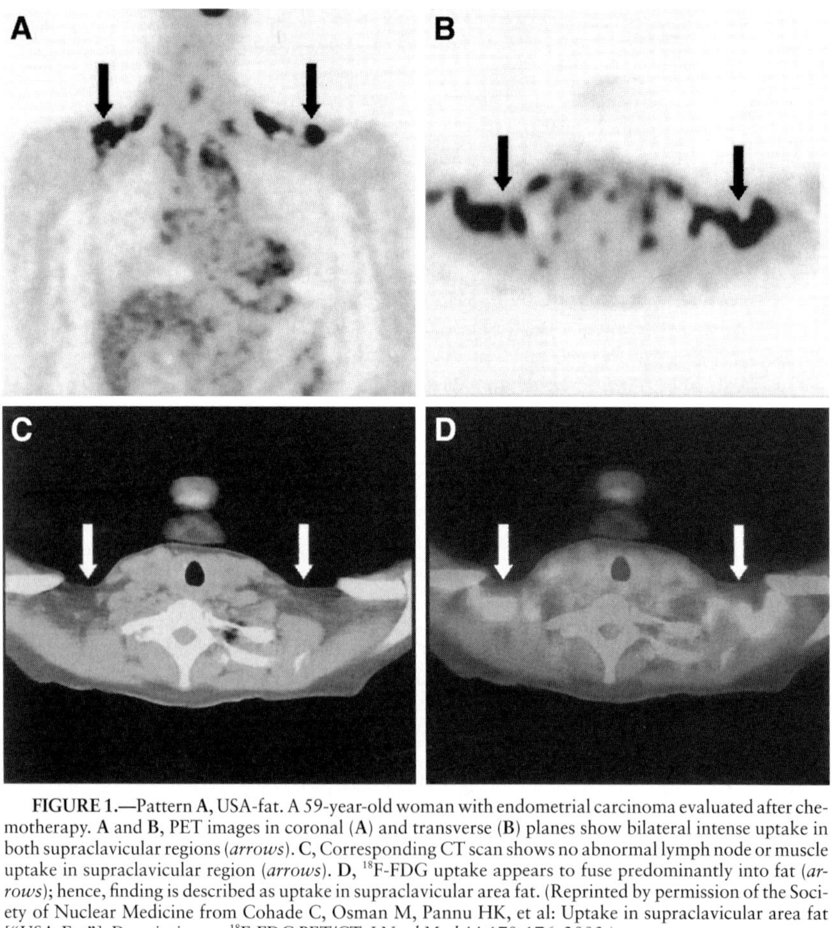

FIGURE 1.—Pattern A, USA-fat. A 59-year-old woman with endometrial carcinoma evaluated after chemotherapy. **A** and **B**, PET images in coronal (**A**) and transverse (**B**) planes show bilateral intense uptake in both supraclavicular regions (*arrows*). C, Corresponding CT scan shows no abnormal lymph node or muscle uptake in supraclavicular region (*arrows*). **D**, ^{18}F-FDG uptake appears to fuse predominantly into fat (*arrows*); hence, finding is described as uptake in supraclavicular area fat. (Reprinted by permission of the Society of Nuclear Medicine from Cohade C, Osman M, Pannu HK, et al: Uptake in supraclavicular area fat ["USA-Fat"]: Description on ^{18}F-FDG PET/CT. *J Nucl Med* 44:170-176, 2003.)

on CT, and pattern C showed uptake localizing to lymph nodes or soft tissue masses on CT.

Results.—Abnormal uptake of ^{18}F-FDG in the supraclavicular region was observed in 49 patients, including 20 patients with muscle uptake (group B) and 15 patients with definite abnormal lymph nodes (group C). However, 14 patients had USA-fat (group A) and foci of very low Hounsfield units observed on CT (Fig 1). These foci were also noted on 68Ge attenuation-corrected images and on nonattenuated-correction images. On PET/CT, uptake in USA-fat manifest typically as bilateral and symmetric, intense, more often multifocal rather than linear, and located in fat. There were no significant differences in age for the 3 groups. Patterns A and C could not be differentiated in terms of intensity; mean standardized uptake value, lean; or maximum standardized uptake value, lean. However, standardized uptake values were significantly lower in group B (muscle uptake) than in the other 2 groups.

Conclusion.—Muscle uptake of ^{18}F-FDG in the supraclavicular region on PET/CT scanning may be caused in most cases by an unrelated process called the USA-fat finding. This finding is probably a reflection of an underlying nonpathologic process that is thought to be in foci of brown fat. This intense supraclavicular uptake should not be misinterpreted as a malignant metastatic process or as muscle uptake.

▶ The uptake seen in the supraclavicular region of some patients undergoing FDG-PET imaging is puzzling. These authors and others have nicely shown that some of the uptake is in fat. This metabolically active fat has been related to the brown fat of hibernation. Some investigators have suggested that it is more common in patients who are cold and shivering at the time of injection.

I have seen this uptake in several patients, and I do not know what the etiology is. My impression is that it is most commonly seen in relatively young women. When scans are repeated several weeks to several months after the initial scan, this supraclavicular area uptake is generally not seen. It may also be seen in combination with symmetrical uptake in the paraspinal region of the thoracic spine. In addition, 2 small focal areas in the posterior cervical region may be seen in many patients. It is important to recognize this abnormal accumulation as a variant that is seen in approximately 2% of the patients.

R. E. Coleman, MD

Accuracy of Image Fusion of Normal Upper Abdominal Organs Visualized With PET/CT

Nakamoto Y, Tatsumi M, Cohade C, et al (Johns Hopkins Univ, Baltimore, Md)
Eur J Nucl Med Mol Imaging 30:597-602, 2003 7–2

Background.—Images obtained by CT scanning require patients to hold their breath or are done quickly to essentially freeze respiratory status. In contrast, PET with the use of FDG are acquired during free breathing over several minutes. The development of PET–CT scanners has allowed for si-

FIGURE 4

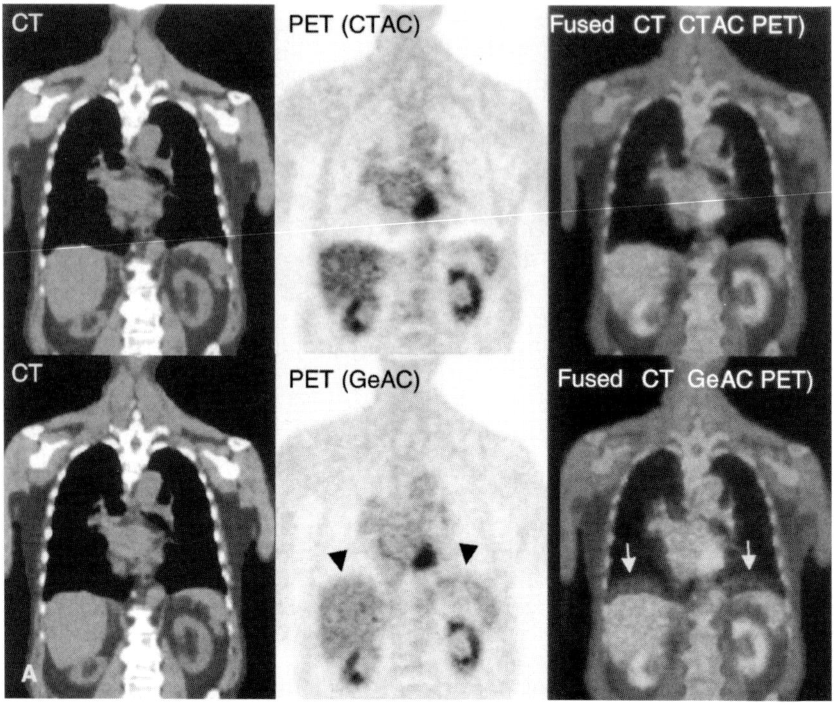

(*Continued*)

multaneous assessment of anatomical and metabolic information. Some PET–CT fusion images have misregistrations in the upper abdomen between PET and CT as a result of respiratory motion, but few data explain the effect of respiratory motion on PET–CT fusion images of the abdominal region. An evaluation of the consistency in measured size and location of FDG-avid upper abdominal organs on both CT and PET was performed with the use of an integrated dedicated PET–CT system.

Methods.—The 46 consecutive inpatients had clinical PET–CT scans indicated by suspected cancer. The CT and PET images attenuation-corrected by both CT (CTAC) and germanium-68 transmission (GeAC) were obtained. When the CT and both sets of PET images were used, the top and bottom, anterior and posterior margins, and right and left margins of each abdominal organ (ie, liver, spleen, and bilateral kidneys) were determined, and differences were assessed.

Results.—Regardless of direction, about 80% of the cases had a difference in the marginal points of less than 10 mm. However, the upper margin of the liver and the lower splenic margin had more than 10-mm differences in more than 30% of cases. On PET compared with CT, the center of the liver

FIGURE 4 (cont.)

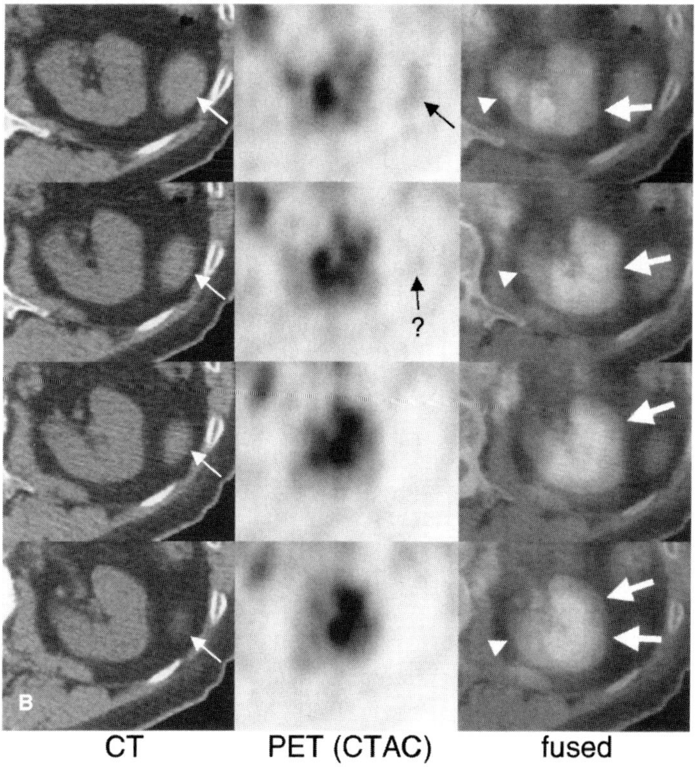

FIGURE 4.—A and B, Representative cases of mismatch of the upper margins of the liver and spleen (A), and the lower margin of the spleen and lateral margin of the left kidney (B). The upper margins of the liver and spleen are seen cranially on the GeAC PET (*A*, *arrowheads*). In the fused image of GeAC PET with CT, severe mismatch of the upper margins of the liver is seen (*A*, *white arrows*), while mismatch between CT and CTAC PET is minimal. In another patient with no mismatch of the upper margin of the spleen, it is possible to trace the lower portion of the spleen in all CT slices (*B*, *white small arrows*), but only the top slice depicts the spleen on CTAC PET (*B*, *black arrow*). In addition, there is mismatch of the lateral margin of the left kidney (*B*, *large white arrows*), whereas good localization in the medial margin was observed (*arrowheads*). *Abbreviations: GeAC*, ^{68}Ge transmission scan-based attenuation correction; *CTAC*, CT-based attenuation correction. (Courtesy of Nakamoto Y, Tatsumi M, Cohade C, et al: Accuracy of image fusion of normal upper abdominal organs visualized with PET/CT. *Eur J Nucl Med Mol Imaging* 30:597-602, 2003.)

tended to be cephalad and to the right, whereas the spleen tended to be cephalad and posterior; in addition, on PET, the center of both kidneys was more often cephalad, posterior, and to the right than on CT. PET values for the size of the organs tended to be slightly larger than CT values; however, the spleen height was slightly underestimated on PET. Kidney thickness was slightly overestimated by PET (Fig 4).

Conclusions.—The differences between PET and CT images in measuring and locating organs in the abdomen were modest but significant. The probable causes include respiratory motion, visualized shape of the organ, and a nonuniform normal interorgan FDG distribution pattern. Differences were slightly greater at the upper liver margin and the lower splenic margin.

▶ Fusion of the PET and CT images on the combined PET–CT system is assumed to be quite accurate. This study documents minor registrations due to physiologic motion. However, the potential for a mismatch must always be kept in mind.

R. E. Coleman, MD

▶ This article has taken an interesting new view on how to assess whether two fused images are indeed looking at the same object. The investigators assess measured sizes of abdominal organs to see whether CT and PET yield similar results. This is an interesting, innovative method for checking superposition accuracy, and admittedly is probably clinically more relevant than looking at fiducial point markers.

I. G. Zubal, PhD

Benefit of Anatomical-Functional Image Fusion in the Diagnostic Work-up of Neuroendocrine Neoplasms

Pfannenberg AC, Eschmann SM, Horger M, et al (Eberhard-Karls-Univ, Tübingen, Germany)

Eur J Nucl Med Mol Imaging 30:835-843, 2003 7–3

Background.—Neuroendocrine tumors (NETs) are rare neoplasms that present as extremely heterogeneous entities. NETs differ in histology, hormone production, and biological and clinical behavior. The majority of these tumors (70%) originate from the pancreas and gut and account for about 2% of all malignant gastrointestinal neoplasms. Symptoms are caused mainly by tumor growth, which indicates an advanced stage of disease. There has been a change in the treatment of NETs over the past decade, with a more aggressive approach to surgery, medical treatment with somatostatin analogues and interferon, and the introduction of tumor-targeted therapy with radiolabeled peptides. Somatostatin receptor scintigraphy (SRS) has become the primary imaging modality for localization of either primary or metastatic NETs. However, SRS does present shortcomings in terms of providing precise anatomical localization of lesions. The use of anatomical-functional image fusion with combined transmission and emission tomography (SPET/CT) in patients with NETs was evaluated.

Methods.—The study group comprised 54 patients with known or suspected NETs who prospectively underwent both tumor scintigraphy with ^{111}In-octreotide (43 patients) or ^{123}I-MIBG (11 patients) and contrast-enhanced high-end spiral CT. Analysis of fused images (SPET/CT) was done on a lesion-by-lesion basis, followed by re-evaluation of SPET and high-end CT by consensus. The reference standard for confirming the presence or absence of malignancy was either histopathologic or clinical evaluation and imaging and follow-up data.

Results.—A total of 120 lesions were identified by CT, scintigraphy, or both, including 4 patients with negative SPET but 8 liver lesions on CT that were determined to be metastases. Six patients were excluded from the final analysis because there was no evidence of tumor, there was a lack of comparison with the reference standard, or the patients were lost to follow-up. In 56 of the 114 evaluated lesions (49%), the results of SPET and CT were concordant, and all of the lesions were interpreted as malignant. In 58 of the 114 lesions (51%), consensus reading of fused images changed the image interpretation of 39 CT scans and 19 SPET studies. The highest accuracy (99%) in classification of NET lesions was obtained with combined analysis of SPET/CT and high-end CT. Therapy was altered in 14 of 50 patients (28%) on the basis of the results of image fusion, including 3 patients who were spared unnecessary surgery because of additional lesions indicating systemic tumor spread.

Conclusions.—The indication from these results is that combined anatomical-functional imaging with SPET/CT and additional visual correlation to high-end CT has a high degree of diagnostic accuracy and provides significantly improved tumor localization and characterization in patients with neuroendocrine tumors.

► More studies are now being performed and reported with the combined SPECT/CT systems. The CT scanner on the combined SPECT/CT device is a low-resolution instrument, but it does provide anatomic information for correlation with the SPECT images. We are going to see more studies demonstrating the value of having a CT scanner on the SPECT device.

R. E. Coleman, MD

Thymic Enlargement and FDG Uptake in Three Patients: CT and FDG Positron Emission Tomography Correlated With Pathology

Wittram C, Fischman AJ, Mark E, et al (Harvard Univ, Boston; New York Univ)

AJR 180:519-522, 2003 7–4

Background.—FDG PET has an important role in the imaging of oncology patients, as in the staging of mediastinal disease from non–small-cell lung cancer (NSCLC). After treatment for NSCLC, a positive finding on FDG PET is a poor prognostic indicator. It has been suggested that the thymus normally takes up FDG in children and adults. However, this has not previously been confirmed pathologically. The results from CT, FDG PET, and pathologic findings in 3 patients were retrospectively reviewed.

Methods.—The review included data from three women, 20 to 44 years old (average, 35 years) who had confirmed normal thymic tissue and available FDG PET and CT scans. All of the patients were asymptomatic with respect to the chest. A mediastinal abnormality was identified on a chest radiograph and confirmed on CT in 1 patient and on staging chest CT in 2 patients. FDG PET images were obtained 5 to 21 days after the CT scans. The CT and FDG PET images were assessed by 2 chest radiologists and a nuclear medicine physician. The longest and shortest perpendicular CT measurements were recorded. Thymic thickness was measured perpendicular to the length of the lobe. The standardized uptake value (SUV) was calculated for each patient using a region of interest that included the highest activity area of the thymus not covering the entire thymus.

Results.—CT in all patients showed a soft-tissue density in the location of the thymus (Fig 1). All of the FDG PET scans depicted increased uptake of FDG in the anterior mediastinum corresponding to the anterior mediastinal

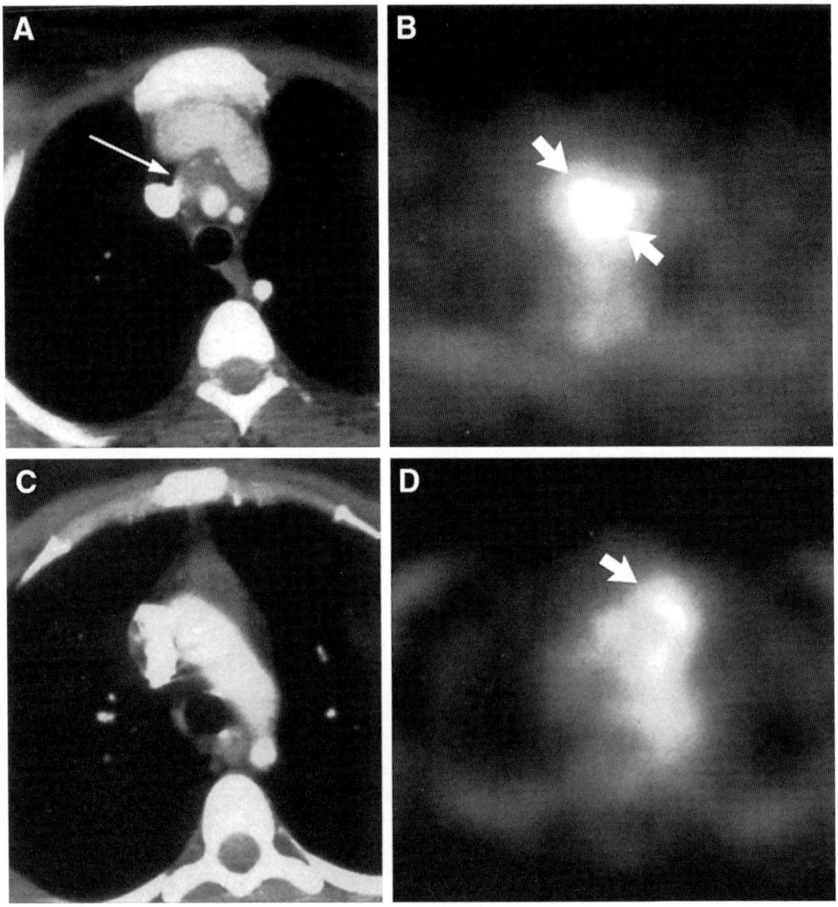

FIGURE 1.—Thymic enlargement in 29-year-old woman. **A**, Contrast-enhanced CT scan of thorax obtained at level of left brachiocephalic vein shows soft tissue (*arrow*) among left brachiocephalic vein anteriorly, superior vena cava laterally, and right brachiocephalic artery and left common carotid artery posteriorly. **B**, Axial FDG positron emission tomography (PET) scan obtained at same level as **A** shows increase in uptake of FDG in soft tissue (*arrows*) compared with mediastinum. **C**, Contrast-enhanced CT scan obtained at level of aortic arch shows thickness of thymus to be 1.5 cm. Note convex lateral margin. **D**, Axial FDG PET scan obtained at same level as **C** shows increase in uptake of FDG in thymus (*arrow*). (Courtesy of Wittram C, Fishman AJ, Mark E, et al: Thymic enlargement and FDG uptake in three patients: CT and FDG positron emission tomography correlated with pathology, *AJR* 180:519-522, 2003. Reprinted with permission from the *American Journal of Roentgenology*.)

soft-tissue opacity seen on CT. The SUVs ranged from 1.1 to 2.2, with an average of 1.8. Histologic examination in all 3 patients found no evidence of malignancy.

Conclusions.—This study found a physiologic uptake of FDG by the thymus in 3 patients with confirmed normal thymic tissue. Standardized uptake values were in the range of thymic neoplasm.

► We frequently see normal thymic uptake in children. Occasionally, we see it in adults. It should not be confused with thymic neoplasia or accumulation in lymphadenopathy.

R. E. Coleman, MD

Prospective Use of Serial Questionnaires to Evaluate the Therapeutic Efficacy of ^{18}F-Fluorodeoxyglucose (FDG) Positron Emission Tomography (PET) in Suspected Lung Cancer

Herder GJ, van Tinteren H, Comans EF, et al (VU Univ, Amsterdam; Comprehensive Cancer Ctr, Amsterdam)

Thorax 58:47-51, 2003 7–5

Background.—PET with FDG is considered an accuracte technique for imaging lung cancer. The effect of FDG PET on the diagnosis and management of clinically problematic patients with suspected non–small-cell lung cancer was reported.

Methods.—One hundred sixty-four patients referred for PET between August 1997 and July 1999 were included in the prospective study. PET was used only for patients in whom noninvasive tests had not identified the source of clinical signs and symptoms. Questionnaires were used to determine the imapct of PET on diagnosis and management. Diagnostic problems were related to unclear radiologic findings in 112 patients, mediastinal staging in 36, and distant staging in 16. Findings on PET were verified by chart review.

Findings.—PET positively affected diagnostic understanding in 84% of the cases. In 26%, diagnostic understanding was improved by PET alone. Referring physicians reported that PET findings prompted management changes in half the patients. The most common change in management after PET was canceled surgery, occurring in 35% of the cases.

Conclusion.—As an adjunct modality, FDG PET is clinically useful for patients with problematic clinical findings. Treatment choice was directly affected in 25% of the patients in this series. Further research is needed to assess the value of the increased confidence associated with PET scanning.

► Several studies have documented the impact of FDG PET on patient management. This study reports a beneficial change of treatment in 50%, with canceled surgery occurring in 35% of the patients. These results are major findings.

R. E. Coleman, MD

Improved Radiologic Staging of Lung Cancer With 2-[^{18}F]-Fluoro-2-Deoxy-D-Glucose–Positron Emission Tomography and Computed Tomography Registration

Aquino SL, Asmuth JC, Alpert NM, et al (Massachusetts Gen Hosp, Boston; Sarnoff Corp, Princeton, NJ)

J Comput Assist Tomogr 27:479-484, 2003 7–6

Purpose.—As new techniques of dual PET-CT scanning are developed, there is a need to document the true effects of image registration on accuracy in cancer detection and staging. An accurate approach to fusion of the 2 datasets and alignment of the anatomic structures should aid radiologic interpretations for cancer staging. A volumetric, nonlinear approach to registration of CT and FDG-PET datasets was evaluated for its effects on detection of nodal disease and on clinical staging of patients with lung cancer.

Methods.—The analysis included 45 patients undergoing sequential CT and FDG-PET for preoperative clinical staging of non–small-cell lung cancer. All underwent subsequent surgical staging with mediastinoscopy, thoracotomy, or both. An automated, volumetric registration algorithm was used to perform registration of the CT and PET datasets. The CT dataset alone, CT and PET side by side, and the CT-PET registration datasets were independently read for the presence of lymph node metastases. The clinical staging results were compared with the findings on surgical staging.

Results.—In each dataset, a total of 130 mediastinal and hilar lymph nodes were analyzed. Sensitivity in the detection of nodal involvement was 74% for CT, 59% to 76% for PET with CT side by side, and 71% to 76% for CT-PET registration. Specificity was 78% for CT, 77% to 89% for PET with CT, and 89% to 96% with CT-PET registration. Positive predictive values were 55%, 48% to 68%, and 70% to 86%, respectively; negative predictive values were 88%, 84% to 91%, and 90% to 91%, respectively.

One independent reader found the registration images more sensitive than PET alone; both readers found CT-PET more specific then PET in detecting the absence of mediastinal lymph node involvement. Both readers found that CT-PET led to improved accuracy, compared with PET.

Conclusions.—In patients undergoing clinical staging for lung cancer, the study technique of registration of CT and FDG-PET datasets is associated with significantly increased specificity for metastatic lymph node involvement. This improvement appears to result from the ability to detect uptake in anatomic structures that, on PET alone, are read as malignant nodes. The registration technique improves radiologic staging, compared with either imaging modality on its own.

► Now that PET-CT systems are available, image registration will be less of an issue. This study using computer-based image registration demonstrates that the registration improved the specificity of detecting metastatic disease. The combined PET-CT scanners will provide better registration, and the initial studies demonstrate that the combined studies are better than either study by itself.

R. E. Coleman, MD

Positron Emission Tomography Scanning With 2-Fluoro-2-Deoxy-D-Glucose as a Predictor of Response of Neoadjuvant Treatment for Non–Small Cell Carcinoma

Cerfolio RJ, Ojha B, Mukherjee S, et al (Univ of Alabama, Birmingham)

J Thorac Cardiovasc Surg 125:938-944, 2003 7–7

Background.—Among patients with non–small cell lung cancer (NSCLC), surgical resection after chemotherapy may be the best strategy only for responders. The abilities of 2-fluoro-2-deoxy-D-glucose positron emission tomography (FDG-PET) and CT to predict this response for the primary tumor and N1 and N2 lymph nodes were determined.

Methods.—Thirty-four patients with NSCLC were prospectively studied. All had had initial FDG-PET scan staging with tissue biopsy, neoadjuvant chemotherapy, repeat FDG-PET scanning, and repeat biopsies.

Findings.—Eleven patients had N2 disease and 7 had N1 disease. Chemotherapy was administered to 27 patients. Seven received chemotherapy plus radiation therapy. Resection was performed in all but 9 patients. In a statistical analysis, FDG-PET scanning was more specific than CT for predicting residual tumor at the primary site. The former also had higher positive and negative predictive values. For paratracheal nodes, FDG-PET scanning was more sensitive and accurate, with greater positive and negative predictive values than CT. In addition, FDG-PET scanning had a greater positive predictive value than CT scanning for the other N2 lymph nodes.

Conclusions.—In patients with NSCLC receiving preoperative chemotherapy, repeat FDG-PET scanning is more specific and has greater positive and negative predictive values than CT scanning. The former is also more sensitive and accurate for paratracheal N2 nodes, though the 2 modalities do not differ significantly in detecting N1 lymph nodes.

► More patients are undergoing preoperative chemotherapy, radiation therapy, or both. If N2 disease after neoadjuvant therapy persists, surgical resection offers little advantage. This study documents that PET is more accurate than CT for evaluating the effects of neoadjuvant therapy.

R. E. Coleman, MD

► Clearly, the next major PET application will be to monitor therapy. Although this article has several flaws, it gives a glimpse at possible future applications of PET scanning in the lung.

H. D. Royal, MD

Prognostic Value of [18F]FDG-PET Imaging in Small Cell Lung Cancer

Pandit N, Gonen M, Krug L, et al (Mem Sloan-Kettering Cancer Ctr, New York)
Eur J Nucl Med 30:78-84, 2003 7–8

Background.—Small cell lung cancer (SCLC) accounts for about 20% of lung cancers. SCLC is clinically aggressive, and the survival rate is poor. The average 2-year survival for SCLC is less than 10%. The staging of SCLC affects survival and treatment decisions. Chest radiography, CT scanning, MRI, thoracoscopy, bone scans, and bone marrow biopsy are routinely used for staging of SCLC. PET FDG has been used in the evaluation of non–small-

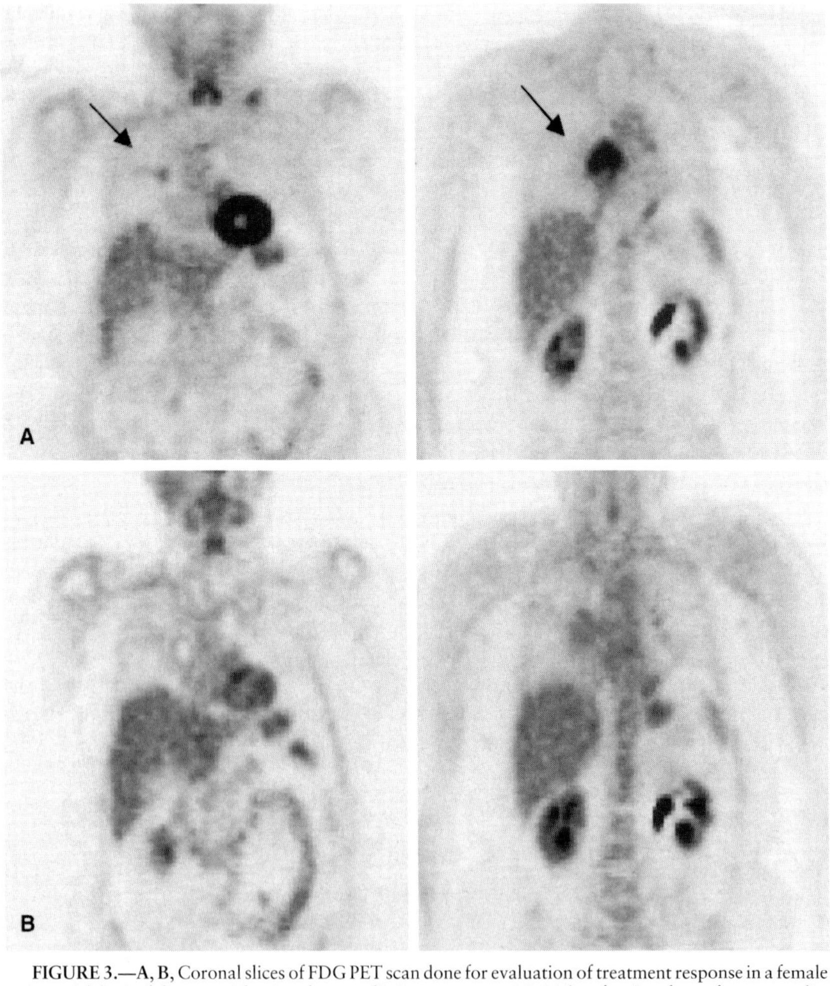

FIGURE 3.—**A, B,** Coronal slices of FDG PET scan done for evaluation of treatment response in a female patient with limited disease, with prior chemoradiation treatment. **A** Initial evaluation showed recurrent disease in the right lung and hilar regions. **B** Post-chemotherapy scan shows a good response with resolution or previously seen lesions. (Courtesy of Pandit N, Gonen M, Krug L, Larson SM: Prognostic value of [18F]FDG-PET imaging in small cell lung cancer. *Eur J Nucl Med* 30:78-84, 2003. Copyright 2003, Springer-Verlag.)

cell lung cancer (NSCLC), and the use of FDG PET has recently been reported in the staging of SCLC. However, the prognostic value of FDG PET imaging for SCLC has not previously been studied. The hypothesis that PET-positive SCLC patients would have a less favorable prognosis than PET-negative patients and that a high standardized uptake value (SUV) would be associated with a poor prognosis was investigated retrospectively.

Methods.—This review included a mixed population of treated and untreated patients' images from 1995 to 2000. Data involving 62 scans from 46 patients (8 untreated and 38 treated patients) were reviewed. Results were correlated with pathologic analyses, CT/MRI findings, and clinical data.

Results.—PET scanning had a sensitivity of 100% with pathologic correlation. Overall survival rate in PET-positive cases was significantly worse than that in PET-negative cases (Fig 3). Correlation of SUV_{max} with survival indicated a significant negative correlation. In the 8 untreated patients, scans were strongly positive; in all of these patients, the scan results were in agreement with the final clinical stage assigned on the basis of conventional methods.

Conclusions.—FDG PET imaging provides prognostic information in treated patients. A positive FDG-PET study and a high SUV_{max} are significantly associated with poor survival. These findings also suggest that FDG PET may aid in staging and follow-up of patients with SCLC.

► Most of the literature on the use of PET in lung cancer has been in non-SCLC. Those of us who have been using PET in SCLC have noted that the uptake in SCLC is at least as great as in non-SCLC. However, there have been very few studies reported in the literature on the use of PET in SCLC. This retrospective study demonstrates the prognostic value of a positive PET scan. Both the subjective interpretation and the SUV were predictive of survival.

R. E. Coleman, MD

Somatostatin Receptor Scintigraphy for Bronchial Carcinoid Follow-up

Fanti S, Farsad M, Battista G, et al (Università degli Studi, Bologna, Italy; Istituto Tumori, Milano, Italy; Istituto Humanitas, Milano, Italy)

Clin Nucl Med 28:548-552, 2003 7–9

Background.—Bronchial carcinoid (BC) accounts for fewer than 5% of all lung tumors and approximately 10% of all carcinoid tumors. BC was once thought to be benign, but it is now recognized as a low-grade, slow-growing neoplasm with the potential for both local invasion and distant metastatic involvement. The age of patients at presentation varies widely, from teenage to elderly, and there is a slight female predominance. There has been no evidence of a relationship between BC and smoking, environmental inhalants, carcinogens, or radiation. The 2 forms of BC are typical and atypical, with typical BC accounting for about 90% of all cases. Typical BC is well differentiated with rare mitoses, pleomorphism, and necrosis. Atypical BC is characterized histologically by increased mitotic activity, nuclear pleomorphism, and disorganization. These more aggressive atypical lesions have a poor prognosis. Somatostatin receptor scintigraphy (SRS) has been used to diagnose BC and is a valuable tool in the accurate staging of lesions. The role of SRS in restaging BC and following up patients after treatment was evaluated.

Methods.—The study group included 31 patients (18 male, 13 female) with confirmed BC who were referred over a period of 7 years. Patients were

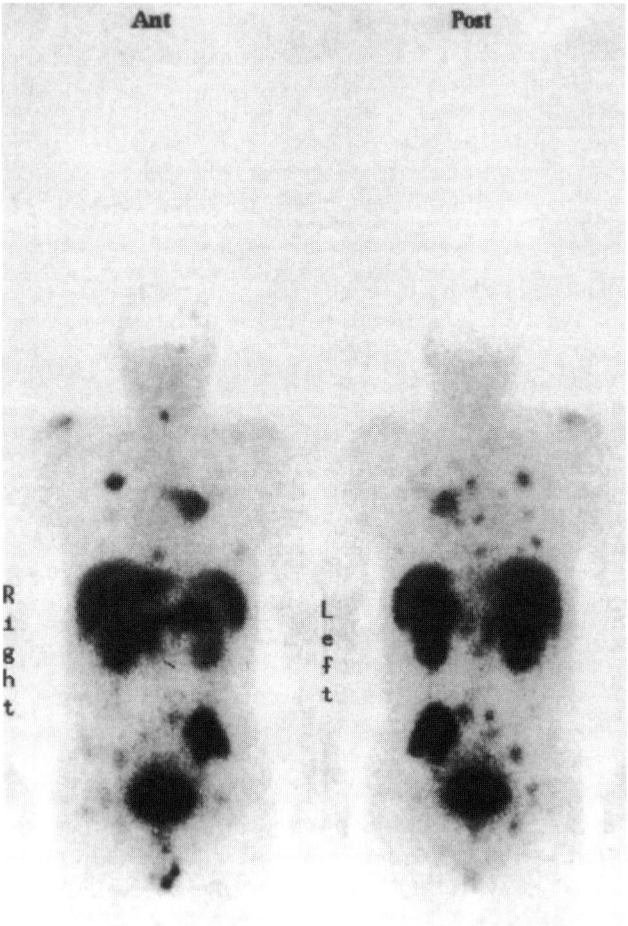

FIGURE 1.—A 58-year-old man was operated on 3 years earlier for BC. CT showed local relapse at the left pulmonary hilum, with several parenchymal nodules. A bone scan with Tc-99m MDP showed several lesions at the ribs, right humerus, left proximal femur, skull, and ilium. SRS revealed several sites of increased uptake in different organs, including the lung and bones, corresponding to previously demonstrated lesions. (Courtesy of Fanti S, Farsad M, Battisti G, et al: Somatostatin receptor scintigraphy for bronchial carcinoid follow-up. *Clin Nucl Med* 28(7):548-552, 2003.)

examined by means of chest radiography (12 studies), chest or abdominal CT (28 scans), chest MRI (2 scans), and liver US (5 scans).

Results.—SRS confirmed the data obtained by other diagnostic procedures in 22 patients (71%) (Fig 1). In 6 patients, SRS showed focal lesions not previously demonstrated. SRS resolved uncertain findings of CT in 2 patients. In 1 patient, SRS showed fewer lesions than did CT. In 8 of 31 patients, important diagnostic information obtained by SRS was not revealed by any of the other imaging procedures.

Conclusions.—These findings show that SRS is a reliable noninvasive method and should be considered as the primary follow-up procedure in patients with BC.

► PET imaging using FDG and planar imaging using MIBG are not very accurate for the detection of bronchial carcinoid tumors. These data suggest that SRS is the appropriate imaging agent for detecting recurrent or metastatic bronchial carcinoid tumors.

R. E. Coleman, MD

Impact of Positron Emission Tomography on the Initial Staging and Therapy in Locoregional Advanced Squamous Cell Carcinoma of the Head and Neck

Schmid DT, Stoeckli SJ, Bandhauer F, et al (Univ Hosp Zurich, Switzerland)

Laryngoscope 113:888-891, 2003 7–10

Background.—Mucosal head and neck squamous cell carcinoma (HNSCC) demonstrates avid uptake of ^{18}FDG on PET. FDG-PET cannot assess the dimensions of a primary tumor because of the lack of anatomic correlation. However, FDG-PET is capable of detecting cervical lymph node and distant metastases or synchronous second primaries with a higher sensitivity and specificity than structural imaging modalities and physical examination. The effects of FDG-PET on staging and radiation treatment planning after a standard diagnostic workup in patients with advanced HNSCC were assessed.

Methods.—This prospective, controlled study enrolled 48 patients (42 men and 6 women) with a mean age of 61 years (range, 35-85 years) who had histologically confirmed, advanced-stage mucosal HNSCC. All the patients underwent FDG-PET after a routine workup that included physical examination, panendoscopy, chest radiographs, and contrast-enhanced, high-resolution helical CT scan (HRCT). Findings of FDG-PET and the initial staging and therapy based on routine workup were compared. End points were the extent of lymph node disease, distant metastases, and second primary tumors.

Results.—The lymph node findings between HRCT and PET were concordant in 41 (85%) of 48 patients. In 3 patients, PET findings caused an upstaging of the tumor in its N category, and in 4 patients PET underestimated the extent of lymph node involvement. PET showed more difficulties in delineating lymph node metastases adjacent to the primary tumor than did HRCT, but PET was superior for the detection of distant and contralateral lymph node metastases. PET suggested distant metastatic lesions in 6 (13%) of 48 patients. Cytologic workup confirmed distant metastases in 2 (4%) of these patients and second primary tumors in 2 patients (4%). PET findings were false-positive in 2 patients (4%) as a result of inflammatory changes.

Conclusions.—Whole-body PET has the capacity for assessment of lymph node involvement, distant metastases, and second primary tumors in a single study in patients with advanced mucosal HNSCC. PET evaluation results in a change of treatment in about 8% of these patients.

► Previous studies have suggested that there is not much difference in the accuracy of PET and CT in the initial staging of patients with head and neck cancer. The advantage of PET for this indication is the ability to detect distant metastatic disease. Two patients with distant metastases were identified, and additional primary tumors in 2 other patients. Overall, PET scan results led to a change in management in 8% of the patients. Compared with the results of PET scanning in other malignancies, this is a small percentage change in management.

R. E. Coleman, MD

FDG-PET for Prediction of Tumour Aggressiveness and Response to Intra-Arterial Chemotherapy and Radiotherapy in Head and Neck Cancer

Kitagawa Y, Sano K, Nishizawa S, et al (Fukui Med Univ, Matsuoka, Japan)

Eur J Nucl Med 30:63-71, 2003 7–11

Background.—Squamous cell carcinoma (SCC) of the head and neck is a histologically distinct, clinically heterogeneous entity that includes multiple anatomical sites with different natural history and clinical behavior. This diversity makes it difficult to accurately predict the efficacy of treatments and the prognosis of patients using conventional clinicopathologic criteria. FDG PET has been used in clinical oncology for the detection and staging of various kinds of malignancies. Previous studies have demonstrated the clinical value of FDG PET in head and neck SCCs for monitoring response to neoadjuvant intra-arterial chemotherapy with concomitant radiotherapy. The potential utility of FDG PET in predicting tumor aggressiveness and response to intra-arterial chemotherapy and radiotherapy in head and neck carcinoma was investigated.

Methods.—The study included 20 patients with SCC of the head an neck. All the patients completed the treatment regimen, and each patient underwent an FDG PET study before and 4 weeks after chemoradiotherapy. Standardized uptake values (SUVs) with an uptake period of 50 minutes were used for quantitative evaluation of regional FDG uptake in the tumor. The pretreatment and posttreatment SUVs were compared with immunohistologically evaluated tumor proliferative potential (MIB-1 and PCNA), tumor cellularity, and other parameters including histologic grade, tumor size and stage, clinical response, and histologic evaluation after therapy.

Results.—All of the neoplastic lesions showed high SUVs (mean, 9.75 mg/mL) before treatment, and these levels decreased significantly after therapy (mean, 2.41 mg/mL). Pretreatment SUV did not correlate with MIB-1, PCNA, cellularity, or other parameters. However, lower posttherapy SUV was significantly correlated with good histologic results after therapy. Compared with moderately differentiated SCCs, well-differentiated SCCs showed significantly lower posttreatment SUV and a larger difference between pretreatment and posttreatment SUVs. Lesions with a high pretreatment SUV exhibited residual tumor cells after treatment in 4 of 15 patients, whereas patients with lesions that manifested a low pretreatment SUV were successfully treated. Four of six tumors with a posttreatment SUV greater than 4 mg/mL had viable tumor cells, while all tumors (14 of 14) with a posttreatment SUV less than 4 mg/mL showed no viable tumor cells. Computational multivariate analysis with multiple regression showed that MIB-1 labeling index, cellularity, the number of MIB-1 labeled tumor cells, and tumor size grade are statistically significant factors contributing to the difference between pretreatment SUV and posttreatment SUV in each patient.

Conclusions.—Pretreatment FDG PET is useful for the prediction of response to treatment, and posttreatment FDG PET is useful in predicting residual viable tumors in patients with squamous cell carcinoma of the head and neck.

► FDG-PET imaging is being used increasingly for the evaluation of the effect of therapy. The data for demonstrating the impact of PET imaging in oncology has been primarily in breast cancer and lymphoma. These investigators now demonstrate that FDG PET is useful in predicting the response to treatment in head and neck cancer. Furthermore, the posttreatment PET is of value in predicting the presence or absence of residual tumor.

R. E. Coleman, MD

Diagnostic and Prognostic Value of [¹⁸F]Fluorodeoxyglucose Positron Emission Tomography for Recurrent Head and Neck Squamous Cell Carcinoma

Wong RJ, Lin DT, Schöder H, et al (Mem Sloan-Kettering Cancer Ctr, New York)

J Clin Oncol 20:4199-4208, 2002 7–12

Background.—The diagnosis and treatment of patients with recurrent head and neck squamous cell carcinoma (HNSCC) are challenging. Treatment of HNSCC, which is the eighth most common malignancy in the United States, often requires a multimodality approach that includes combinations of surgery, radiation, and chemotherapy. This treatment frequently causes significant edema or fibrosis of normal tissues, which may obscure the early detection of recurrent disease and make subsequent salvage treatment

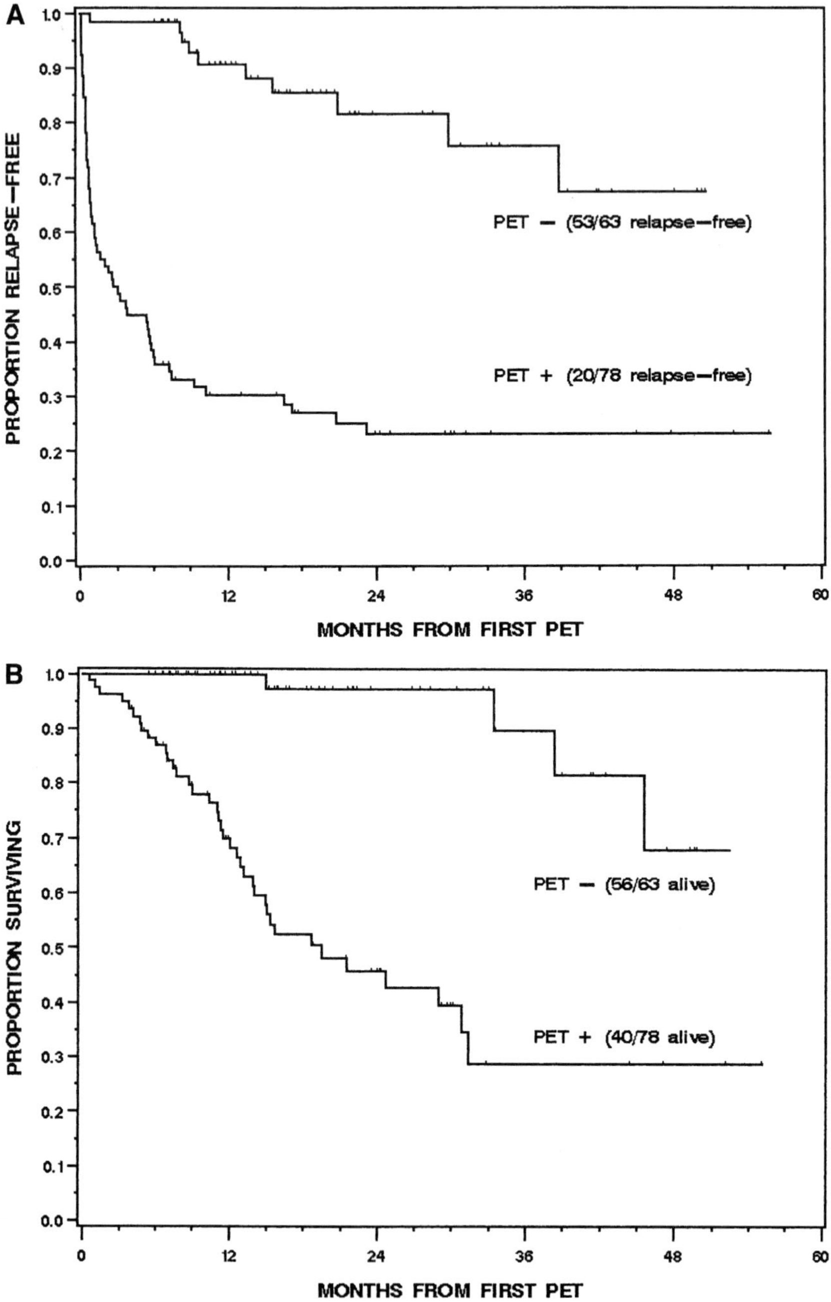

FIGURE 3.—Kaplan-Meier relapse-free survival and overall survival probabilities for PET-negative and PET-positive patients. (Courtesy of Wong RJ, Lin DT, Schöder H, et al: Diagnostic and prognostic value of [^{18}F] Fluorodeoxyglucose positron emission tomography for recurrent head and neck squamous cell carcinoma. *J Clin Oncol* 20(20):4199-4208, 2002. Reprinted by permission from the American Society of Clinical Oncology.)

more difficult. The diagnostic accuracy and prognostic value of FDG PET for patients with HNSCC were investigated.

Methods.—A retrospective review was conducted of 143 patients with previously treated HNSCC who underwent 181 PET scans from 1996 to 2001 for detection of recurrent disease. Disease recurrence within 6 months was the criterion for assessing the true disease status at PET.

Results.—Equivocal sites were considered positive, a specification that yielded an overall sensitivity of 96% and a specificity of 72% for the detection of recurrence by PET. PET was highly sensitive and specific at regional and distant sites, while at local sites, the sensitivity was high but the specificity was low because of false-positive findings. Twenty percent of all false-positive PET scans occurred at sites of known inflammation or infection. The mean area under the curve for a receiver operator characteristic (ROC) based on standardized uptake value (SUV) was 0.882. A time-dependent, multivariate proportional hazards model identified PET interpretation, SUV, and physical examination as independent predictors of relapse-free survival and overall survival (Fig 3). An increase in SUV by 1 unit increased the relative risk (RR) of relapse by 11% and the RR of death by 14%. A positive PET interpretation was associated with a 4-fold increase in the RR of relapse and a 7-fold increase in the RR of death.

Conclusions.—PET is a highly sensitive method for the detection of recurrent HNSCC. PET provided important prognostic information for relapse-free and overall survival.

► The diagnostic and prognostic information from FDG-PET imaging has been demonstrated in several cancers. In this study, the authors demonstrate the high sensitivity of PET for detecting HNSCC. The specificity was also high at regional and distant sites. Both the qualitative interpretation and SUV evaluation demonstrated a significant impact on both relapse-free survival and overall survival.

R. E. Coleman, MD

Functioning Pulmonary Metastases of Thyroid Cancer: Does Radioiodine Influence the Prognosis?

Hindié E, Mellière D, Lange F, et al (Hôpital Saint-Antoine, Paris Cedex; Hôpital Henri Mondor, Créteil, France; Hôpital Saint-Louis, Paris; et al)

Eur J Nucl Med Mol Imaging 30:974-981, 2003 7–13

Purpose.—Functioning pulmonary metastases are a common and potentially fatal occurrence in patients with differentiated thyroid cancers. Iodine-131 has long been used to treat functioning pulmonary metastases, as well as for "preventive" ablation of residual thyroid tissue and in scanning for unsuspected metastases. However, there is continued debate over the benefits of ^{131}I for this group of patients. The prognostic impact of ^{131}I therapy for patients with functioning pulmonary metastases of thyroid cancer was evaluated.

Methods.—The retrospective study included 509 patients treated for thyroid cancer from 1970 through 1995, during which time a consistent approach to ^{131}I treatment was followed. Total thyroidectomy followed by ^{131}I ablation was used in 74% of patients. In 20 patients who developed functioning pulmonary metastases, regular ^{131}I therapy was continued as long as the patients had persistent ^{131}I uptake. Three patients required pulmonary resection, whereas 4 underwent local treatment for bone lesions. The patients were followed up through 2001, with an average 12.7-year follow-up in 17 surviving patients.

Findings.—In all but one of the patients with functioning pulmonary metastases, the lesions were detected on the immediate postoperative ^{131}I scan. When the pulmonary lesions were detected, findings on chest x-rays were negative in 11 patients; in 56%, serum thyroglobulin levels did not indicate the presence of metastases. Of the 11 radiographically negative patients, 1 died with recurrent cancer in the neck, and 2 continued to have pulmonary ^{131}I uptake. The remaining 8 patients were in continued apparent remission after ^{131}I therapy, receiving an average cumulative ^{131}I activity of 338 mCi. Of the 9 radiographically positive patients, 2 died, 5 were still receiving ^{131}I, and 2 were in remission; the average cumulative ^{131}I activity received in this group was 939 mCi. Ten-year survival was 84%.

Conclusions.—This experience shows good outcomes with ^{131}I therapy in patients with functioning pulmonary metastases of thyroid cancer. Even in the presence of advanced disease, long-term survival is possible with continued ^{131}I treatments. Patients with radiographically occult metastases detected on the postoperative ^{131}I scan have better outcomes than those whose lesions are visible on chest x-ray films.

▶ These are interesting data. Anyone treating patients with thyroid cancer should read this article in its entirety.

R. E. Coleman, MD

In-111 DTPA-Octreotide Scintigraphy for Disease Detection in Metastatic Thyroid Cancer: Comparison With F-18 FDG Positron Emission Tomography and Extensive Conventional Radiographic Imaging

Sarlis NJ, Gourgiotis L, Guthrie LC, et al (NIH, Bethesda, Md)
Clin Nucl Med 28:208-217, 2003 7–14

Background.—Authorities disagree on the value of ^{111}In-DTPA octreotide scintigraphy (SRS) for detecting metastatic thyroid carcinoma (TCA). The sensitivities of ^{111}In-based SRS, FDG PET, and extensive conventional radiographic imaging (CRI) in patients with this disease were compared.

Methods.—Twenty-one patients, aged a mean of 56.4 years, with aggressive TCA underwent SRS, FDG PET, and CRI. To obtain concordance rates between different pairs of techniques, the ratio of the number of lesions positive with both techniques was divided by the sum of the total number of le-

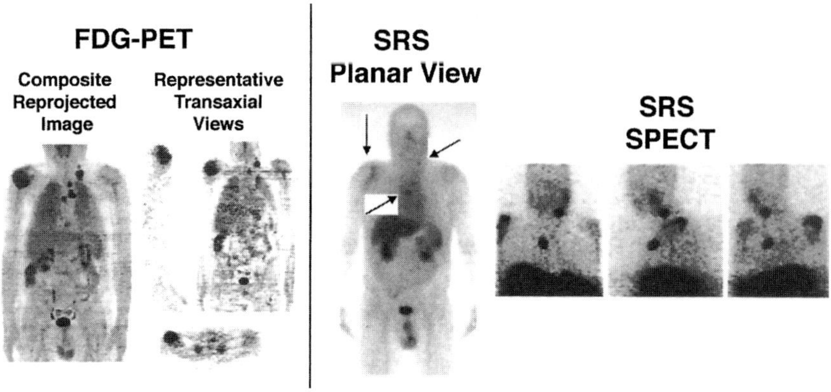

FIGURE 3.—Findings of FDG PET (**left-hand panels**) and ^{111}In-DTPA octreotide scintigraphy (*SRS*) (**right-hand panels**) in 1 patient. (Courtesy of Sarlis NJ, Gourgiotis L, Guthrie LC, et al: In-111 DTPA-octreotide scintigraphy for disease detection in metastatic thyroid cancer: Comparison with F-18 FDG positron emission tomography and extensive conventional radiographic imaging. *Clin Nucl Med* 28(3):208-217, 2003.)

sions positive with the first technique plus the total number of lesions positive with the second technique and multiplied by 200.

Findings.—The combined use of all 4 modalities detected 105 lesions presumed to be caused by metastatic deposits. The sensitivity of SRS was 49.5% and of FDG PET, 67.6%. Lesion detection concordance rates were 80.8% for CRI versus FDG PET; 74.2% for CRI versus SRS; and 58.6% for FDG PET versus SRS (Fig 3). Scintigraphy identified 5 unexpected lesions not detected by CRI or FDG PET. In 2 representative patients, there was a positive association between the percentage of lesional ^{111}In-DTPA octreotide uptake and the standard uptake value in 8 concordant lesions.

Conclusion.—In this series, SRS had only a moderate sensitivity for detecting metastatic TCA. However, SRS may reveal lesions that otherwise would not be detected by CRI or FDG PET.

► FDG PET was approved in April 2003 for coverage by Medicare for patients with previously well-differentiated TCA that is no longer I-131 avid and with elevation of thyroglobulin levels. This study documents the superiority of FDG PET over somatostatin receptor scintigraphy in the detection of metastatic lesions. However, somatostatin receptor scintigraphy may detect lesions not detectable on the FDG PET scan.

R. E. Coleman, MD

Whole Body ^{18}FDG-PET and the Response of Esophageal Cancer to Induction Therapy: Results of a Prospective Trial

Downey RJ, Akhurst T, Ilson D, et al (Mem Sloan-Kettering Cancer Ctr, New York; Singapore Gen Hosp; Toronto Gen Hosp)

J Clin Oncol 21:428-432, 2003 7–15

Introduction.—Combined modality regimens, especially chemoradiotherapy followed by surgery, are reported to increase median survival and 5-year survival rates in patients with esophageal cancer. Whole-body ^{18}FDG-PET imaging, performed before and after induction therapy, was prospectively evaluated for its ability to measure response to therapy in patients with esophageal cancer.

Methods.—Thirty-nine patients (34 men and 5 women) were enrolled in a single-institution clinical trial between April 1997 and April 1999. After conventional staging, all patients underwent PET imaging, then induction therapy, followed by repeat CT and PET imaging. The PET scans imaged patients from the orbito-meatal line to the pelvis. Seventeen patients underwent R_0 esophagectomy after induction therapy and were followed up either to recurrence, to death, or through a disease-free interval of at least 24 months.

Results.—The median age of the patients was 59 years; 26 had adenocarcinoma and 13 had squamous cell carcinoma. All 17 patients who underwent esophagectomy had been treated with concurrent Taxol/CDDP and radiotherapy (50.4 Gy). After standard staging studies and before therapy, PET imaged undetected sites of metastatic disease in 6 patients (15%). Restaging (including PET) after induction therapy did not identify any patients with disease progression or with loco-regionally unresectable disease at exploration. During induction therapy, the median decrease in the standardized uptake value was 59%. Two-year disease-free and overall survival rates after R_0 esophagectomy were 38% and 63%, respectively, among patients who had a less than 60% decrease in the standardized uptake value. For patients with decreases greater than 60%, these rates were 67% and 89%, respectively.

Conclusion.—Between 10% and 20% of patients with newly diagnosed esophageal cancer will have metastatic disease detected by PET that is missed by other imaging modalities. Thus, PET should be a standard component of the initial evaluation in patients with esophageal cancer. Repeating PET scanning after induction therapy is useful in assessing the effectiveness of the initial therapy.

► FDG-PET imaging is assuming an important role in the management of patients with esophageal cancer. This study from Memorial Sloan-Kettering Cancer Center nicely demonstrates the utility of PET imaging. In this study of 39 patients, 6 (15%) had distant metastatic disease identified on the initial PET scan. On the post–induction therapy scan, no new sites of metastatic disease were demonstrated. When stratified by a change in standardized uptake value of greater or less than 60%, a greater than 60% decrease in standardized uptake value was associated with a greater 2-year disease-free and overall survival.

R. E. Coleman, MD

Metastasis to Regional Lymph Nodes in Patients With Esophageal Squamous Cell Carcinoma: CT versus FDG PET for Presurgical Detection—Prospective Study

Yoon YC, Lee KS, Shim YM, et al (Sungkyunkwan Univ, Seoul, Korea)
Radiology 227:764-770, 2003 7–16

Background.—Patients who have early stage squamous cell carcinoma and undergo surgical treatment have excellent 5-year survival rates (57% to 78%); however, those with advanced but potentially resectable esophageal cancer who undergo surgery plus neoadjuvant chemotherapy, radiotherapy, or both have a 5-year survival rate of 20% to 30%. Accurate staging is key, and resectability and disease stage is essential in choosing appropriate treatment and in evaluating the patient's response to the initial treatment. FDG PET is reportedly more sensitive than CT in detecting primary tumors and distant metastases. The role of PET in detecting nodal metastases remains controversial, however. The accuracy of FDG PET and CT in detecting primary tumor and metastases to individual lymph node groups and for nodal staging was evaluated prospectively in patients with biopsy-proved squamous cell carcinoma of the esophagus.

Methods.—Seventy-eight men and 3 women (age range, 31-90 years; mean age, 63 years) were evaluated by CT and FDG PET before undergoing esophagectomy and lymph node dissection. All visible and palpable lymph nodes in the surgical fields were removed. A comparison of the accuracy of CT and FDG PET in detecting metastasis to lymph nodes was carried out.

Results.—Of the 81 patients, 2 were found to have carcinoma in situ, 13 were found to have T1 cancer, 22 were found to have T2 cancer, 42 were found to have T3 cancer, and 2 were found to have T4 cancer. On CT, 65 of the 81 patients (80%) had their primary tumor correctly diagnosed; on FDG PET, 74 patients (91%) had their primary tumor identified accurately. CT missed 2 cases of carcinoma in situ, 9 cases of T1 cancer, 3 cases of T2 cancer, and 2 cases of T3 cancer; FDG PET missed 1 case of carcinoma in situ and 6 cases of T1 cancer. Both modalities missed 1 case of carcinoma in situ and 5 cases of T1 cancer. Of the 677 nodal groups assessed, 96 were positive for malignancy on pathologic evaluation. CT detected 11% of the metastatic nodal groups, and FDG PET identified 29. CT had 28 false-positive interpretations, which yielding a specificity of 95%; FDG PET had 56 false-positive interpretations which yielded a specificity of 90%. CT proved significantly more specific in detecting metastases to lymph nodes. FDG PET's accuracy in depicting malignant lymph node groups was 82%, whereas that for CT was 83%. Overall, the accuracy of CT for nodal staging was 49%, and that for FDG PET was 62%.

Conclusions.—In depicting metastases to lymph nodes in patients with squamous cell carcinoma of the esophagus, FDG PET scans were significantly more sensitive than CT. CT had greater specificity because FDG PET had many false-positive interpretations. Thus, caution is advisable in using FDG PET, particularly when chronic inflammatory pulmonary disease may be present and in areas in which chronic inflammatory diseases are endemic.

► FDG PET was more sensitive than CT in the detection of primary esophageal carcinomas: PET detected 91% and CT detected 80% of the primary cancers. Ninety-six nodal groups in 46 patients were positive for malignancy. CT detected 11 of the 96 nodal groups, whereas PET detected 29 of the 96 nodal groups. There were 28 false-positive interpretations by CT and 56 false-positive interpretations by FDG-PET imaging. Thirty-two of the 56 false-positive PET interpretations related to hilar activity.

These data support the results of previously published studies. This study does represent a rather large patient population that was carefully studied.

R. E. Coleman, MD

Potential Impact of [^{18}F]3'-deoxy-3'-fluorothymidine Versus [^{18}F]fluoro-2-deoxy-D-glucose in Positron Emission Tomography for Colorectal Cancer

Francis DL, Visvikis D, Costa DC, et al (Middlesex Hosp, London; Hammersmith Hosp, London)

Eur J Nucl Med Mol Imaging 30:988-994, 2003 7–17

Objective.—Fluorine-18-labeled FDG is widely used as a tracer for PET studies in patients with cancer. ^{18}FDG offers high sensitivity, but problems with specificity have prompted attempts to develop new tracers. The novel tracer [^{18}F]3'-deoxy-3'-fluorothymidine (^{18}FLT) visualizes cellular proliferation by a different mechanism, namely, entering the DNA synthesis salvage pathway. ^{18}FLT and ^{18}FDG were compared for PET imaging in patients with colorectal cancer.

Methods.—The prospective study included 17 patients with colorectal cancer who had a total of 50 primary or metastatic lesions, identified by CT scanning. All patients underwent PET with both ^{18}FLT and ^{18}FDG. Uptake of the 2 tracers was compared semiquantitatively with the use of standardized uptake values in normal tissues and malignant lesions.

Results.—Both tracers demonstrated 6 of 6 primary tumors, although ^{18}FDG uptake was approximately twice as high as ^{18}FLT uptake. There were no differences in uptake by lung and peritoneal lesions; FLT PET demonstrated 5 of 6 lung lesions and 6 of 6 peritoneal lesions. On analysis of the 32 colorectal liver metastases, visualization rates for the 2 tracers differed significantly: 34% for ^{18}FLT versus 97% for ^{18}FDG. Uptake of the 2 tracers was not significantly correlated. ^{18}FLT was highly sensitive for detection of extrahepatic lesions, but was not sensitive in demonstrating liver metastases (Fig 5).

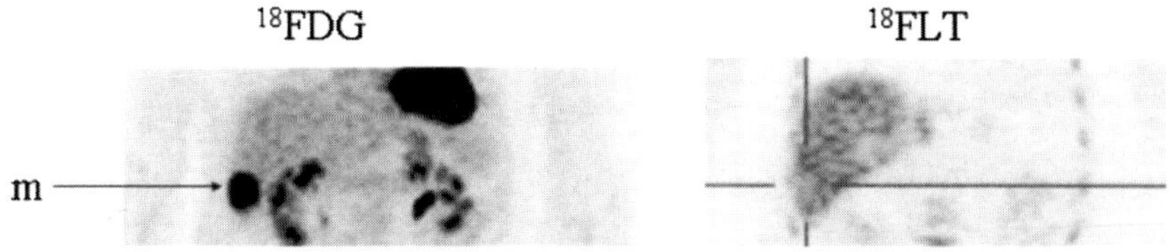

FIGURE 5.—Liver metastases (*m*) displaying high uptake of ^{18}FDG. The corresponding area in the ^{18}FLT image displays lower activity in comparison to the background normal liver. (Courtesy of Francis DL, Visvikis D, Costa DC, et al: Potential impact of [^{18}F]3'-deoxy-3'-fluorothymidine versus [^{18}F]fluoro-2-deoxy-D-glucose in positron emission tomography for colorectal cancer. *Eur J Nucl Med Mol Imaging* 30:988-994, 2003.)

Conclusions.—The new PET tracer ^{18}FLT shows lower uptake values than the standard tracer ^{18}FDG. The 2 tracers visualize different processes, and thus there is no correlation between their retention values. Because of its low sensitivity for hepatic metastases, ^{18}FLT is unlikely to be of value in the imaging of patients with colorectal cancer. Further studies are needed to examine its use as a predictor of survival and response to chemoradiotherapy.

▶ Although FDG is an excellent radiopharmaceutical for imaging cancer, more sensitive and specific radiopharmaceuticals will be welcomed. FLT is a new tracer that images cellular proliferation, and may have advantages over FDG. In this nice study comparing FLT and FDG in patients with colorectal cancer, FLT accumulates less in the lesions than does FDG. FLT demonstrated poor sensitivity in the detection of liver metastases.

R. E. Coleman, MD

A Case-controlled Study of 18-Fluorodeoxyglucose Positron Emission Tomography in the Detection of Pelvic Recurrence in Previously Irradiated Rectal Cancer Patients

Moore HG, Akhurst T, Larson SM, et al (Mem Sloan-Kettering Cancer Ctr, New York)

J Am Coll Surg 197:22-28, 2003 7–18

Background.—Although effective for detecting locally recurrent colorectal cancer, the accuracy FDG-PET for detecting rectal cancer recurrence in an irradiated pelvis has not been systematically studied.

Study design.—Records of surgically resected rectal cancer patients who underwent FDG-PET imaging at least 6 months after external beam radiation therapy (EBRT) were reviewed (Fig 1). Cases (n = 19) were defined as scans from patients in whom a pelvic recurrence was confirmed (histologically, n = 14; radiologic follow-up, n = 5). Controls (n = 41), defined as scans from patients without clinical or radiologic evidence of pelvic recurrence, were compared with cases for the time interval between completion of EBRT and FDG-PET imaging (RT/PET interval, mean 25.1 months vs 27.5 months, respectively), as well as EBRT dose (mean 5084 cGy vs 5062 cGy, respectively). All 60 FDG-PET scans were iteratively reconstructed and re-

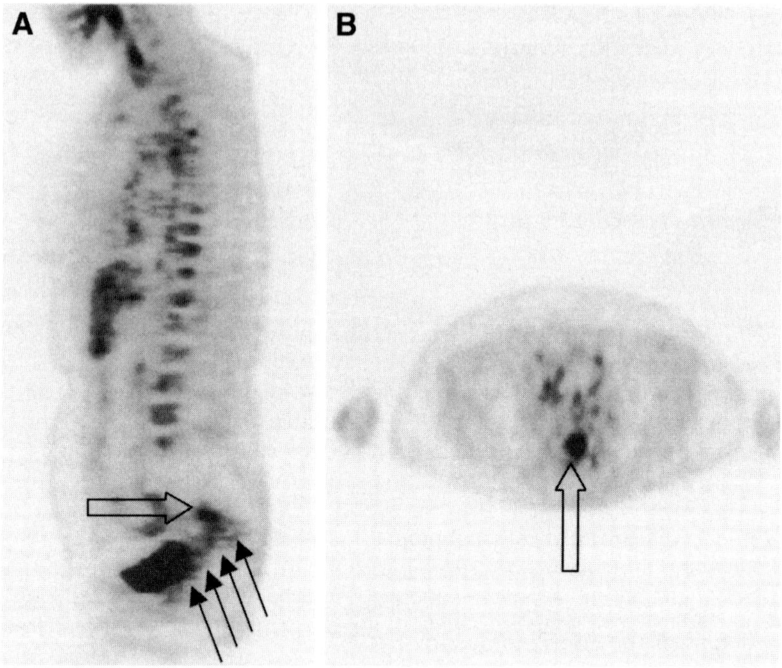

FIGURE 1.—False-positive FDG-PET scan. Sagittal (**A**) and transaxial (**B**) slices of a 53-year-old woman with rising CEA. Note focal uptake in the region of the rectum (*open arrows*), which appears diffusely inflamed (*closed arrows*). Note also the absence of marrow uptake in the sacrum secondary to earlier administration of radiotherapy. Clinical follow-up has revealed no evidence of local recurrence. *Abbreviation: FDG-PET*, Fluorine-18 fluorodeoxyglucose positron emission tomography. (Courtesy of Moore HG, Akhurst T, Larson SM, et al: A case-controlled study of 18-flurodeoxyglucose positron emission tomography in the detection of pelvic recurrence in previously irradiated rectal cancer patients. *J Am Coll Surg* 197:22-28. Copyright 2003, the American College of Surgeons.)

interpreted by a single nuclear medicine physician blinded to original FDG-PET interpretation and disease status. Certainty of disease was scored on a 5-point scale (1 to 5), with scores greater than or equal to 4 considered positive.

Results.—FDG-PET correctly identified 16 of 19 recurrences, for a sensitivity of 84% and a specificity of 88%. Overall accuracy was 87%. Positive predictive value was 76%, and negative predictive value was 92%. Positive predictive value and accuracy improved in scans performed more than 12 months after EBRT.

Conclusions.—Our preliminary data suggest that FDG-PET is an accurate modality for detecting pelvic recurrence of rectal cancer after full-dose EBRT. Its reliability appears to improve with time, perhaps because of resolution of early postradiation inflammation.

► The inflammation resulting from radiation therapy may be FDG avid. Previous studies have suggested that false-positive abnormalities may occur up to 6 months after the completion of radiation therapy in patients with rectal cancers. This study includes patients whose FDG-PET scans were performed at least 6 months after EBRT, and the investigators found an overall accuracy of 87%. The accuracy was improved if the scans were obtained more than 1 year after the radiation therapy. Thus, false-positive studies from inflammation related to irradiation can occur even out to 1 year after treatment.

R. E. Coleman, MD

Impact of Metaiodobenzylguanidine Scintigraphy on Assessing Response of High-Risk Neuroblastoma to Dose-Intensive Induction Chemotherapy

Kushner BH, Yeh SDJ, Kramer K, et al (Mem Sloan-Kettering Cancer Ctr, New York)

J Clin Oncol 21:1082-1086, 2003 7–19

Introduction.—Metaiodobenzylguanidine (MIBG) scintigraphy is recommended as part of the disease status assessment for patients with neuroblastoma (NB), according to the International Neuroblastoma Response Criteria. However, questions remain about the value of routine MIBG scanning in the clinical management of patients with NB. The use of MIBG scanning in assessing the response of high-risk NB to dose-intensive induction chemotherapy was reported.

Methods.—The study included 162 patients with high-risk NB undergoing MIBG scintigraphy to assess their response to dose-intensive induction chemotherapy, before starting consolidative therapy. Imaging was performed with iodine-131 in 99 patients and with iodine-123 in 63 patients. Other staging modalities included CT, ^{99m}Tc bone scanning, bone marrow histologic examination, and urine catecholamine measurement. The induction chemotherapy regimen included high-dose cyclophosphamide and cisplatin/etoposide. Ninety patients received dose-intensive therapy at the study cancer center from the time of diagnosis, whereas 72 were initially treated elsewhere before referral for intensified therapy. The effects of the MIBG scans on the classification of patient response to this induction therapy protocol were analyzed.

Results.—For patients receiving dose-intensive therapy from the time of diagnosis, the inclusion of MIBG scans in the response assessment was associated with a significant increase in the rate of incomplete responses, from 15.5% to 22%. In this group, the rate of complete remission/very good partial remission (CR/VGPR) was 78%. In contrast, in the referral group, the results of MIBG led to a change in response classification for only one patient. This group had a CR/VGPR rate of 43%. Of 38 patients with histologic evidence of NB in bone marrow specimens, 15 had no signs of bone marrow involvement on MIBG scanning. In contrast, 5 patients with no histologic evidence of NB in bone marrow had MIBG uptake consistent with bone marrow involvement.

Conclusions.—For patients receiving dose-intensive chemotherapy from the time of NB diagnosis, MIBG scintigraphy should be a required part of disease status assessment, along with extensive bone marrow evaluation. In contrast, for patients receiving standard-dose chemotherapy before referral for intensified therapy, MIBG scans provide no further information beyond the results of other staging modalities. With the high rates of major disease regression achieved with dose-intensive induction therapy, comprehensive evaluation is essential to ensure accurate assessment of disease status in patients with NB.

► Iodine-131 MIBG is used for the diagnosis and treatment of neuroendocrine tumors. Iodine-123 has imaging advantages that are particularly important in children being evaluated for NB. This study documents the importance of MIBG imaging in the evaluation of patients who are being treated with dose-intensity induction therapy for high-risk NB. An interesting finding of this study is that the ^{99m}Tc bone scan did not contribute to the management of the patient who had MIBG scans.

R. E. Coleman, MD

Pilot Study of Iodine-131–Metaiodobenzylguanidine in Combination With Myeloablative Chemotherapy and Autologous Stem-cell Support for the Treatment of Neuroblastoma

Yanik GA, Levine JE, Matthay KK, et al (Univ of Michigan, Ann Arbor; Univ of California, San Francisco)

J Clin Oncol 20:2142-2149, 2002 7–20

Background.—Children with relapsed or metastatic neuroblastoma continue to have a poor survival rate. The feasibility of a novel regimen combining ^{131}I-MIBG and myeloablative chemotherapy with autologous stem-cell rescue was assessed.

Methods.—The study included 12 patients with neuroblastoma. Five were treated after relapse, and 7 after induction therapy. For all patients, treatment consisted of ^{131}I-MIBG, 12 mCi/kg on day −21, followed by carboplatin, 1500 mg/m^2; etoposide, 800 mg/m^2; and melphalan, 210 mg/m^2, administered from day −7 to −4. On day 0, autologous peripheral-blood stem cells or bone marrow were infused.

Results.—Patients tolerated the infusion and myeloablative chemotherapy well. The main nonhematopoietic toxicity was grade 2 to 3 oral mucositis, which occurred in all the patients. Median times to neutrophil and platelet engraftment were 10 and 28 days, respectively. Three of the 8 patients with metastatic disease achieved complete response and 2 had a partial response by day 100 after transplantation.

Conclusions.—Treatment with ^{131}I-MIBG combined with myeloablative chemotherapy and hematopoietic stem cell rescue is a feasible treatment strategy in children with neuroblastoma. The toxicity associated with it was acceptable in the current series. Further research on this novel approach is warranted.

► Radionuclide therapy is having an increasingly important role in the practice of nuclear medicine. MIBG has been used for treating neuroendocrine tumors for many years in only a few centers. This pilot study demonstrates the feasibility of using MIBG therapy in combination with other therapy. The toxicity of the combined therapy was considered acceptable, and the results in this small population are similar to the results of other trials involving this malignant tumor.

R. E. Coleman, MD

Evaluation of F18-Deoxyglucose Positron Emission Tomography (FDG-PET) to Assess the Nature of Neurogenic Tumours

Cardona S, Schwarzbach M, Hinz U, et al (Univ of Heidelberg, Germany; German Cancer Research Ctr, Heidelberg, Germany)

Eur J Surg Oncol 29:536-541, 2003 7–21

Aims.—Benign neurofibromas and malignant peripheral nerve sheath tumours (MPNST) commonly develop in patients with neurofibromatosis. Differentiation of benign from malignant tumours by conventional preoperative imaging is unreliable. FDG-PET is a non-invasive technique for biological tumour evaluation. The aim of this study was to assess the value of FDG-PET in patients with neurogenic tumours suspicious for MPNST.

Methods.—Benign and malignant neurogenic soft tissue tumours were prospectively evaluated by computed tomography or magnetic resonance imaging. Three-dimensional qualitative and quantitative FDG-PET was performed. Standard uptake value (SUV) was analyzed with respect to histological diagnosis and follow-up data.

Results.—Twenty-five neurogenic soft tissue tumours were included. FDG-PET identified all primary ($n=6$) and recurrent MPNST ($n=7$). Benign lesions ($n=12$) did not demonstrate high FDG uptake. The SUV was significantly higher in MPNST (median 2.9; range 1.8-12.3), than in benign tumours (median 1.1; range 0.5-1.8) ($P < 0.001$). At a cut-off value of 1.8 SUV measured 1 h post-injection FDG-PET distinguished between MPNST and benign neurogenic tumours with 100% sensitivity and 83% specificity.

Conclusions.—FDG-PET allows discrimination of benign from malignant neurogenic tumours. This should be particularly useful in patients with neurofibromatosis as FDG-PET may help to avoid multiple surgical procedures for benign tumours.

► Very few studies have been performed with FDG-PET in patients with benign neurofibromas and MPNST. This study demonstrates that PET is highly accurate in differentiating benign from malignant neurogenic tumors. More data are needed.

R. E. Coleman, MD

Usefulness of Semiquantitative FDG-PET in the Prediction of Brain Tumor Treatment Response to Gamma Knife Radiosurgery

Lee J-K, Liu R-S, Shiang H-R, et al (Natl Yang-Ming Univ, Taiwan; Taipei Veterans Gen Hosp, Taiwan)

J Comput Assist Tomogr 27:525-529, 2003 7–22

Background.—In patients undergoing gamma knife radiosurgery (GKRS) for benign or malignant brain tumors, the treatment effect is usually monitored with MRI. However, changes in tumor size may not correspond to changes in tumor metabolism. The use of FDG-PET to predict brain tumor responses to GKRS was analyzed.

Methods.—The prospective study included 18 patients (median age, 40 years) undergoing GKRS for histologically documented glioma. The most common diagnosis was grade 2 astrocytoma; 13 patients had previously undergone surgery, whereas 5 were initially treated with GKRS. Six to 8 months after GKRS, the patients underwent FDG-PET, followed within a mean of 10 days by correlative MRI scans. Fused PET-MRI images were used calculate the tumor-to-cortex (T/C) and tumor-to-white matter (T/WM) FDG uptake ratio. The metabolic findings were compared with tumor response as assessed by morphologic changes in tumor size on MRI.

Results.—At a mean follow-up of 29 months, MRI indicated partial remission in 4 tumors and stable disease in 6 tumors (group 1), and progressive disease in 8 tumors (group 2). Mean T/C ratio values were 0.65 in group 1 and 0.84 in group 2. Values for T/WM were 1.29 and 1.76, respectively. Both values were significantly different between the 2 response groups (Fig 2).

Conclusions.—In patients undergoing GKRS for glioma, FDG-PET may be a useful predictor of treatment response. The FDG-PET patterns of glu-

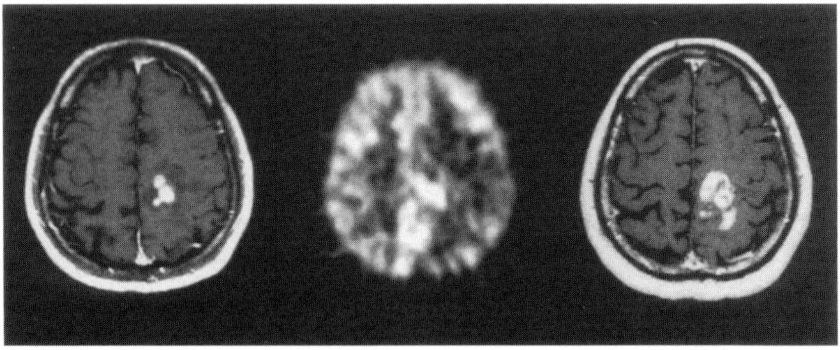

FIGURE 2.—Anaplastic astrocytoma in a 59-year-old woman (patient 6). **Left**, Seven months after gamma knife radiosurgery (GKRS), axial MR image shows a lesion in the left parietal lobe. **Middle**, Corresponding axial FDG-PET image. The tumor-to-cortex (T/C) ratio is 0.93. The tumor-to-white matter (T/WM) ratio is 1.85. **Right**, Thirty-three months after GKRS, the tumor shows progressive change on axial MR image. (Courtesy of Lee J-K, Liu R-S, Shiang H-R, et al: Usefulness of semiquantitative FDG-PET in the prediction of brain tumor treatment response to gamma knife radiosurgery. *J Comput Assist Tomogr* 27(4):525-529, 2003.)

cose metabolism at 6 to 8 months after GKRS correspond well to MRI-measured changes in tumor size at longer-term follow-up.

▶ GKRS is a high radiation dosed technique to treat primary and secondary brain tumors. Very few studies have been performed with FDG-PET to determine the effect of GKRS on subsequent FDG-PET scans. Certainly, radiation necrosis after therapy may be FDG avid.

The authors found that FDG-PET obtained 6 to 8 months after GKRS was predictive of treatment response.

R. E. Coleman, MD

Methionine Positron Emission Tomography of Recurrent Metastatic Brain Tumor and Radiation Necrosis After Stereotactic Radiosurgery: Is a Differential Diagnosis Possible?

Tsuyuguchi N, Sunada I, Iwai Y, et al (Osaka City Univ, Japan; Saiseikai Ibaragi Hosp, Osaka, Japan; Osaka Gen Hosp, Japan)

J Neurosurg 98:1056-1064, 2003 7–23

Background.—In evaluating metastatic brain tumors, CT, MRI, SPECT have all proved useful, but differentiating between a tumor recurrence and radiation necrosis still presents difficulties once brain tumors have been treated with radiotherapeutic methods. The clinical usefulness of L-[methyl-^{11}C]methionine (MET) used in conjunction with PET was evaluated in this application.

Methods.—The 21 patients were being investigated for suspected recurrent metastatic brain tumors or radiation injury, for which MET–PET scans were used. All had had stereotactic radiosurgery and contrast-enhanced MR examinations before nuclear medicine assessment. Results were compared with findings in 20 healthy volunteers. The region of interest was defined as the portion of the tumor with the highest accumulation of MET; the ratio of tumor tissue to normal tissue (T/N) was obtained by determining the mean counts of radioisotope per pixel in the tumor divided by the mean counts per pixel in normal gray matter. The accuracy of MET–PET scanning was determined by correlating the findings with the results of histologic analysis or with the subsequent clinical course and MRI findings.

Results.—Viable tumor cells were found in 11 cases on histologic examination. Ten cases were identified as necrosis because the patients had stable neurologic symptoms and no massive enlargement of the lesion after 5 months. No significant differences were found between the healthy volunteers and patients with tumors in terms of the measurements of standardized uptake values (SUVs) in the frontal lobe. The T/N ratio varied from 1.74 to 3.58, and the SUV varied from 1.58 to 4.99 in the 8 patients who had MET–PET scans before treatment. Significant differences in the T/N ratio and SUV were noted between patients having a recurrence of cancer and those having radiation necrosis. The mean T/N ratio of the radiation necrosis group was 1.15, and that in the tumor recurrence group was 1.62. The mean SUV in the necrosis group was 1.78, and that in the tumor necrosis group was 2.5. No high accumulation was found with the use of MET–PET studies in 2 cases of recurrence, but visible accumulation was found in 2 necrosis cases. The sensitivity of MET–PET scanning in detecting a tumor recurrence was 77.8%, and the specificity was 100%.

Conclusions.—Significant differences were found between patients with a tumor recurrence and those with radiation necrosis when MET–PET scanning. The specificity of this method was 100%, and its sensitivity was 77.8%. The MET–PET results matched those identified on clinical diagnosis and helped to differentiate between these 2 diagnoses.

► The differentiation of a recurrent tumor from necrosis after therapy is a difficult clinical problem that is not clarified by contrast enhanced MRI or CT scanning or FDG PET imaging. FDG PET is frequently metabolically active after stereotactic radiosurgery and after instillation of radiolabeled monoclonal antibody for therapy in postoperative cavities. This study suggests that MET may be helpful in that differential diagnosis. More data are needed.

R. E. Coleman, MD

Value of F-18 Fluorodeoxyglucose Positron Emission Tomography for Predicting the Clinical Outcome of Patients With Aggressive Lymphoma Prior to and After Autologous Stem-Cell Transplantation

Filmont J-E, Czernin J, Yap C, et al (Univ of California, Los Angeles)

Chest 124:608-613, 2003 7–24

Introduction.—The most important factor influencing the success rate of autologous stem-cell transplantation (ASCT) in patients who have failed standard chemotherapy for lymphoma is the tumor response to salvage chemotherapy. A variety of imaging tests provide prognostic information after ASCT. The predictive value of CT was compared with that of FDG-PET in patients with lymphoma who underwent salvage chemotherapy and ASCT.

Methods.—Twelve patients had Hodgkin disease (HD) and 31 had non-Hodgkin lymphoma (NHL). In group 1 (6 patients with HD and 14 with NHL), FDG-PET was performed at a median of 3.8 weeks after the start of salvage chemotherapy but before high-dose chemotherapy, and at a median interval of 7 weeks before ASCT. Patients in group 2 (6 with HD and 17 with NHL) had FDG-PET performed within a median interval of 2.4 months after ASCT. Patients were followed up for at least 6 months after ASCT.

Results.—After a median period of 13.3 months, 8 patients in group 1 were disease free, and 12 had relapsed or died. The PET findings were true negative in 7 of 8 patients, and true positive in 11 of 12 who relapsed after ASCT. Nine patients in group 2 were disease-free after a median period of 16.5 months, and 14 had relapsed. In group 2, PET findings were true negative in 8 of 9 patients, and true positive in 13 of 14 who relapsed. Positive predictive values of PET were 92% in group 1 and 93% in group 2; negative predictive values were 88% and 89%, respectively. The predictive accuracy values of CT were 58% and 67% for groups 1 and 2, respectively; corresponding values for PET were 90% and 91% (Fig 1).

Conclusion. The use of FDG PET, either before or after ASCT can accurately predict the long-term outcome of patients with aggressive lymphoma. Imaging with CT had poor specificity and was thus unable to reliably predict disease-free survival. The accuracy of FDG-PET makes it the imaging modality of choice in patients with aggressive lymphoma eligible for ASCT.

▶ The results of studies using FDG-PET to evaluate the effect of therapy are now appearing and are quite positive. Gallium scanning has been previously

FIGURE 1

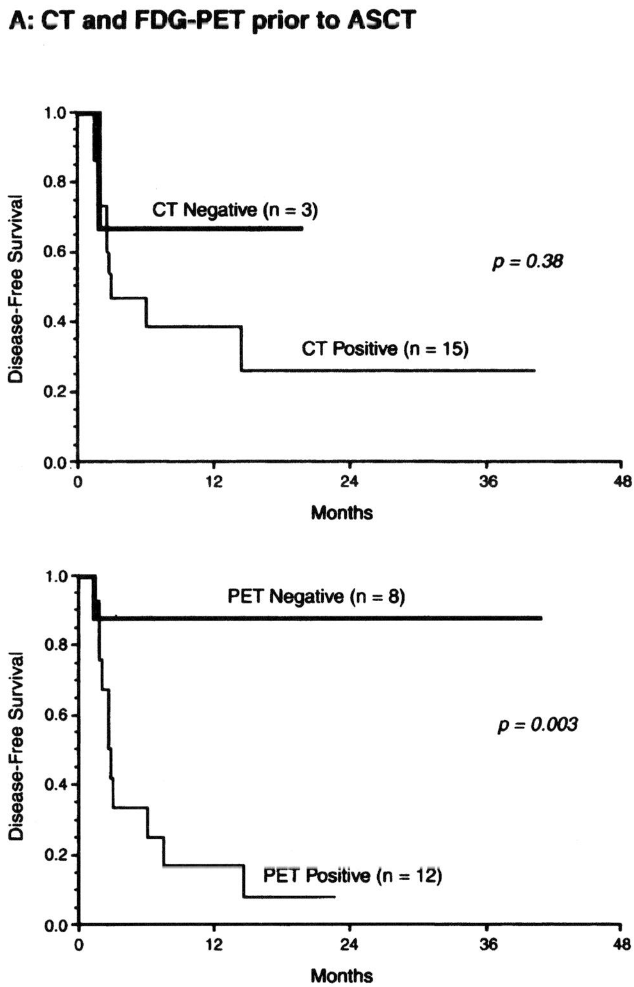

(*Continued*)

FIGURE 1 (cont.)

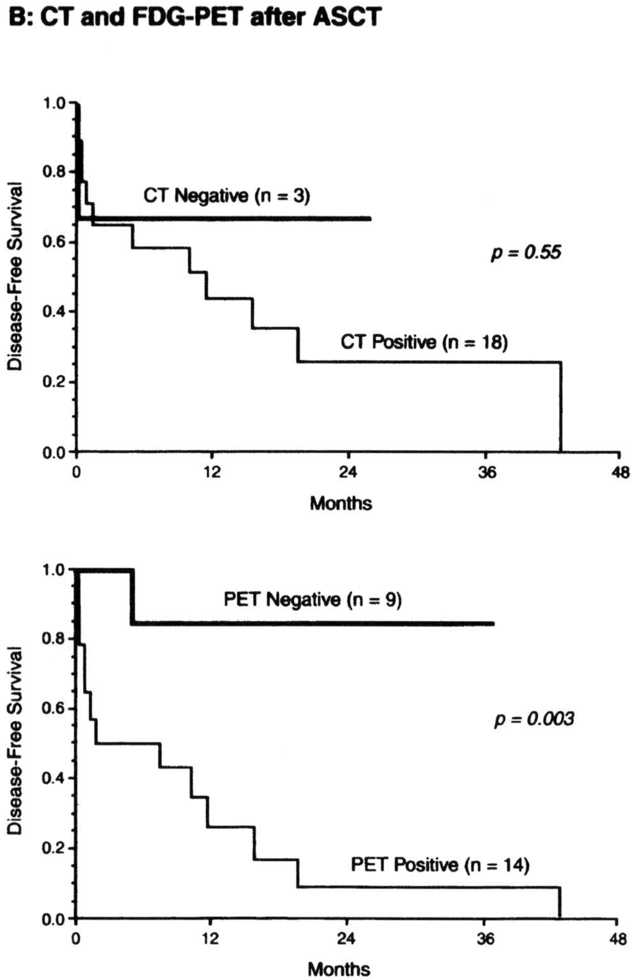

FIGURE 1.—Kaplan-Meier estimates for disease-free survival in patients with lymphoma by CT and FDG-PET imaging results obtained prior to ASCT (**top, A**) and after ASCT (**bottom, B**). *Abbreviation: ASCT*, Autologous stem-cell transplantation. (Courtesy of Filmont J-E, Czernin J, Yap C, et al: Value of F-18 fluorodeoxyglucose positron emission tomography for predicting the clinical outcome of patients with aggressive lymphoma prior to and after autologous stem-cell transplantation. *Chest* 124:608-613, 2003.)

used to determine whether the patient was likely to have a complete remission. The results of this study suggest that FDG-PET is highly accurate in predicting the outcome of patients who undergo salvage chemotherapy or ASCT. Furthermore, PET was more accurate than CT in determining disease-free survival.

R. E. Coleman, MD

18F-Fluoro-Deoxy-Glucose Positron Emission Tomography (18F-FDG-PET) for Assessment of Enteropathy-Type T Cell Lymphoma

Hoffmann M, Vogelsang H, Kletter K, et al (Univ of Vienna)

Gut 52:347-351, 2003 7–25

Background.—Enteropathy-type T cell lymphoma (ETCL), an aggressive lymphoma, accounts for less than 1% of non-Hodgkin's lymphomas. This lymphoma may be seen de novo or may arise in patients with long-standing or untreated celiac disease (CD). The potential of ^{18}F-FDG PET for imaging ETCL was investigated.

Methods.—Five patients with ETCL and 12 with CD who had undergone ^{18}F-FDG PET at 1 center during a 2-year period were included in the retrospective analysis. Material for histologic reevaluation was available for all

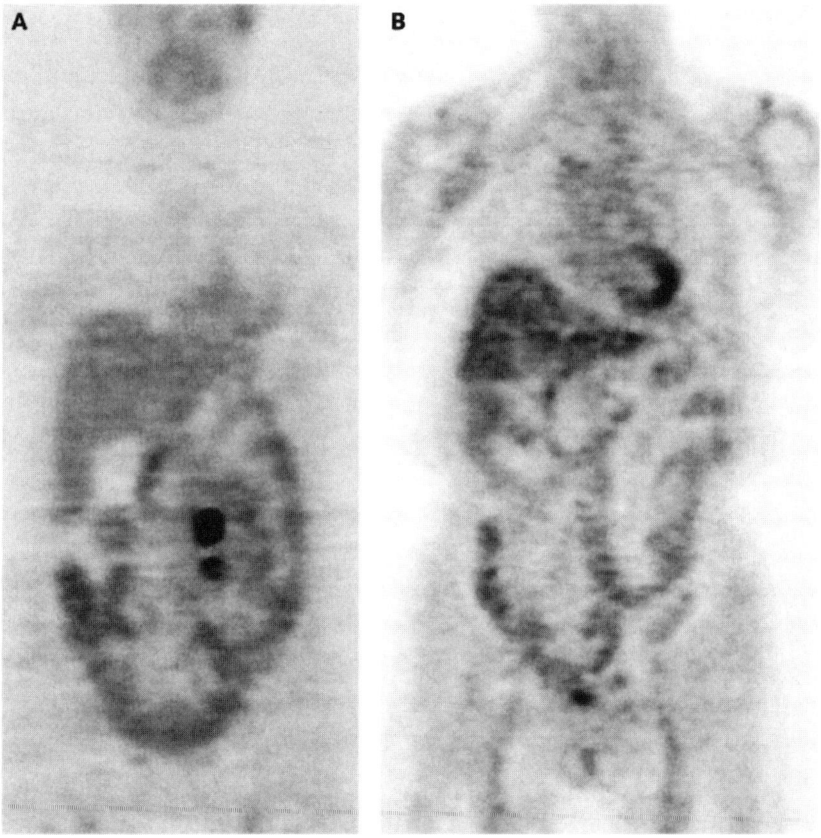

FIGURE 2.—A, Coronal ^{18F}-FDG PET image of a 60-year-old woman suffering from enteropathy-type T cell lymphoma showing 2 lesions with elevated FDG uptake (standard uptake value, 7.7). B, Coronal ^{18}F-FDG PET image of a 74-year-old woman suffering from refractory sprue showing diffuse intestinal FDG uptake (standard uptake value, 2.2). (Courtesy of Hoffman M, Vogelsang H, Kletter K, et al: 18F-fluoro-deoxy-glucose positron emission tomography (18F-FDG-PET) for assessment of enteropathy-type T cell lymphoma. *Gut* 52:347-351, 2003. With permission from the BMJ Publishing Group.)

patients. Whole body ^{18}F-FDG PET scans were done 40 minutes after 300 to 380 Mbq of ^{18}F-FDG was injected. Standard uptake values (SUVs) were calculated for areas with focally increased FDG uptake and diffusely increased intestinal ^{18}F-FDG accumulation.

Findings.—Four of the 5 patients with ETCL underwent imaging before cytotoxic treatment, and 1 had regular PET scanning for follow-up. All 4 patients imaged before therapy showed substantially increased intestinal ^{18}F-FDG uptake (Fig 2). The maximal mean SUV was 7.15. In the patient imaged after treatment, no pathologic ^{18}F-FDG uptake was identified. This correlated with normal duodenal mucosa, as evidenced by repeated biopsies and conventional imaging techniques. Of the 12 patients with CD, 4 had no increased intestinal ^{18}F-FDG uptake, and 5 had minor diffuse intestinal ^{18}F-FDG accumulation. The mean SUV was 3.4. No SUV could be determined in the remaining 3 patients with diffuse intestinal ^{18}F-FDG uptake. Patients with ETCL had notably higher SUVs than those with CD, regardless of CD activity at the time of imaging.

Conclusion.—^{18}F-FDG PET is potentially useful for diagnosing and imaging ETCL. This modality may enable early diagnosis in patients with long-standing CD in whom ETCL is developing, as ^{18}F-FDG does not appear to accumulate significantly in the gut of patients with CD, regardless of the level of disease activity.

► I was unfamiliar with ETCL prior to reviewing this article. FDG PET is quite accurate in characterizing most lymphomas, and this one is no exception. PET appears to be able to differentiate intestinal lymphoma from CD.

R. E. Coleman, MD

Positron Emission Tomography With ^{11}C-Acetate and ^{18}F-FDG in Prostate Cancer Patients

Fricke E, Machtens S, Hofmann M, et al (Hannover Med School, Germany)
Eur J Nucl Med Mol Imaging 30:607-611, 2003 7–26

Background.—Many advances have been made in the imaging of prostate cancer, but the diagnostic capabilities remain unsatisfactory in light of the rising incidence of this disease. ^{18}F-FDG PET has proved useful in corroborating distant metastases, but little ^{18}F-FDG accumulates in primary prostate cancers cells. It was hypothesized that carbon-11 acetate (^{11}C-acetate) PET might be more useful because ^{11}C-acetate might possibly be taken up more intensely than ^{18}F-FDG by prostate tumor tissue.

Methods.—The 25 patients who were evaluated were being followed up after primary prostate cancer and had a suspected relapse or metastatic disease. All underwent investigation with the use of ^{11}C-acetate, and 15 patients also underwent ^{18}F-FDG PET. While they were being evaluated, 14 patients were receiving anti-androgen treatment.

Results.—Twenty-one patients had lesions depicted with positive contrast medium: 10 were found in the patients having ^{18}F-FDG PET and 20 were found in those having ^{11}C-acetate investigations. ^{18}F-FDG identified 53 lesions, and ^{11}C-acetate identified 74. The median standardized uptake values (SUVs) were 1.4 for ^{18}F-FDG and 3.2 for ^{11}C-acetate, which was a statistically significant difference. Diagnostic scans were obtained in 70% of the patients with the use of ^{11}C-acetate and in only 43% of those with the use of ^{18}F-FDG. In 75% of the cases with lymph node metastases, these lesions were identified with the use of ^{11}C-acetate; ^{18}F-FDG identified only 30% of them. Distant metastases were identified in 50% of the affected cases with the use of ^{11}C-acetate and in 75% with the use of ^{18}F-FDG. The tumor marker prostate-specific antigen and ^{11}C-acetate SUVs correlated positively, as did prostate-specific antigen and ^{18}F-FDG SUVs.

Conclusions.—The number of patients in this study was small, but ^{11}C-acetate PET appeared to have clinical significance when used in investigations of patients with prostate cancer. Combining it with ^{18}F-FDG PET may be a desirable protocol for these patients.

► Better methods for imaging prostate cancer are needed. Carbon-11 acetate appears to be a promising imaging agent. Our facility has used fluorine-18 fluorocholine, and it is also a promising agent.

In this study, FDG PET seems to be superior to carbon-11 acetate in detecting distant metastases, whereas the carbon-11 acetate was better than FDG for detecting a local recurrence and regional lymph node metastases. Several other institutions, including Washington University in St. Louis and University of California-Los Angeles are performing studies with carbon-11–labeled acetate in prostate cancer.

R. E. Coleman, MD

Comparison of [^{18}F]Fluorocholine and [^{18}F]Fluorodeoxyglucose for Positron Emission Tomography of Androgen Dependent and Androgen Independent Prostate Cancer

Price DT, Coleman RE, Liao RP, et al (Duke Univ, Durham, NC)

J Urol 168:273-280, 2002 7–27

Background.—The metabolic assessment of cancer includes PET imaging, commonly using the radiotracer FDG. However, the low cellular uptake rate in prostate cancer limits the value of FDG in this patient population. The efficacy of a novel choline analogue, ^{18}F-fluorocholine (FCH), for detecting androgen-dependent and androgen-independent prostate cancer and its metastases was investigated.

Methods.—Cultured prostate cancer cells LNCaP and PC-3 were used in the study. The cellular uptake of FCH and FDG in these cells was compared. In addition, FCH and FDG were injected into nude mice xenografts, and uptake in various organs was documented. Eighteen patients with androgen-dependent or androgen-independent prostate cancer also underwent FCH and FDG PET.

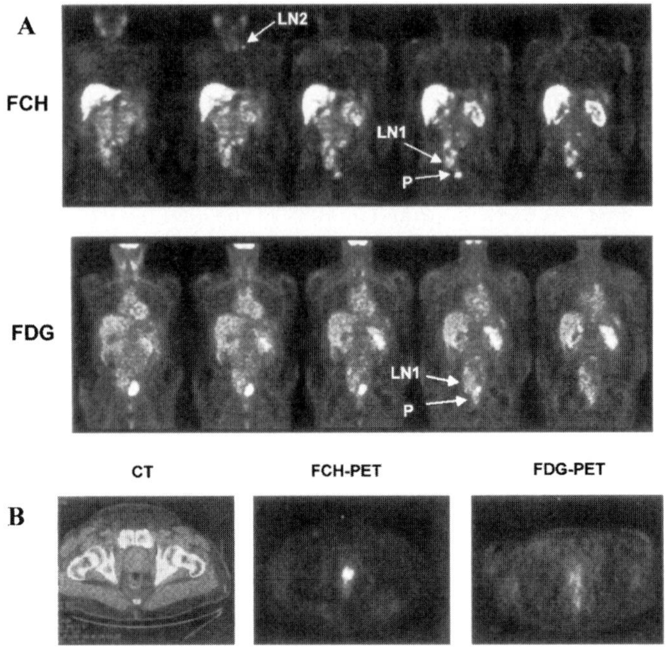

FIGURE 3.—Patient with hormone naïve metastatic prostate cancer. A, FDG and ^{18}F-fluorocholine (FCH) coronal images (12.9-mm slice thickness). FCH shows high uptake in prostate (*P*), right retroperitoneal adenopathy (*LN1*) and supraclavicular focus (*LN2*) suggestive of disease in lymph node (standardized uptake values, 5.2 to 5.7). FDG demonstrates intense bladder accumulation but moderate uptake in prostate (standardized uptake value, 2.2) and retroperitoneal adenopathy (standardized uptake value, 2.3). No focal uptake is evident in left neck. B, Comparison of transaxial CT, FCH, and FDG PET at prostate level. FCH scan revealed focal uptake in left neck, and FCH uptake in prostate was more focal and intense than was FDG uptake. (Courtesy of Price DT, Coleman RE, Liao RP, et al: Comparison of [^{18}F]fluorocholine and [^{18}F]fluorodeoxyglucose for positron emission tomography of androgen dependent and androgen independent prostate cancer. *J Urol* 168:273-280, 2002.)

Findings.—Compared with FDG uptake, FCH uptake was 849% greater in androgen-dependent and 60% greater in androgen-independent cells. Adding hemicholinium-3 thirty minutes before radiotracer was administered inhibited FCH uptake by 79% and 70% in LNCaP and PC-3 cells, respectively. However, FDG uptake was not affected significantly. Nude mice xenografts demonstrated that FDG uptake was equal to or greater than FCH uptake. However, clinical imaging in patients showed 2- to 4-fold higher FCH uptake in those with androgen-dependent and androgen-independent prostate carcinoma (Fig 3). In primary tumors, osseous metastases, and soft tissue metastases, FCH detected more lesions than did FDG.

Conclusion.—These data suggest that FCH is preferable to FDG for PET studies of prostate carcinoma. Further research is needed to verify these findings in a greater number of patients.

► New radiopharmaceuticals are needed for PET imaging of prostate cancer. FCH and C-11 acetate are 2 tracers that are being evaluated for their utility in diagnosis and staging of prostate cancer. In vivo and in vitro data demonstrate that FCH is better than FDG in the detection of prostate cancer. More studies are under way to further evaluate this tracer.

R. E. Coleman, MD

The Role of PET Scanning in the Dectection of Recurrent Cervical Cancer

Havrilesky LJ, Wong TZ, Secord AA, et al (Duke Univ, Durham, NC)

Gynecol Oncol 90:186-190, 2003 7–28

Objectives.—FDG PET has recently been established as a sensitive and specific method of detecting lymph node metastases in newly diagnosed cervical cancer. Little is known about the efficacy of PET for detecting recurrent disease. We evaluated the potential role of FDG PET in the context of suspected recurrent cervical cancer.

Methods.—The records of patients undergoing PET scan to evaluate for cervical cancer recurrence between July 1998 and February 2002 were reviewed. Radiographic findings were classified as negative, suspicious, or equivocal. PET scan findings were compared to available clinical data to classify each PET result as a true positive, true negative, false positive, or false negative. Clinical proof of recurrence consisted of a tissue biopsy revealing recurrent cancer within 3 months of the PET scan. Clinical proof of no evidence of disease consisted of a negative tissue biopsy within 3 months or no clinical evidence of recurrence within 6 months after the PET scan.

Results.—Twenty-eight patients underwent 37 PET scans. Twenty-nine cases among 22 patients were clinically evaluable for recurrence status. Median age was 42, and stage distribution was IB 1 ($n = 3$), IB2 ($n = 4$), IIA ($n = 1$), IIB ($n = 10$), IIIB ($n = 9$), IVB ($n = 1$). Histologic types included squamous ($n = 23$) adenocarcinoma ($n = 4$) and unknown ($n = 1$). There were 12 true positive PET scans, 13 true negatives, 2 false positives, and 2 false negatives. The sensitivity and specificity of FDG PET for detecting recurrent cervical cancer were 85.7 and 86.7%, respectively. The positive and negative predictive values were 85.7 and 86.7%, respectively.

Conclusions.—Whole-body FDG PET is a sensitive and specific tool for the detection of recurrent cervical cancer in patients who have clinical findings suspicious for recurrence. A larger prospective trial will determine whether this modality should be used routinely in conjunction with, or in lieu of, other imaging studies to detect recurrent disease in a broader population of cervical cancer patients.

► More studies on the utility of PET in evaluation of cervical cancer are now being performed. These studies are determining the utility of PET in staging and restaging cervical cancer. This study further documents the ability of FDG-PET imaging to detect recurrent cervical cancer.

R. E. Coleman, MD

Usefulness of ^{18}F-Fluorodeoxyglucose Positron Emission Tomography to Detect Para-aortic Lymph Nodal Metastasis in Advanced Cervical Cancer With Negative Computed Tomography Findings

Lin WC, Hung YC, Yeh LS, et al (China Med College Hosp, Taichung, Taiwan; Natl Taiwan Univ Hosp, Taipei; Shin Kong Wu Ho-Su Mem Hosp, Taipei, Taiwan)

Gynecol Oncol 89:73-76, 2003 7–29

Objective.—In advanced cervical cancer, it has been reported that progression-free survival is significantly related to para-aortic lymph node metastasis. Computed tomography (CT) has been widely used for clinical staging, but its sensitivity for lymph nodal metastasis is low. Therefore, this prospective study was undertaken to evaluate ^{18}F-fluorodeoxyglucose positron emission tomography (FDG-PET) in detecting para-aortic lymph nodal metastasis in patients with locally advanced cervical carcinoma when CT findings were negative.

Methods.—Fifty women with advanced cervical cancer confined to the pelvis with negative abdominal CT findings were included in this study. After 10 mCi of FDG was administered intravenously, the abdomens were scanned by PET. Para-aortic lymph node metastases were diagnosed as present or absent according to a standardized staging procedure (Fig 1).

Results.—Retroperitoneal surgical exploration revealed 14 patients with para-aortic lymph nodal metastasis. Two patients had false-negative FDG-

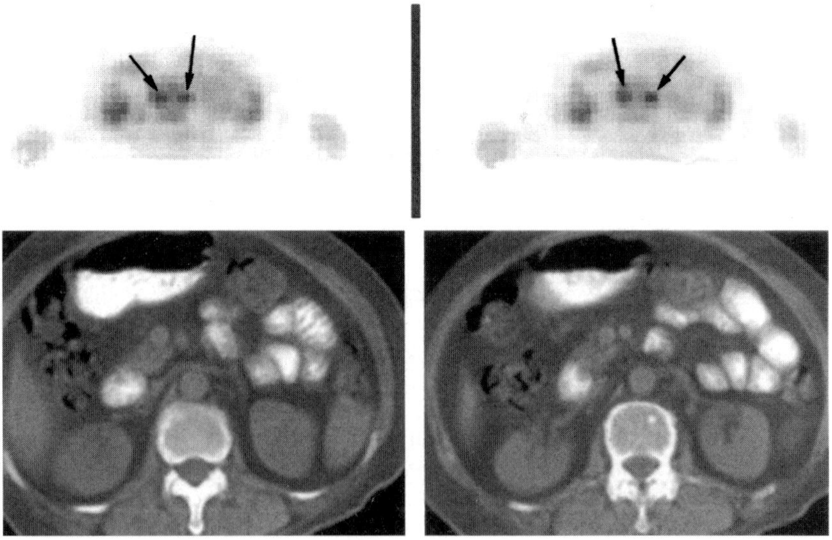

FIGURE 1.—A patient with positive pathological results of para-aortic lymph node metastases had positive abdominal ^{18}F-fluorodeoxyglucose positron emission tomography findings (*arrows*, **upper row**) but negative abdominal computed tomographic findings (**lower row**). (Reprinted with permission of the publisher from Lin WC, Hung YC, Yeh LS, et al: Usefulness of ^{18}F-fluorodeoxyglucose positron emission tomography to detect para-aortic lymph nodal metastasis in advanced cervical cancer with negative computed tomography findings. *Gynecol Oncol* 89:73-76. Copyright 2003 by Elsevier Science Inc.)

PET findings and the other two patients had false-positive FDG-PET findings.

Conclusion.—Overall, FDG-PET imaging had a sensitivity of 85.7%, a specificity of 94.4%, and an accuracy of 92%. When abdominal CT findings are negative, the use of FDG-PET can accurately detect para-aortic lymph nodal metastatis in patients with advanced cervical cancer.

► This study validates the use of PET in the identification of para-aortic lymph node metastasis when CT findings are negative. Perry Grigsby and colleagues from Washington University School of Medicine in St Louis have documented the prognostic impact of the findings on PET.

R. E. Coleman, MD

Positron Emission Mammography: Initial Clinical Results

Levine EA, Freimanis RI, Perrier ND, et al (Wake Forest Univ, Winston-Salem, NC; PEM Technologies Inc, Bethesda, Md; Seleon gmbh, Freiburg, Germany; et al)

Ann Surg Oncol 10:86-91, 2003 7–30

Background.—The detection of small cancers is one of the major goals of breast imaging, as it allows the initiation of treatment when the outlook is most favorable. It is useful to demonstrate the extent of such cancers for surgical planning and to identify other foci of tumor in the breast. However, these tasks cannot be reliably accomplished with mammography and US, primarily due to the limitation of conventional imaging to anatomical depictions. Functional imaging, as with PET, may permit the better characterization of mammographically occult disease, recognition of benign lesions, and detection of unsuspected tumors. Currently available PET devices are not well suited to the imaging of small breast cancers. However, positron emission mammography (PEM) could improve the imaging of these lesions. An initial experience with PEM in women scheduled for stereotactic breast biopsy was reported.

Methods.—A total of 16 patients were recruited from a surgical clinic. Patients were injected with 10 mCi of 2-^{18}F-FDG. One hour after injection, patients were positioned on the stereotactic biopsy table and imaged with a PEM scanner before the stereotactic biopsy was performed. Imaging findings were reviewed and compared with pathologic results.

Results.—A total of 18 lesions were imaged. PEM images were analyzed by drawing a region of interest at the biopsy site and comparing the count density in that region with the background. A lesion-to-background ratio of greater than 2.5 appeared to be a good indicator of malignancy, with a sensitivity of 86%, specificity of 91%, and overall diagnostic accuracy of 89% (Fig 4). There were no adverse events associated with PEM imaging.

Conclusion.—PEM is safe and feasible for imaging of small lesions in the breast and supports the further development of this imaging modality. In this

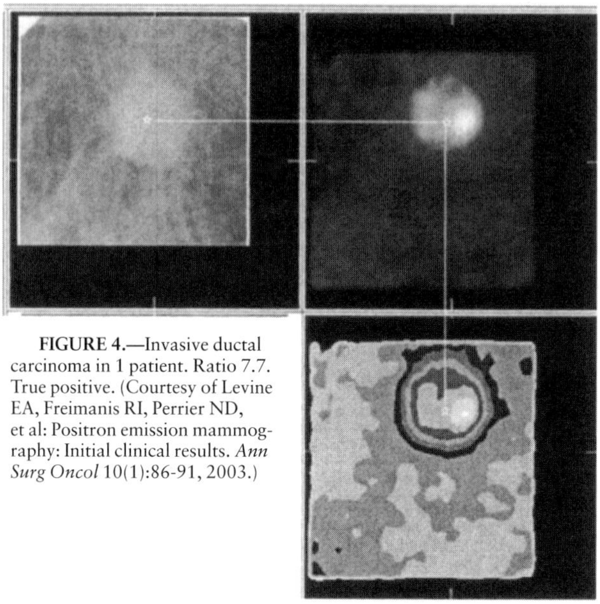

FIGURE 4.—Invasive ductal carcinoma in 1 patient. Ratio 7.7. True positive. (Courtesy of Levine EA, Freimanis RI, Perrier ND, et al: Positron emission mammography: Initial clinical results. *Ann Surg Oncol* 10(1):86-91, 2003.)

study, lesion-to-background ratios of greater than 2.5 were found to be a useful threshold value for the identification of positive (malignant) results.

▶ The best method for FDG imaging of the breast is still being evaluated. The authors use a device that is mounted on a stereotactic breast biopsy system for imaging the breast. A good diagnostic accuracy is shown in this study of selected patients. We are evaluating a different device. Our initial results have been quite good. PEM has the possibility of being able to detect lesions not seen on mammography.

R. E. Coleman, MD

Effect of Radioisotope Sentinel Node Mapping in Patients With cT1 N0 M0 Lung Cancer

Sugi K, Kaneda Y, Sudoh M, et al (Natl Sanyo Hosp, Ube, Yamaguchi, Japan; Yamaguchi Univ, Ube, Japan)

J Thorac Cardiovasc Surg 126:568-573, 2003 7–31

Background.—Application of the sentinel node concept to lung cancer is still controversial. Patients with peripheral small lung cancers would gain the most benefit from this concept, if it were valid. We sought to determine whether it is possible to choose between limited lymph node sampling and systematic lymphadenectomy from the distribution of sentinel lymph nodes in patients with node-negative disease on the basis of imaging.

Methods.—Sixty-five consecutive patients with cT1 N0 M0 non–small cell lung cancer were enrolled. A radioisotope tracer (4 mCi of technetium-

99m tin colloid, 2.0 mL) was injected in the vicinity of the tumor before surgical intervention with computed tomographic guidance. The radioactivity of each resected lymph node was measured separately with a hand-held gamma probe after complete tumor resection. Sentinel nodes were identified, and the accuracy of sentinel node mapping was examined. Whether the location of the sentinel node depended on the site of the primary tumor was also examined.

Results.—Of the 65 patients, 3 were excluded because of the final pathologic results. Successful radionuclide migration occurred in 39 (62.9%) of the 62 patients. There was 1 (2.6%) false-negative result among 39 patients with a sentinel node, and therefore the sensitivity was 90%, and the specificity was 100%. The most common sentinel lymph nodes were at level 12 (46.7%), followed by level 11 (18.3%), the mediastinum (16.7%), and level 10 (11.7%).

Conclusion.—The sentinel node concept is valid in patients with cT1 N0 M0 lung cancer. The lobar lymph nodes were identified as sentinel nodes more frequently than other lymph nodes. We need to make further efforts to increase the sentinel node identification rate. However, we believe that if sentinel nodes are identified, sentinel node mapping can allow the accurate intraoperative diagnosis of pathologic N0 status in patients with cT1 N0 M0 lung cancer.

► These authors demonstrate that intraoperative sentinel lymph node mapping is highly accurate in evaluating patients with stage 1 lung cancer. Because of the regulations in Japan related to rooms where radiopharmaceuticals can be administered, the radiopharmaceutical was not administered under CT guidance but was documented by CT after administration. This method of administration may have accounted for the somewhat low success rate of the procedure. The interest in sentinel node mapping continues to increase.

R. E. Coleman, MD

Sentinel Lymph Nodes With Technetium-99m Collodial Rhenium Sulfide in Patients With Esophageal Carcinoma

Kato H, Miyazaki T, Nakajima M, et al (Gunma Univ, Maebashi, Japan)

Cancer 98:932-939, 2003 7–32

Introduction.—The value of sentinel lymph node biopsy in breast carcinoma has been examined extensively, but there are few clinical studies of sentinel lymph nodes in patients with esophageal squamous cell carcinoma. The feasibility of using technetium-99m colloidal rhenium sulfide to detect sentinel lymph nodes was assessed in 25 consecutive patients with thoracic esophageal squamous cell carcinomas.

Methods.—Patients were 20 men and 5 women with a median age of 62 years. None had received preoperative treatment, and all were considered to have resectable disease. The day before radical esophagectomy, patients had technetium-99m colloidal rhenium sulfide injected into the submucosa at 4 sites around the primary tumor. Sentinel lymph nodes were defined as hot lymph nodes identified by 2 surgeons at the time of lymphoscintigraphy. After surgery, the lymph nodes were prepared for pathologic evaluation with cytokeratin (CK) staining.

Results.—Fifty-seven sentinel lymph nodes were detected in 23 (92%) patients (mean, 2.3 lymph nodes per patient). The accuracy of sentinel lymph nodes was 91.3%, the sensitivity was 86.7%, and the false-negative rate was 8.7%. The number of sentinel lymph nodes was significantly associated with tumor location, lymph node status, pathologic stage, and the number of metastatic lymph nodes. Patients with advanced tumor status had a greater number of sentinel lymph nodes. No correlation was found between the number of sentinel lymph nodes and histologic grade or patient gender. Occult metastasis was detected by CK staining in 56% of patients and in 1.7% of lymph nodes. The 2 patients with false-negative results on routine pathologic evaluation were found to have occult metastases. When CK staining was used, the accuracy of sentinel lymph node evaluation was 100%.

Conclusion.—Sentinel lymph node mapping was found to be a feasible technique in patients with esophageal squamous cell carcinoma. Accuracy is improved by analysis of the sentinel lymph nodes based on CK immunohistochemistry.

▶ I was unaware of the use of sentinel lymph node studies in esophageal carcinoma. The results look promising.

R. E. Coleman, MD

Lymphoscintigraphic Visualization of Internal Mammary Nodes With Subtumoral Injection of Radiocolloid in Patients With Breast Cancer

Shimazu K, Tamaki Y, Taguchi T, et al (Osaka Univ, Japan)

Ann Surg 237:390-398, 2003 7–33

Background.—Anatomic studies have shown retromammary lymphatic communication between the breast gland and the internal mammary basin as well as the axillary basin. Experience with sentinel lymph node (SLN) biopsy suggests that some lymph—particularly from the subtumoral parenchyma—drains into both the internal mammary and axillary nodes. Subtumoral radiocolloid injection was evaluated for its utility in lymphoscintigraphic visualization of the internal mammary nodes and SLN biopsy in women with breast cancer.

Methods.—Technetium-99m tin colloid was injected into various sites of the breast in 196 women with T1-2 N0 breast cancer on the day before surgery. Immediately before surgery, blue dye was injected. In 41 patients (group A), both radiocolloid and blue dye were injected peritumorally; 70 patients (group B) received periareolar radiocolloid and peritumoral blue dye; 45 patients (group C) received intradermal radiocolloid and periareolar blue dye; and 40 patients (group D) received subtumoral radiocolloid and intradermal blue dye. The authors compared (1) visualization of "hot spots"

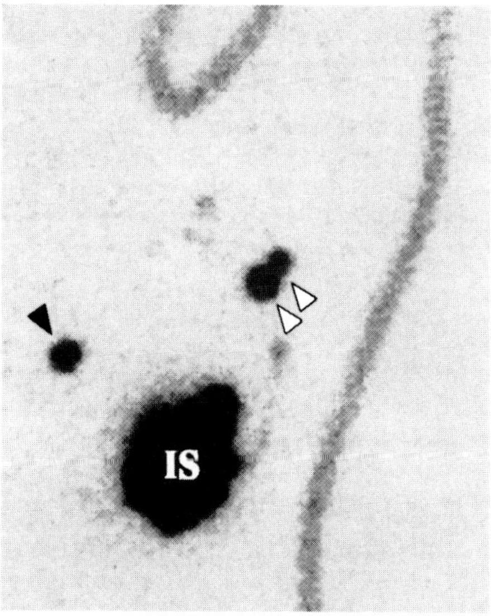

FIGURE 1.—Lymphoscintigram. Focal accumulations of radioactivity (not spots) are evident in both axillary (*white arrowheads*) and internal mammary (*black arrowhead*) basins. This patient with a tumor in the lower outer quadrant received radiocolloid injection into the subtumoral parenchyma. *Abbreviation: IS*, Injection site. (Courtesy of Shimazu K, Tamaki Y, Taguchi T, et al: Lymphoscintigraphic visualization of internal mammary nodes with subtumoral injection of radiocolloid in patients with breast cancer. *Ann Surg* 237 (3):390-398, 2003.)

in the internal mammary chain with the various methods of radiocolloid injection and (2) the concordance between blue-dye and radiocolloid visualization of axillary nodes in the 4 groups. In a separate analysis, findings from 1297 patients who had previously undergone extended radical mastectomy with internal mammary node dissection were reviewed to assess the relation between vertical tumor location (i.e., superficial vs. deep) and axillary and internal mammary node metastases.

Findings.—Lymphoscintigraphy showed "hot spots" in the internal mammary region in 2% of patients in group A, 4% in group B, 0% in group C and 38% in group D (Fig 1). The group D patients—who received subtumoral radiocolloid and intradermal blue dye—had a significantly lower concordance rate between the 2 techniques for detecting SLNs in the axillary basin. No patient in group D had the same SLN detected by both radiocolloid and blue dye. In the review of patients who underwent extended radical mastectomy, those with deep tumors were significantly more likely to have axillary and internal mammary metastases than were those with superficial tumors.

Conclusions.—A retromammary lymphatic pathway seems to exist between the deep portion of the breast and both the axillary and internal mammary lymphatic basins. This retromammary pathway seems to be separate from the superficial pathway. The findings indicate that in patients undergoing SLN biopsy, injecting radiocolloid in the subtumoral location in addition to other locations will enhance staging in both the axillary and internal mammary nodes.

► Studies are now showing that the injection technique can result in differences in the distribution of the radiopharmaceutical for identifying sentinel lymph nodes. These investigators found that a subtumoral and a more superficial injection was needed to identify both axillary and internal mammary lymph nodes.

R. E. Coleman, MD

Sequential Dermal-Peritumoral Radiocolloid Injection for Sentinel Node Biopsy for Breast Cancer: The University of Florida Experience

Feezor RJ, Kasraeian A, Copeland EM III, et al (Univ of Florida, Gainesville)

Am Surg 68:684-688, 2002 7–34

Background.—Sentinel lymph node (SLN) biopsy is quickly becoming the standard of care for patients with small breast tumors. The optimal radiocolloid injection technique, however, has yet to be identified. Reported is a single-institution experience with sequential dermal-peritumoral radiocolloid injection.

Methods.—The medical records of 118 patients who underwent SLN biopsy for clinical stage Tis, T1, T2, and N0 cancer were retrospectively reviewed. At 12 to 18 hours before surgery, 0.5 to 1.0 mCi 50:50 filtered/unfiltered technetium sulfur colloid was injected into the dermis overlying the tumor or 3- to 4-mCi of radiocolloid was injected peritumorally 30 minutes later. Dynamic lymphoscintigraphy was performed, and the topographic location of all imaged lymph nodes was marked on the skin. The following morning, a handheld gamma probe was used to identify and then remove all SLNs, which included all lymph nodes with radioactivity counts of 10% or more of the ex vivo count of the most radioactive SLN. Radioactive internal mammary (IM) nodes were noted but not removed.

Findings.—The SLN detection rate was 98.5% (3 IM nodes) for dermal injection, 83.3% (1 IM node) for peritumoral injection, and 100% (14 IM nodes) for sequential dermal-peritumoral injection ($P < .05$, dermal-peritumoral vs dermal).

Conclusions.—Sequential injection of 50:50 filtered/unfiltered technetium sulfur colloid preparation, first in the dermis over the tumor and then around the tumor, quickly and accurately labels SLNs, and the labeling persists until surgery the following morning. Identification of nonaxillary SLNs may allow more accurate breast cancer staging and may affect the delivery of IM node irradiation.

► Several different radiopharmaceuticals and injection techniques have been utilized in breast lymphoscintigraphy. This article describes using a mixture of filtered and unfiltered Tc-99m sulphur colloid and recommends a sequential dermal-peritumoral injection the day before surgery. I think that each facility needs to determine which radiopharmaceutical and injection technique works best for it.

R. E. Coleman, MD

Lymphoseek: A Molecular Radiopharmaceutical for Sentinel Node Detection

Wallace AM, Hoh CK, Vera DR, et al (Univ of California, San Diego, La Jolla)

Ann Surg Oncol 10:531-538, 2003 7–35

Background.—Lymphoseek (previously ^{99m}Tc-diethylenetriamine pentaacetic acid [DTPA]-mannosyl-dextran) is a new radiopharmaceutical that accumulates in lymphatic tissues by binding to a receptor on the surface of macrophages. This substance is composed of a dextran backbone to which multiple unites of mannose and DTPA are synthetically attached. The mannose units are substrates for receptor recognition and binding, and the DTPA units serve as attachment sites for labeling the macromolecule with ^{99m}Tc. Previous preclinical studies with Lymphoseek have shown that it possesses the properties needed for imaging of the sentinel lymph node. A phase 1 clinical trial compared Lymphoseek with filtered [^{99m}Tc] sulfur colloid (fTcSC) for detection of the sentinel lymph node in patients with breast cancer.

Methods.—A total of 12 women (age, 42-71 years) with breast cancer were randomly assigned to a 3-hour imaging protocol with peritumoral/subdermal injections (0.5 mCi) of either Lymphoseek or 0.2 μm of fTcSC. Serial images were then obtained from each patient for 180 minutes. Sentinel nodes were excised within 4.2 to 7.3 hours of administration and were assayed on a dose calibrator.

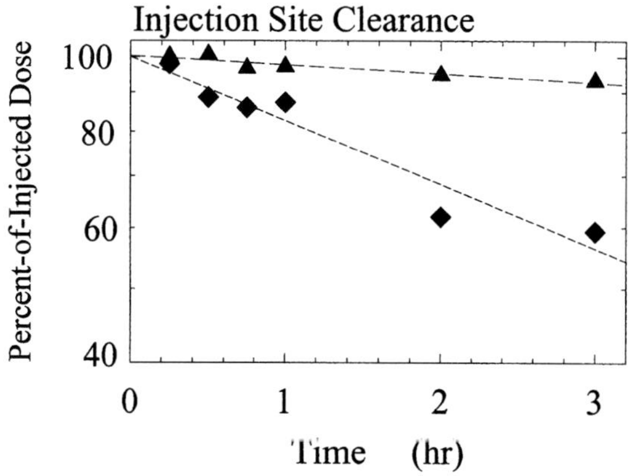

FIGURE 2.—Clearance of radioactivity from the injection site of 2 sentinel node cases. Lymphoseek (*diamond*, subject 2) exhibited a half-life of 3.23 ± 0.47 hours. Filtered [^{99m}Tc] sulfur colloid (*triangle*, subject 1) exhibited a half-life of 15.4 ± 5.10 hours. (Courtesy of Wallace AM, Hoh CK, Vera DR, et al: Lymphoseek: A molecular radiopharmaceutical for sentinel node detection. *Ann Surg Oncol* 10(5):531-538, 2003.)

Results.—Lymphoseek demonstrated a significantly faster rate of injection site clearance (Fig 2). The mean Lymphoseek clearance half-time was 2.72 ± 1.57 hours compared with 49.5 ± 38.5 hours for fTcSC. No difference was seen in the primary sentinel node uptake of Lymphoseek and fTcSC. However, Lymphoseek showed a lower mean number of sentinel nodes per study than did fTcSC and a higher concordance with Lymphazurin.

Conclusions.—Lymphoseek, a new molecular receptor-binding agent, demonstrated faster injection site clearance and equivalent primary sentinel node uptake in this comparison with fTcSC.

► Lymphoscintigraphy is being used widely for several malignancies, primarily of which are breast cancer and malignant melanomas. fTcSC has become the standard radiopharmaceutical that is used in most centers. This novel imaging agent may have some advantages over fTcSC. More data will need to be obtained to understand the potential role of this radiopharmaceutical as compared with the presently used pharmaceutical.

R. E. Coleman, MD

8 Musculoskeletal

Introduction

Radionuclide bone scanning is one of the most commonly performed procedures in most nuclear medicine departments. Single rib abnormalities are not uncommon on a radionuclide bone scan, and the best method for evaluating those abnormalities has not been clearly defined. Rib films have been particularly useless in my experience. Thin-section reformatted computed tomography does appear to be useful in characterizing these lesions.

FDG-PET is being utilized in the evaluation of musculoskeletal lesions. Although Medicare has not developed a policy for coverage of FDG-PET in musculoskeletal lesions, the data continues to build that PET is useful in certain circumstances.

R. Edward Coleman, MD

Solitary Hot Spots in the Ribs on Bone Scan: Value of Thin-Section Reformatted Computed Tomography to Exclude Radiography-Negative Fractures

Niitsu M, Takeda T (Univ of Tsukuba, Tennodai, Ibaraki, Japan)

J Comput Assist Tomogr 27:469-474, 2003 8–1

Objective.—For patients with extraskeletal cancers undergoing bone scanning, solitary hot spots in the ribs are a common finding. In many cases, it is difficult to tell whether these rib hot spots represent metastases. The use of thin-section, reformatted helical CT scans to exclude rib fractures in patients with solitary scintigraphic hot spots in the ribs was evaluated.

Methods.—The study included 47 patients with solitary hot spots in the ribs as their initial abnormal scintigraphic finding. All patients had known extraskeletal malignancies, most frequently involving the lung, breast, or urinary tract. In each case, the results of plain x-ray films were negative or indeterminate. Within 3 weeks after the suspicious bone scan result, helical CT scanning was performed, followed by creation of thin-section reformatted images. The appearance of these reformatted images was analyzed and compared with the patients' final outcomes, based on a mean follow-up of 20 months.

Results.—The final diagnosis was rib fracture in 17 cases, with CT findings including a transverse fracture line in 7 cases, a fracture line with focal

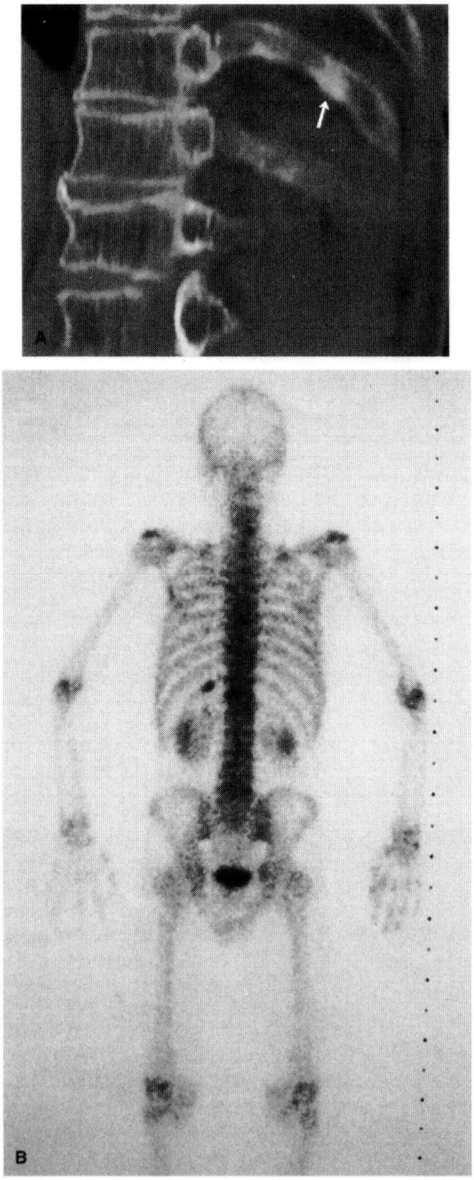

FIGURE 4.—A 72-year-old man with urinary bladder cancer. The reformatted CT demonstrates a fracture line with bulged cortex and internal sclerosis of the left eleventh posterior rib (*arrow*, **A**). A solitary hot spot at the left eleventh rib is demonstrated in a dorsal view of a whole-body scintigram (**B**). This rib deformity was classified as a fracture with callus formation. (Courtesy of Niitsu M, Takeda T: Solitary hot spots in the ribs on bone scan: Value of thin-section reformatted computed tomography to exclude radiography-negative fractures. *J Comput Assist Tomogr* 27(4):469-474, 2003.)

sclerosis in 2, and a fracture with callus formation in 8 (Fig 4). In these patients, the hot spots resolved on repeated bone scans. Intramedullary focal osteosclerosis was noted in 14 ribs, usually disappearing on repeated scans. Eight ribs showed no abnormalities, and all of these hot spots resolved. Four metastases were identified, showing bone destruction with mass formation or intramedullary osteolysis/osteosclerosis. Another 4 ribs showed intramedullary lesions with a cystic appearance, which was unchanged on follow-up scans.

Conclusions.—Thin-section, reformatted helical CT images are useful in demonstrating or excluding the presence of fractures in cancer patients with solitary scintigraphic hot spots in the ribs. The CT scans can show subtle fracture lines and cortical deformities where radiographs are normal. Used to exclude fractures in this common clinical situation, helical CT can play an important role in avoiding unnecessary additional tests.

▶ Solitary rib abnormalities are not uncommonly found on radionuclide bone imaging. The likelihood that a solitary rib abnormality is related to metastatic disease is 10% to 17%. We have found dedicated x-rays of the ribs to not be very helpful.

This study demonstrates the value of thin-section reformatted tomography to characterize the rib abnormalities. The thin-section reformatted helical CT depicted small, radiographically occult rib fractures by demonstrating fracture lines and cortical deformities. The helical CT did contribute to the differential diagnosis of these lesions; thus, this may be the best method for evaluating these abnormalities.

R. E. Coleman, MD

---

^{18}FDG PET Scanning of Benign and Malignant Musculoskeletal Lesions

Feldman F, van Heertum R, Manos C (Columbia Univ, New York; New York Presbyterian Hosp)

Skeletal Radiol 32:201-208, 2003 8–2

Background.—Since the development of clinical PET scanning in the 1990s, its use has expanded to include a variety of organ systems. However, the use of PET in musculoskeletal applications has not been extensively explored. ^{18}F-FDG is a favored metabolic tracer for clinical PET scanning. The technique, applications, and advantages of ^{18}FDG PET scanning were described in the detection, analysis, and management of musculoskeletal lesions.

Methods.—A total of 45 patients aged 9 to 81 years (19 males and 26 females) underwent radiography, routine radionuclide scanning, CT, or MRI of clinically suspected active benign or malignant musculoskeletal lesions. Region of interest (ROI) 3×3 pixel image analysis of transverse whole-body images with a slice thickness of 3.37 mm generated Maximum Standard Uptake Values (Max SUV). A cutoff of 2.0 was used to distinguish benign from malignant lesions.

Results.—SUV ROI analysis was performed in 39 studies. The overall sensitivity for differentiating malignant from benign osseous and nonosseous lesions was 91.7%, the overall specificity was 100%, and the accuracy was 91.7%. All the aggressive lesions had a Max SUV of greater than 2.0. The differences in data distinguishing benign from malignant lesions and aggressive from benign lesions were statistically significant. However, there was no statistically significant difference in distinguishing aggressive from malignant lesions.

Conclusions.—^{18}FDG PET provides unique information for evaluating the metabolism of musculoskeletal lesions. PET scanning for musculoskeletal lesions may prove to be cost-effective because residual, recurrent, or metastatic tumors can be documented simultaneously on a single whole-body scan.

▶ More data are needed on the utility of FDG PET scanning in the evaluation of musculoskeletal lesions. In this study, PET was quite accurate in differentiating benign from malignant lesions. We have seen positive PET scans in benign conditions such as Paget disease, fibrous dysplasia, enchondroma, and pigmented villonodular synovitis.

R. E. Coleman, MD

Prognostic Value of Bone Scan in Patients With Metastatic Prostate Cancer Treated Initially With Androgen Deprivation Therapy

Rigaud J, Tiguert R, Le Normand L, et al (CHU Hôtel Dieu, Nantes, France)
J Urol 168:1423-1426, 2002 8–3

Background.—Androgen deprivation therapy used as palliation for prostate cancer can control symptoms and prolong life. Whether the extent of disease seen on bone scans correlates with survival in men with prostate cancer metastases treated with androgen deprivation was investigated.

Methods.—Eighty-six patients with bone metastases were followed up from September 1988 to September 1999. All were treated initially with androgen deprivation alone. Medical records were reviewed for clinical, pathologic, and radiologic data. The patients were divided into 2 groups based on metastasis grade as seen on bone scans obtained at diagnosis: those with metastases on the axial skeleton (group 1) and those with bone metastases on the appendicular skeleton (group 2). Patients were also stratified according to Soloway and Crawford et al classifications.

Findings.—Groups 1 and 2 did not differ in patient age, biopsy Gleason score, serum prostate-specific antigen, or clinical stage. The median survival was 53 months in group 1 and 29 months in group 2. Survival was better among those with axial disease than among those with appendicular bone metastases. No differences among Soloway and Crawford et al strata were noted.

Conclusion.—Classifying bone scans according to axial or appendicular metastases is helpful for determining patient prognosis. Patients with axial metastases on the initial scan have a better prognosis than those with appendicular metastasis.

► The finding of a worse prognosis in patients who have appendicular involvement from metastatic prostate cancer has not been something that I have previously considered. In the 86 patients included in this study, 23 had appendicular involvement, and those patients with appendicular involvement had a significantly worse prognosis than those who had axial disease only.

R. E. Coleman, MD

Are Serial Bone Scans Useful for the Follow-up of Clinically Localized, Low to Intermediate Grade Prostate Cancer Managed With Watchful Observation Alone?

Yap BK, Choo R, Deboer G, et al (Univ of Toronto)

BJU Internatl 91:613-617, 2003 8–4

Background.—At the present time, no consensus exists as to how to monitor disease progression in patients with clinically localized prostate cancer (CLPC) who choose watchful observation. Bone scintigraphy is often used as 1 of the tools in this surveillance; however, the predictive value of serial bone scans for detection of the development of new bone metastasis has never been prospectively evaluated in patients with CLPC being managed by watchful observation. The predictive value of this approach was assessed in this population of patients with low to intermediate grade prostate cancer.

Methods.—This prospective, single-arm study assessed the feasibility of a watchful observation protocol with selective delayed intervention for patients with CLPC. All patients had stages T1b to T2bN0M0 cancer, a Gleason score of 7 or less, and a prostate-specific antigen (PSA) level of 15 ng/mL or less. All patients were managed expectantly as long as they did not meet predetermined criteria of clinical, histologic, or PSA progression. Bone scintigraphy was repeated every year for the first 2 years, then every 2 years thereafter if the patient continued to be treated with watchful observation. Patients with PSA levels greater than 15 ng/mL underwent bone scintigraphy every year.

Results.—A total of 224 patients were enrolled. A total of 449 bone scans (150 baseline and 299 in follow-up) were obtained over a median follow-up of 30 months. All 299 follow-up scan results were negative for bone metastasis. The true rate of positive follow-up bone scan results was estimated to be 0% to 1%. A total of 171 patients had at least 1 follow-up bone scan. Of these patients, 52% had 1 follow-up scan, 31% had 2 follow-up scans, 10% had 3 follow-up scans, 4.7% had 4 follow-up scans, and 2.3% had 5 or more follow-up scans. The PSA levels corresponding to all follow-up bone scans were 214 scans at PSA levels less than 10 ng/mL, 61 scans at levels of 10 to 14.9 ng/mL, 18 scans at levels of 15 to 19.9 ng/mL, and 6 scans at levels of 20 ng/mL or greater. The probability of a negative bone scan result was estimated at 88% to 100% when the PSA threshold of 15 ng/mL was used.

Conclusions.—This study found that the probability of positive findings on serial bone scans in untreated, localized, low to intermediate grade prostate cancer was low when the follow-up PSA level remained less than 15 ng/mL. Omitting bone scans in these patients would provide significant cost savings and would reduce the psychological and physical burden of disease. However, the role of serial bone scintigraphy for patients with follow-up PSA levels of more than 15 ng/mL remains undefined and in need of further study.

► The role of bone scans in patients with prostate cancer continues to be evaluated. In patients who have localized and low to intermediate grade prostate cancer and a PSA level less than 15 ng/mL, bone scans do not detect metastatic disease. It has been demonstrated in some studies that a positive bone scan was very likely in men when the pretreatment PSA level was less than 10 ng/mL; however, in other studies, the pretreatment PSA level was even 20 ng/mL. Recent data suggest that the rate of change of the PSA level may be a better predictor of metastatic disease than is the absolute value.

R. E. Coleman, MD

Pelvic Insufficiency Fracture After Pelvic Irradiation in Uterine Cervix Cancer

Huh SJ, Kim B, Kang MK, et al (Sungkyunkwan Univ, Seoul, Korea)
Gynecol Oncol 86:264-268, 2002 8–5

Background.—The advent of megavoltage has helped to reduce the incidence of osseous complications after pelvic irradiation. However, pelvic insufficiency fractures remain an important late complication. The incidence of pelvic insufficiency fractures is unknown in patients being treated with irradiation for cervical cancer and endometrial carcinoma, but several recent studies have reported an incidence of symptomatic pelvic fractures of 3% to 6%. Because these fractures are uncommon and frequently misinterpreted, the clinical features of pelvic insufficiency fractures were investigated.

Methods.—Clinical examinations were performed in 463 patients treated between 1994 and 2000 for uterine cervix cancer. All patients had been treated with 10 or 15 mV photons and 50.4 to 55.8 Gy in 28 fractions with adjuvant intent (235 patients) in addition to high-dose-rate brachytherapy (24 Gy in 6 fractions) for curative treatment (228 patients). The median follow-up was 38 months.

Results.—A total of 8 patients (1.7%) had pelvic insufficiency fractures 7 to 19 months after treatment (Fig 1). Of these patients, 7 were treated with curative intent, and 1 was treated with adjuvant intent. All the patients were postmenopausal and complained of moderate to severe pelvic pain (Fig 2). The pain resolved after 1 to 11 months with conservative therapy. Two patients also had radiation proctitis.

Conclusions.—In women who have been treated with radiotherapy for cervical cancer and who subsequently report pain, bony destruction and

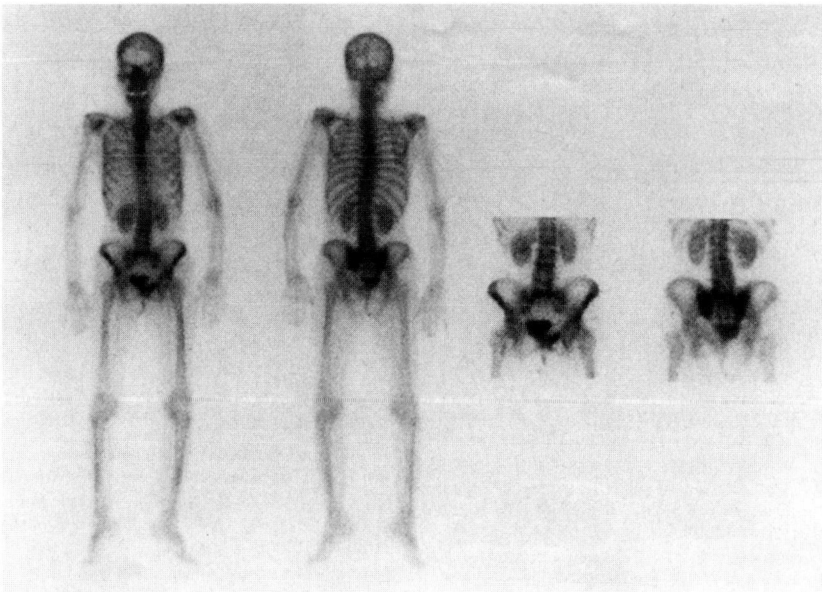

FIGURE 1.—Bone scan showing the H-shaped sacral fracture and hot uptake on left pubic ramus. (Reprinted by permission of the publisher, courtesy of Huh SJ, Kim B, Lee JE, et al: Pelvic insufficiency fracture after pelvic irradiation in uterine cervix cancer. *Gynecol Oncol* 86:264-268. Copyright 2002 by Elsevier Science Inc.)

fractures may be indicative of a late radiation effect rather than osseous metastasis. Pelvic insufficiency fractures are more commonly seen in patients treated with curative intent rather than in those who undergo radiotherapy as a postoperative adjuvant therapy.

► Pelvic insufficiency fractures are often difficult to differentiate from metastatic disease. The bone scan shows increased activity in both metastases and insufficiency fractures. The radiographic findings may be identical between the 2 processes. These fractures may occur from osteopenia alone but seem to be more frequent in patients who have had pelvic irradiation. A biopsy may be misleading in these patients. The clinical and imaging findings should be taken in concert to determine the cause of the abnormalities.

R. E. Coleman, MD

A
B
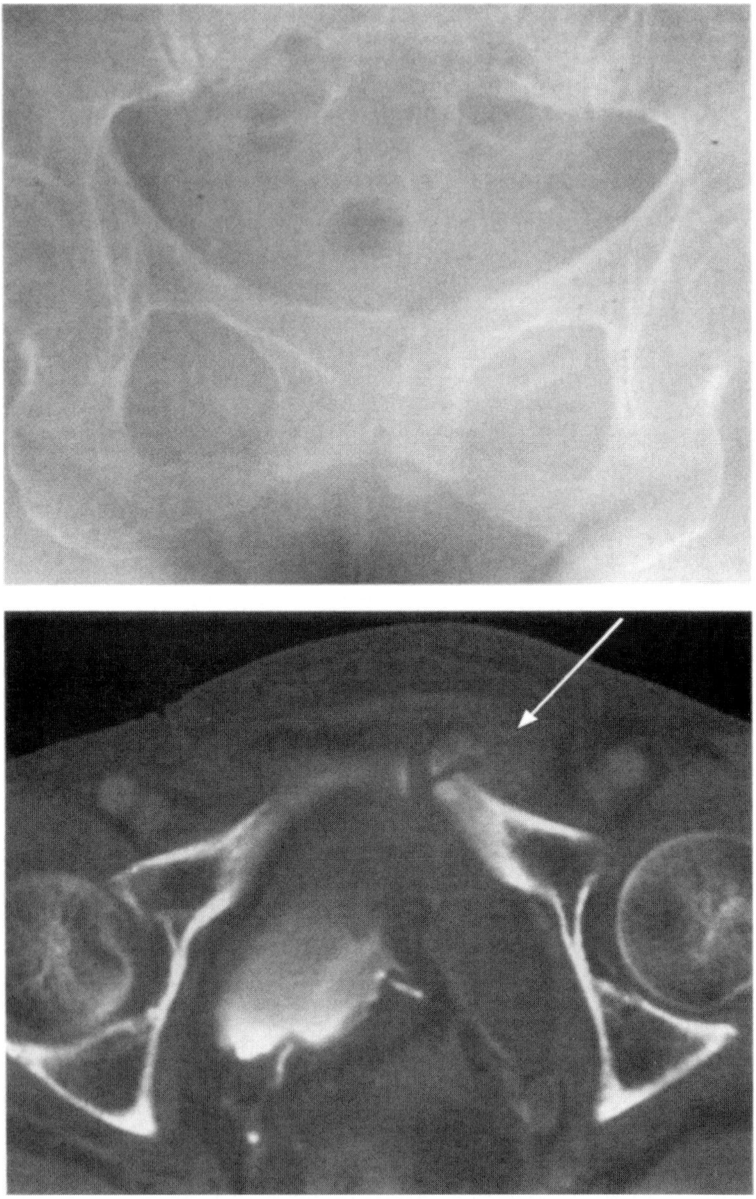

FIGURE 2.—A, Plain pelvic radiograph 16 months after radiotherapy shows a fracture, sclerosis, and fragmentation of the left pubic bone. B, CT scan of the pelvis showing fracture line and surrounding callus formation on left superior pubic ramus. (Reprinted by permission of the publisher, courtesy of Huh SJ, Kim B, Lee JE, et al: Pelvic insufficiency fracture after pelvic irradiation in uterine cervix cancer. *Gynecol Oncol* 86:264-268. Copyright 2002 by Elsevier Science Inc.)

Metastatic Breast Carcinoma to Bone Disguised by Osteopoikilosis
Kennedy JG, Donahue JR, Aydin H, et al (Weil Cornell Med School, New York)
Skeletal Radiol 32:240-243, 2003 8–0

Background.—Osteopoikilosis is a rare osteosclerotic bone dysplasia with typical radiographic features of sclerotic densities in multiple foci throughout the axial and appendicular skeleton. Osteopoikilosis is asymptomatic, with unaltered bone chemistry; the distinctive radiographic findings are usually diagnostic. Diagnosis of osseous metastases is made not only on the basis of radiologic appearance but also on clinical symptoms supported by biochemical parameters. In breast cancer cases, up to 70% of metastases are skeletal. Bony metastases from primary breast carcinoma may be lytic, blastic, or of mixed radiologic appearance. Bone scintigraphy will show an increased uptake with both osteoblastic and osteoclastic activity. In addition, the changes in bony metabolism will be evident as altered biochemical profiles. A case in which there were none of these diagnostic features was presented.

Case Report.—Woman, 59, with a history of lobular breast carcinoma was seen by the orthopaedic service for evaluation of possible bony metastasis. The patient had been on a 3-month course of chemotherapy before presentation and was considered to be in remission from primary breast disease. The patient was asymptomatic. A radiograph of the pelvis showed multiple well-circumscribed sclerotic lesions throughout the pelvic and vertebrae. CT showed a similar pattern without evidence of bony destruction. Technetium bone scan showed no increase in uptake by multiple lesions. The patient had no systemic symptoms and had normal blood parameters. An iliac crest bone biopsy indicated metastatic disease in addition to osteopoikilosis.

Conclusions.—As demonstrated by this case report, current imaging techniques may not be capable of distinguishing metastatic bone cancer in the setting of preexisting osteopoikilosis. In such cases, the final diagnosis can only be made histologically after core biopsy.

► We need to keep in mind the limitations of bone scans. An interesting case with 2 bone diseases, neither of which was detected by bone imaging.

R. E. Coleman, MD

Prospective Two Year Follow Up Study Comparing Novel and Conventional Imaging Procedures in Patients With Arthritic Finger Joints

Backhaus M, Burmester GR, Sandrock D, et al (Humboldt Univ of Berlin)

Ann Rheum Dis 61:895-904, 2002 8–7

Background.—The treatment options for patients with rheumatoid arthritis (RA) now include targeted treatments that halt clinical progression of the disease and the process of joint destruction. These newer and more expensive treatments are greatly dependent on the early and reliable diagnosis of RA. Conventional radiography is the current standard imaging technique for detection and quantification of destructive joint processes in arthritis, although its sensitivity limits utility in demonstrating early arthritic joint lesions. US and MRI are alternative imaging modalities for demonstrating early arthritis.

This study is the first long-term investigation comparing conventional radiography, 3-phase bone scintigraphy, US, and 3-dimensional MRI with precontrast and dynamic postcontrast examination in the detection of early arthritis. The purpose of the follow-up study was to use different modalities to monitor the course of erosions during treatment with disease-modifying antirheumatic drugs and to determine whether the radiographically occult changes by MRI and US in the initial study would manifest on conventional radiographs 2 years later.

Methods.—The initial study included 49 patients with various forms of arthritis. The metacarpophalangeal, proximal interphalangeal, and distal interphalangeal joints (for a total of 14 joints) of the more severely affected hand as determined in the first study of 49 patients were examined twice. The follow-up study divided the patients into 2 groups and included 2 examinations. Follow-up group I included 28 subjects (392 joints) without radiographic signs of destructive arthritis (Larsen grades 0 to 1) of the investigated hand and wrist. Group II served as the control group and included 21 patients (294 joints) with radiographs showing erosions (Larsen grade 2) of the investigated hand or wrist, or both, at the initial examination.

Results.—Radiography at 2 years detected only 2 erosions in 2 patients in group I and 10 additional erosions in 9 patients in group II. The initial MRI had already detected both erosions in group I and 7 of the 10 erosions in group II. Initial US had detected 1 erosion in group I and 4 of the 10 erosions in group II. Thus, 3-dimensional MRI and US demonstrated an increase in erosions compared with the initial investigation. Both groups showed significant clinical improvement in synovitis and tenosynovitis, which was also evident on MRI and US. There was a significant difference between the decrease in soft tissue lesions as demonstrated by clinical findings, MRI, and US and the significant increase in erosive bone lesions, which were evident mainly on MRI and US.

Conclusion.—In patients with RA of the finger joints, erosive bone lesions were increased at 2-year follow-up despite clinical improvement and a regression of inflammatory soft tissue lesions. These findings suggest that conventional radiography alone has limitations in the intermediate-term follow-up of treatment. US is highly sensitive for the detection of inflammatory soft tissue lesions; however, dynamic 3-dimensional MRI is more sensitive in the differentiation of minute erosions.

► There appears to be a renewed interest in the use of radionuclide bone imaging for evaluating arthritis. In this study, radionuclide bone imaging was found to be a good screening modality, but its low specificity resulted in its not being suitable for the detection of early erosions. We are now doing a study evaluating various imaging modalities for the detection of knee osteoarthritis.

R. E. Coleman, MD

FDG PET Imaging Guided Re-evaluation of Histopathologic Response in a Patient With High-Grade Sarcoma

Vernon CB, Eary JF, Rubin BP, et al (Univ of Washington, Seattle)
Skeletal Radiol 32:139-142, 2003 8–8

Background.—Before chemotherapy, FDG PET is used to assess the metabolic activity of intermediate- to high-grade soft tissue sarcomas. MRI and FDG PET are then repeated after chemotherapy to determine response to treatment. The authors of this study recently encountered a patient with discrepant findings between the final histologic diagnosis and PET results. This case was described.

Case Report.—Man, 55, diagnosed as having a pleomorphic intermediate-grade sarcoma, underwent 3 cycles of neoadjuvant chemotherapy. During treatment, the patient's pain resolved, and tumor size decreased significantly. Pathologic analysis indicated a 95% response. However, the PET scan result indicated a 15% reduction in maximum standardized uptake variable. This discrepancy prompted a reevaluation of the gross specimen compared with the FDG PET images. Reexamination revealed a peripheral nodule, which correlated with the FDG PET focus of high tumor uptake and minimal re-

TABLE 1.—^{18}F-FDG PET Standardized Uptake Variable (*SUV*) results. Region A, tumor peripheral nodule, the region of greatest FDG uptake (value reflects reported maximum SUV); region B, tumor region excluding peripheral nodule (value reflects maximum SUV for this area); region C, full tumor region (value reflects average SUV over this area)

	Tumor Region A	Tumor Region B	Tumor Region C
Baseline	14.2	6.2	3.2
Post-chemotherapy cycle 2	12.4	3.1	2.9
Pre-resection	12.0	2.5	2.5
%SUV response	15	60	22

(Courtesy of Vernon CB, Eary JF, Rubin BP, et al: FDG PET imaging guided re-evaluation of histopathologic response in a patient with high-grade sarcoma. *Skeletal Radiol* 32:139-142, 2003.)

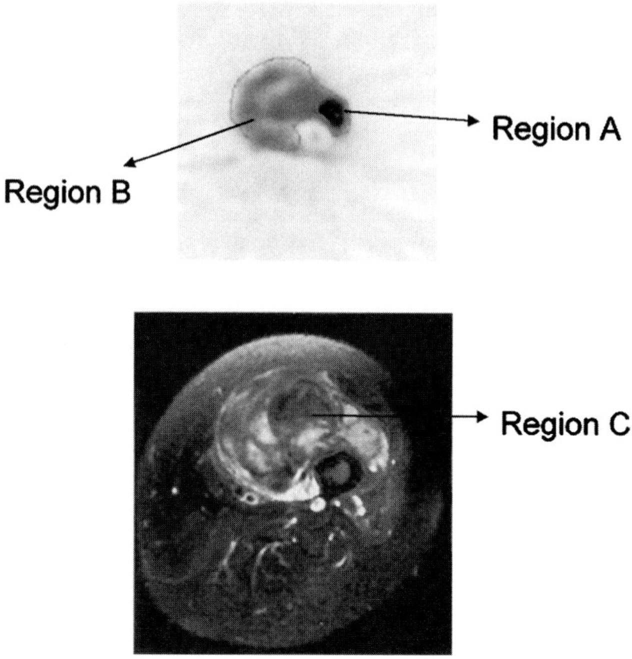

FIGURE 3.—PET scan and MR images identifying the corresponding regions in Table 1. *Region A*, tumor peripheral nodule, the region of greatest FDG uptake (value reflects the reported maximum standardized uptake variable (SUV_{max}); *region B*, tumor region excluding the peripheral nodule (value reflects SUV_{max} for this area); *region C*, full tumor region (value reflects average SUV over this area). (Courtesy of Vernon CB, Eary JF, Rubin BP, et al: FDG PET imaging guided re-evaluation of histopathologic response in a patient with high-grade sarcoma. *Skeletal Radiol* 32:139-142, 2003. Copyright, Springer-Verlag.)

sponse. Histologic evaluation of sections of this nodule demonstrated viable tumor with no treatment effect (Table 1 and Fig 3).

Conclusion.—In this patient, discrepant results between the final histologic diagnosis and percent change in maximum standardized uptake variable prompted further investigation. The discrepancy was attributed to the heterogeneity of the tumor and its response to treatment. Thus, FDG PET imaging plays an important role in the assessment of tumor metabolic activity and response to neoadjuvant chemotherapy in patients with sarcomas.

► FDG PET imaging is used to follow the effect of therapy in several cancers. Janet Eary and colleagues at the University of Washington have had extensive experience using FDG PET in sarcoma. This case report describes a discordancy in the PET results and pathologic findings. However, with further reviewing of PET scans and pathologic specimens, the discordancy was found to be related to the tumor heterogeneity.

R. E. Coleman, MD

Carbon-11 Choline Positron Emission Tomography in Musculoskeletal Tumors: Comparison With Fluorine-18 Fluorodeoxyglucose Positron Emission Tomography

Yanagawa T, Watanabe H, Inoue T, et al (Gunma Univ, Maebashi, Japan)
J Comput Assist Tomogr 27:175-182, 2003 8–9

Background.—FDG is used as a tracer in PET for various kinds of neoplasms. FDG PET has been used in musculoskeletal tumor systems to detect metastatic and recurrent tumors, to evaluate the effects of chemotherapy, to grade tumor malignancy, and to differentiate malignant from benign lesions. A new tracer, carbon-11 choline, has recently been introduced in oncology investigations using PET. However, the role of choline PET in musculoskeletal tumor evaluation has not been investigated. The utility of choline PET was compared with that of FDG PET in the evaluation of musculoskeletal tumors.

Methods.—The study included 33 patients who were evaluated with both choline PET and FDG PET. Standardized uptake values (SUVs) were used for evaluation of the lesions. Receiver operating characteristic (ROC) curve analysis was used to determine the appropriate cutoff value and compare the 2 PET studies. The binomial test was used to compare the sensitivities between choline PET and FDG PET.

Results.—A significant correlation was noted between choline PET and FDG PET for all lesions (Fig 1). The mean SUVs for malignant tumors were significantly higher that those for benign lesions in both choline PET and FDG PET. When a cutoff value of 2.7 was used for choline SUVs, the sensitivity for correctly diagnosing malignancy was 92.3%, with a specificity of

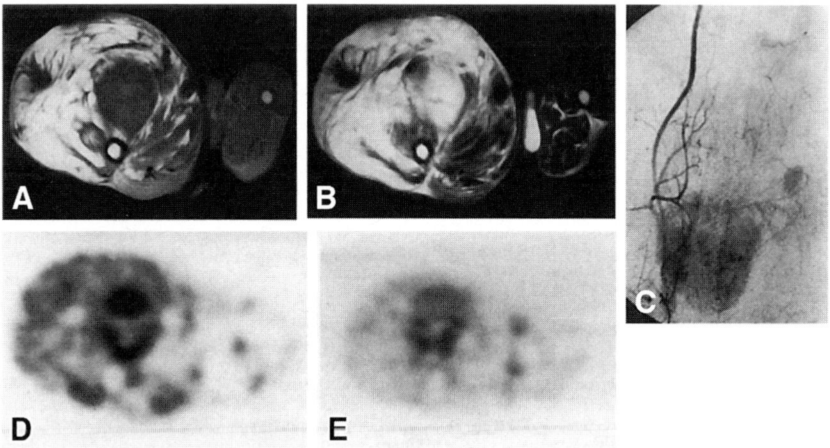

FIGURE 1.—An 83-year-old man (lesion 9) with liposarcoma in his right thigh. T1-weighted (**A**) and T2-weighted (**B**) magnetic resonance images. Angiography (**C**), choline positron emission tomography (PET) (**D**) and fluorine-18 fluoro-2-deoxy-D-glucose PET (**E**) analyses. (Courtesy of Yanagawa T, Watanabe H, Inoue T, et al: Carbon-11 choline positron emission tomography in musculoskeletal tumors: Comparison with fluorine-18 fluorodeoxyglucose positron emission tomography. *J Comput Assist Tomogr* 27:175-182, 2003.)

90% and an accuracy rate of 90.9%. With the use of a cutoff value of 3.3% for SUVs in FDG PET, the sensitivity was 84.6% with a specificity of 80%, for an accuracy rate of 81.8%. The ROC curve analyses showed that the mean area under the curve of choline PET was significantly greater than that for FDG PET. No significant difference was seen in sensitivity and specificity between choline PET and FDG PET analysis, using either the binomial test or the McNemar test.

Conclusions.—These findings suggest that choline PET may not be inferior to FDG PET for the differentiation of malignant from benign musculoskeletal tissues. Choline PET had several advantages, including a shorter examination time and little retention in the bladder. Thus, choline PET may be useful for preoperative planning for musculoskeletal tumors, particularly for lesions around the hip joints.

► Carbon-11 choline and F-18 fluorocholine are being evaluated in several different malignancies. Choline is incorporated into cell membranes, and previous studies have demonstrated both carbon-11 choline and F-18 fluorocholine studies are more sensitive than FDG in detecting metastatic prostate cancer.

A limitation of FDG PET imaging is its accumulation in inflammatory processes. It appears from the results of this study that C-11 choline may have less accumulation in inflammatory processes, such as sarcoidosis. More data are needed.

R. E. Coleman, MD

9 Inflammation and Infection

Introduction

Gallium-67 citrate and white blood cells labeled with In-111 or Tc-99m have been the mainstay of the nuclear medicine imaging techniques for the detection of infection and inflammation. New techniques are becoming available. FDG is being utilized in evaluation of infectious and inflammatory processes, and the role of FDG-PET imaging is still being determined. The initial results appear to be promising in specific circumstances.

Granulocyte scintigraphy with labeled antibodies is starting to appear more in the literature, and the initial results appear promising. We still need more studies to document the efficacy of this new technology.

R. Edward Coleman, MD

Uptake of ^{18}Fluorodeoxyglucose in the Cystic Fibrosis Lung: A Measure of Lung Inflammation?

Labiris NR, Nahmias C, Freitag AP, et al (McMaster Univ, Hamilton, Ont, Canada)

Eur Respir J 21:848-854, 2003 9–1

Introduction.—^{18}FDG PET has been widely used to assess cellular energy metabolism in studies of cancer and neurologic and cardiac disease. Relatively few studies have assessed its use in the lung. Various lung diseases involve an inflammatory process, particularly involving neutrophils. The use of FDG PET to assess neutrophil activation, and thus inflammation, in the lungs of patients with cystic fibrosis was assessed.

Methods.—Ten adult CF patients with chronic pulmonary *Pseudomonas aeruginosa* infection were studied. All received a bolus IV injection of ^{18}FDG, followed by a 90-minute dynamic acquisition over the midsternal region of the lung. Uptake of ^{18}FDG in the right lung was evaluated by using a Patlak plot, then converted into glucose utilization values. The scans were repeated after a 28-day course of inhaled tobramycin therapy in 8 patients.

Results.—The patients' mean baseline sputum neutrophil level was 14 × 10^6 cells/mL. Of these, 7 patients had a normal or slightly reduced pulmonary glucose utilization rate. The mean rate was 1.33 μmol/g/h, compared with 2.82 μmol/g/h in 3 controls with clinically inactive sarcoidosis. Tobramycin therapy resulted in no change in pulmonary glucose utilization or sputum neutrophil count.

Conclusions.—This FDG PET study found no evidence of increased lung glucose utilization in patients with CF, despite their elevated sputum neutrophil levels. Thus, FDG PET does not appear to be a useful tool for assessment and monitoring of pulmonary inflammation in CF.

► The accumulation of FDG in inflammatory processes in patients who have malignancy is considered false-positive accumulation. This "false-positive" accumulation might be a way to diagnose inflammatory disease. Preliminary studies in small numbers of patients suggest that it might be useful in detecting abscesses, active osteomyelitis, and infections in total joint prostheses.

In this study of patients with cystic fibrosis and high sputum neutrophil levels, lung glucose utilization was not increased. The results were not those that were anticipated by the authors, and I am also surprised by these results. It seems to me that inflammatory lung disease does have more FDG accumulation than normal lung.

R. E. Coleman, MD

Clinical Value of Gallium-67 Scintigraphy in Assessment of Disease Activity in Wegener's Granulomatosis

Slart RHJA, Jager PL, Poot L, et al (Groningen Univ, The Netherlands)

Ann Rheum Dis 62:659-662, 2003 9–2

Background.—The cause of Wegener's granulomatosis (WG) is unknown. WG is characterized by necrotizing vasculitis and granulomatous lesions that primarily affect the upper and lower respiratory tract. The diagnosis of active pulmonary and paranasal involvement in patients with WG can be difficult. Antineutrophil cytoplasmic antibodies (ANCAs) directed against proteinase-3 or myeloperoxidase in plasma are considered to be a useful tool for diagnosis of WG; however, the presence of these antibodies is not strictly related to disease activity. Gallium-67 (^{67}Ga) scintigraphy is commonly used in the detection of malignant lymphoma or inflammatory lesions such as sarcoidosis. The diagnostic value of gallium-67 scintigraphy in patients with WG with suspected granulomatous inflammation of the paranasal and chest regions was evaluated.

Methods.—This retrospective study evaluated the diagnostic contribution of chest and head planar gallium scans in 40 cases of suspected vasculitis disease activity in 28 patients with WG. Scans were classified as showing normal or increased uptake for each region. The gold standard for the presence of WG activity was histologic proof or response to treatment.

Results.—WG activity was confirmed in 8 cases (20%), with pulmonary locations in 3 cases, paranasal location in 4 cases, and both locations in 1 case (Fig 2). Gallium scans showed an increase in gallium uptake in all of

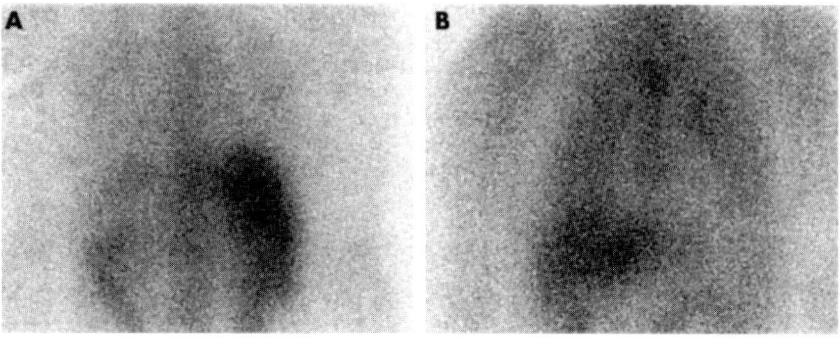

FIGURE 2.—Gallium scan; anterior chest view of normal uptake in a patient without WG activity (**A**) and increased uptake (**B**) in a patient with active WG. Active WG in the lung was histologically proved in the patient shown in **B**. (Courtesy of Slart RHJA, Jager PL, Poot L, et al: Clinical value of gallium-67 scintigraphy in assessment of disease activity in Wegener's granulomatosis. *Ann Rheum Dis* 62:659-662, 2003. BMJ Publishing Group.)

these patients (sensitivity 100%). Gallium scans were negative for the pulmonary area in 23 of 36 scans (specificity 64%) and negative for paranasal activity in 13 of 16 scans (specificity 81%) in episodes without WG activity. The positive predictive value of WG activity for the lungs and paranasal region was 24% and 63%, respectively, and the negative predictive value was 100% for both regions. False-positive findings were caused by bacterial or viral infections.

Conclusions.—This study found gallium scans to be clinically useful in assessing disease activity in Wegener's granulomatosis because a negative scan virtually excludes active WG. Gallium scintigraphy of the chest and nasal region has a high sensitivity for the detection of disease activity in WG; however, specificity was lower because of positive scans in cases of bacterial or viral infections.

► The number of gallium scans that we perform at our institution has decreased dramatically over the last several years. This decrease has primarily resulted because FDG imaging has replaced gallium imaging in lymphoma. We have not performed gallium imaging for the detection of inflammatory processes recently.

This article reminds me of previous work that we and others did to show that gallium was able to determine the activity of pulmonary disease in sarcoidosis.

R. E. Coleman, MD

Noninvasive Assessment of Crohn's Disease Activity: A Comparison of ^{18}F-Fluorodeoxyglucose Positron Emission Tomography, Hydromagnetic Resonance Imaging, and Granulocyte Scintigraphy With Labeled Antibodies

Neurath MF, Vehling D, Schunk K, et al (Univ of Mainz, Germany)
Am J Gastroenterol 97:1978-1985, 2002 9–3

Objectives.—Detection of disease activity in Crohn's disease (CD) is of crucial importance for diagnosis and management of the disease. Noninvasive methods for monitoring are desirable and comprise hydromagnetic resonance imaging (hydro-MRI) and leukocyte scintigraphy. In addition, a recent case report indicated the potential of FDG-PET to assess CD activity. However, comparative prospective studies are lacking.

Methods.—Between February, 1999 and August, 2000, 59 patients with CD were enrolled in a prospective study to assess disease activity by FDG-PET, hydro-MRI, and immunoscintigraphy with anti-nonspecific cross-reacting antigen 95 antigranulocyte antibodies. In 28 of these patients, colonoscopy could be performed. Twelve patients with irritable bowel syndrome and 20 tumor patients without gut inflammation served as controls. Results were compared by statistical analysis.

Results.—FDG-PET detected 127 pathological findings (average maximum standardized uptake value = 4.4 ± 1.1) in the terminal/neoterminal ileum (37), small bowel (24), and colon (66) of 54 patients with CD, whereas no pathological findings were seen in five patients with CD, the control patients with irritable bowel syndrome, and the tumor patients without gut inflammation. In contrast, examination with hydro-MRI or granulocyte antibodies detected less pathological findings in CD patients. Forty-five of the detected foci were accessible to endoscopic verification. The correlation of the foci with endoscopic findings showed a high specificity (>89%) of all three methods to detect inflamed areas in the terminal ileum and colon of patients with CD, although analyses by hydro-MRI and granulocyte antibody scan had strikingly lower sensitivities (40.9% and 66.7%) than FDG-PET analysis (85.4%).

Conclusions.—FDG-PET appears to be a reliable noninvasive tool for simultaneous detection of inflamed areas in the small and large bowel of patients with CD. FDG-PET can be used to detect disease activity in the terminal ileum and colon of CD patients with high sensitivity and specificity.

► An area of potential utilization of FDG PET is in evaluating inflammatory processes. Very few data are in the literature on the use of FDG PET in inflammatory processes. This study demonstrates the superiority of FDG imaging over MRI and granulocyte antibody scanning in the detection of active inflammatory disease in CD. Further studies will be needed to determine whether FDG PET can monitor disease activity in these patients.

R. E. Coleman, MD

LeukoScan for Imaging Infection in Different Clinical Settings: A Retrospective Evaluation and Extended Review of the Literature

Gratz S, Schipper ML, Dörner J, et al (Philipps Univ, Marburg, Germany; Georg August Univ, Göttingen, Germany; Dept of Nuclear Medicine, Stuttgart, Germany)

Clin Nucl Med 28:267-276, 2003 9–4

Background.—The use of radiolabeled autologous leukocytes has provided the gold standard for nuclear medicine imaging of patients with infection. However, demand is increasing for novel imaging techniques for mixed patient populations who do not have sufficient clinical signs and symptoms to establish a diagnosis. The current study determined the overall diagnostic accuracy of ^{99m}Tc-labeled antigranulocyte monoclonal antibody Fab' fragments (LeukoScan) for routinely detecting bone and soft tissue infections.

Methods.—The study included 138 patients with fever of unknown origin and possible endocarditis, infection of arthroplastic joints, arthritis, peripheral and central bone infections, soft tissue infection, appendicitis, pericarditis, or vascular graft infection. Imaging was done after injection of 555 to 925 Mbq ^{99m}Tc-labeled antigranulocyte monoclonal antibody Fab' fragments.

Findings.—Imaging results were true positive in 63 of 81 lesions. Overall, the sensitivity was 76% and the specificity was 84%. In patients with arthritis, all 7 foci were detected. Results were false-negative in 3 of 9 infections of the femoral bone and in 3 of 8 periprosthetic infections of long bones. Good

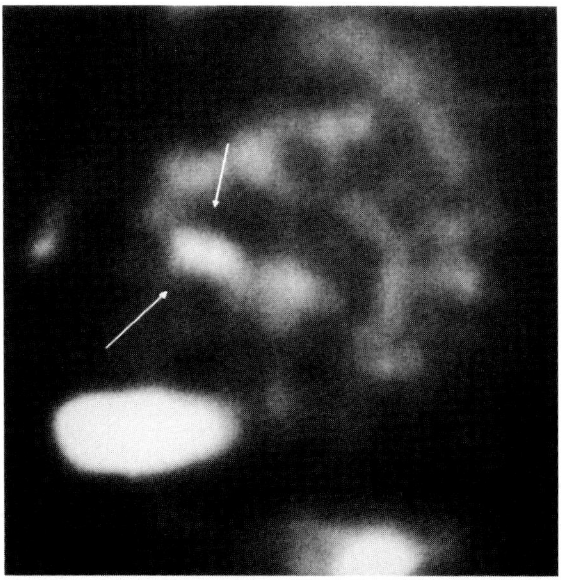

FIGURE 1.—A 56-year-old patient had endocarditis of the mechanical aortic prosthetic valve. (Courtesy of Gratz S, Schipper ML, Dörner J, et al: LeukoScan for imaging infection in different clinical settings: A retrospective evaluation and extended review of the literature. *Clin Nucl Med* 28(4):267-276, 2003.)

results were documented in 5 of 6 soft tissue infections, 4 of 6 endocarditis cases, 3 of 4 atypical cases of appendicitis, 2 of 2 infected vascular grafts, and the case of pericarditis (Fig 1). In all 8 patients with subacute and chronic infections of the spine, photopenic regions were seen. Including photopenic lesions in the diagnostic criteria resulted in an 88% sensitivity and a 67% specificity.

Conclusion.—Acute infections of peripheral bones and soft tissues can be imaged using ^{99m}Tc-labeled antigranulocyte monoclonal antibody Fab' fragments. The false-negative rate is high in patients with chronic infections. Including photopenic lesions in the spine as diagnostic, criteria for localizing disease increases the sensitivity but decreases the specificity of this imaging technique.

▶ We are still searching for a better agent for imaging infection. Gallium-67 citrate and leukocyte imaging have assumed a role in detection of infection. However, these agents certainly have their limitations. It is not clear to me that this agent has any advantages over the agents that we are presently utilizing.

R. E. Coleman, MD

10 Endocrinology

Introduction

PET imaging is having a profound impact on all of nuclear medicine. Its greatest utilization has been in malignancy, but there is increasing work on potential uses in benign disease. The use of PET for evaluating the thyroid was recently approved by the Center for Medical Services under rather restricted conditions. PET imaging is reimbursed in thyroid cancer for patients with rising thyroglobulin and negative ^{131}I scans. It seems likely that these indications will be expanded in the light of increasing numbers of studies supporting the role of PET in thyroid disease. I have included several PET articles in this issue of the YEAR BOOK that evaluate thyroid nodules, differentiation of benign from malignant thyroid disease and the use of PET in dosimetry. The other major growth area in thyroid disease is the use of recombinant human TSH, which is being intensively studied for its role in the preparation of patients with thyroid cancer for treatment. Other diagnostic modalities also are being applied to thyroid disease including magnetic resonance spectroscopy. Although these modalities are not widely used at this time we may see broader use in the future.

A number of articles on the parathyroid are included. However, there really is not any revolutionary information being published anymore about evaluation of hyperparathroidism with nuclear medicine techniques. Unfortunately, nuclear medicine suffers from a plethora of techniques and a lack of uniform approach to the various procedures used.

A few other articles are included here that are addressed include pancreatic disease and disease associated with somatastatin receptors as well as adrenal cortical disease. Reviewing these articles in their totality, it appears that even though endocrinology was one of the earliest clinical applications of nuclear medicine, there is still a great more to be learned and done in this particular area.

M. Donald Blaufox, MD, PhD

Improving the Yield of Preoperative Parathyroid Localization: Technetium Tc 99m–Sestamibi Imaging After Thyroid Suppression

Royal RE, Delpassand ES, Shapiro SE, et al (Univ of Texas, Houston)
Surgery 132:968-975, 2002 10–1

Background.—Preoperative localization is essential for successful directed, minimally invasive or reoperative parathyroidectomy. Standard technetium Tc 99m-sestamibi imaging is the most sensitive modality for localization. We reviewed our experience with ^{99m}Tc-sestamibi imaging and specifically investigated the effect of thyroid suppression on repeat imaging of patients who had initially nonlocalizing scans.

Methods.—The records of patients who underwent ^{99m}Tc-sestamibi imaging during evaluation for primary hyperparathyroidism were reviewed (Fig 2). A subset of patients with initially nonlocalizing scans underwent thyroid suppression with either thyroxin or liothyronine and then had their scans repeated.

Results.—Ninety-nine patients with primary hyperparathyroidism underwent ^{99m}Tc-sestamibi imaging followed by parathyroidectomy (initial

A.

B.

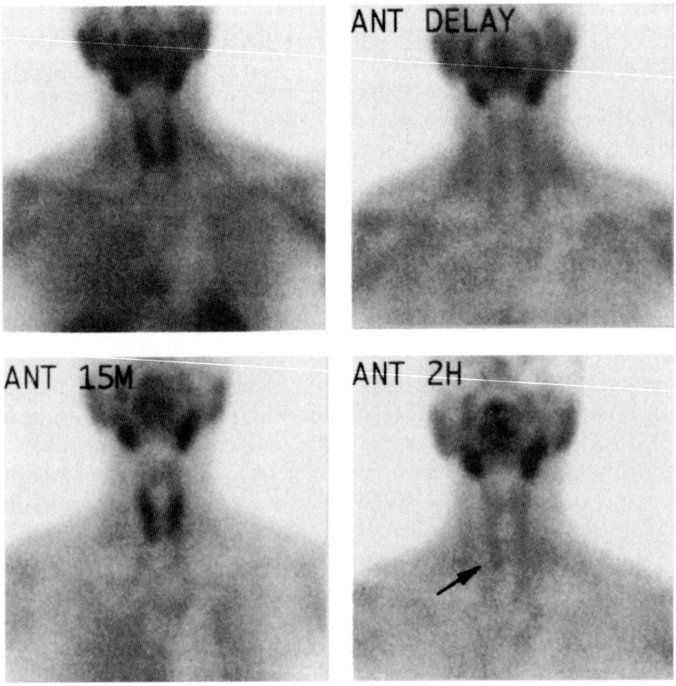

FIGURE 2.—Immediate (**left**) and delayed (**right**) anterior planar ^{99m}Tc-sestamibi images obtained from a patient before (**A**) and after (**B**) thyroid suppression. Persistent sestamibi uptake near the right lower pole of the thyroid is seen after thyroid suppression, consistent with a parathyroid adenoma in this location (*arrow*). (Reprinted by permission of the publisher courtesy of Royal RE, Delpassand ES, Shapiro SE, et al: Improving the yield of preoperative parathyroid localization: Technetium Tc 99m-sestamibi imaging after thyroid suppression. *Surgery* 132:968-975. Copyright 2002 by Elsevier.)

operation, 78; reoperation, 21). Successful parathyroid localization was obtained on standard imaging in 67 patients. Fourteen of 32 patients who had nonlocalizing ^{99m}Tc-sestamibi imaging studies underwent an additional scan after thyroid suppression. In 10 of 14 patients (71%), repeat ^{99m}Tc-sestamibi imaging after thyroid suppression successfully localized abnormal parathyroid tissue.

Conclusions.—Thyroid suppression may improve the yield of ^{99m}Tc-sestamibi imaging in patients with hyperparathyroidism who have an initially nonlocalizing study. This diagnostic strategy may be helpful in patients motivated to undergo a directed, minimally invasive operation, as well as in the evaluation of patients for reoperative parathyroidectomy.

► ^{99m}Tc- sestamibi imaging is widely used for the preoperative localization of parathyroid adenomas. The test does not successfully localize all abnormal parathyroid tissue. This study suggests that patients with suspected abnormalities of parathyroid tissue that are normal on the initial study should have the study repeated with thyroid suppression. An alternative might be to perform all studies with thyroid suppression. These results need to be confirmed. The planar images that are included in the article are not very convincing regarding the benefit of doing thryoid suppression, but SPECT images were also obtained and were not included in the article.

R. E. Coleman, MD

Fluorine-18-Fluorodeoxyglucose Positron Emission Tomography in the Preoperative Assessment of Thyroid Nodules in an Endemic Goiter Area

Kresnik E, Gallowitsch HJ, Mikosch P, et al (Univ of Klagenfurt, Austria)

Surgery 133:294-299, 2003 10–2

Background.—The aim of this study was to evaluate the usefulness of ^{18}F-FDG PET in the preoperative assessment of suspicious thyroid nodules.

Methods.—A total of 43 patients were examined before surgical resection. In all patients, imaging was obtained at 70 minutes after the intravenous administration of 180 MBq ^{18}F-FDG. Standard uptake values (SUVs) were calculated (Fig 2).

Results.—A total of 16 patients with thyroid carcinomas (11 papillary, 3 follicular, 2 anaplastic), 23 thyroid adenomas (11 microfollicular, 10 Hurthle cell, 2 macrofollicular), and 4 patients with degenerative goiter were found. ^{18}F-FDG uptake in Hurthle cell adenoma, thyroid cancer, microfollicular adenoma, degenerative goiter, and macrofollicular adenoma was 4.4 ± 2.2, 3.7 ± 1.9, 1.6 ± 0.3, 1.2 ± 0.2, and 0.9 ± 0.1, respectively. Significant differences were observed between thyroid carcinomas and both micro follicular adenomas and degenerative goiters ($P < 0.05$), and between Hurthle cell adenomas and both microfollicular adenomas as well as degenerative goiter ($P < 0.05$). For diagnosis of thyroid carcinoma, 100% sensitivity, 63% specificity, and 100% negative predictive value was found when a cutoff value for SUV of 2 was used.

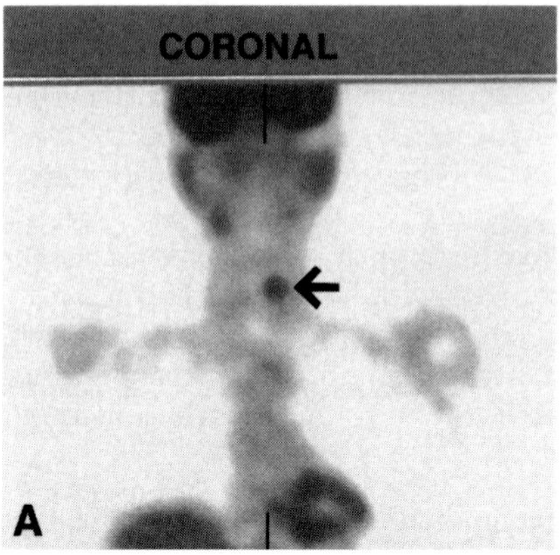

FIGURE 2.—A 63-year-old woman with a tumor in the left lobe of the thyroid. Histology revealed a papillary carcinoma of 1.2 cm in diameter. **A**, ^{18}F-FDG PET shows increased tracer uptake in the tumor (*arrow*; standard uptake value, 3.03). (Reprinted by permission of the publisher courtesy of Kresnik E, Gallowitsch HJ, Mikosch P, et al: Fluorine-18-fluorodeoxyglucose positron emission tomography in the preoperative assessment of thyroid nodules in an endemic goiter area. *Surgery* 133:294-299. Copyright 2003 by Elsevier.)

Conclusions.—Our results indicate that thyroid carcinomas, in contrast to most benign thyroid nodules, demonstrate significantly increased glucose metabolism. ^{18}F-FDG PET is unlikely to differentiate successfully all benign tumors from malignant tumors, but it can help select patients who need surgery, especially if cytology is inconclusive or malignancy cannot be excluded.

► The use of PET in the preoperative evaluation of thyroid nodules is probably not going to be practical. However, this article is useful in helping to understand the significance of hot nodules that are occasionally seen on PET imaging for other conditions. It supports the concept that these nodules are frequently malignant. During the year 2003, Medicare in the United States approved FDG imaging in patients with thyroid cancer. The conditions under which it is approved concerns those patients who have a rising thyroglobulin level and a negative ^{131}I scan. This is a reasonable indication and is likely to be the primary indication for using FDG PET in thyroid cancer for some time, unless information is developed to show that it has a use in another group of patients.

M. D. Blaufox, MD, PhD

Teflon-Induced Granuloma: A False-Positive Finding With PET Resolved With Combined PET and CT

Yeretsian RA, Blodgett TM, Branstetter BF IV, et al (Univ of Pittsburgh, Pa)
AJNR Am J Neuroradiol 24:1164-1166, 2003 10–3

Background.—Patients who have undergone thyroidectomy may have recurrent laryngeal nerve injury. The standard treatment for this injury was, until recently, Teflon injection for vocal cord medialization. However, Teflon injections have fallen out of favor because of a well-established propensity to cause reactive granulomas. Presented was a patient with a history of thyroid cancer who had significantly increased and unilateral ^{18}F-FDG uptake in the larynx caused by Teflon thyroplasty.

Case Report.—Man, 77, with a history of well-differentiated follicular carcinoma of the thyroid was referred to a PET facility. The patient had undergone total thyroidectomy 6.5 years earlier. Postoperatively, he had recurrent left laryngeal nerve paralysis for which he underwent Teflon injection into the paralyzed vocal cord. Six month before this presentation, findings of repeat ^{131}I scintigraphy were negative, the thyroid-stimulating hormone level exceeded 150 IU/mL, and the thyroglobulin level was 97 ng/mL. Combined PET and CT showed significantly increased and unilateral FDG uptake in the neck, localized to the left vocal cord and presumably the result of a Teflon-induced granuloma (Fig 1).

Conclusion.—Awareness of Teflon-induced granuloma as a potential source of false-positive PET interpretation and the use of combined PET and

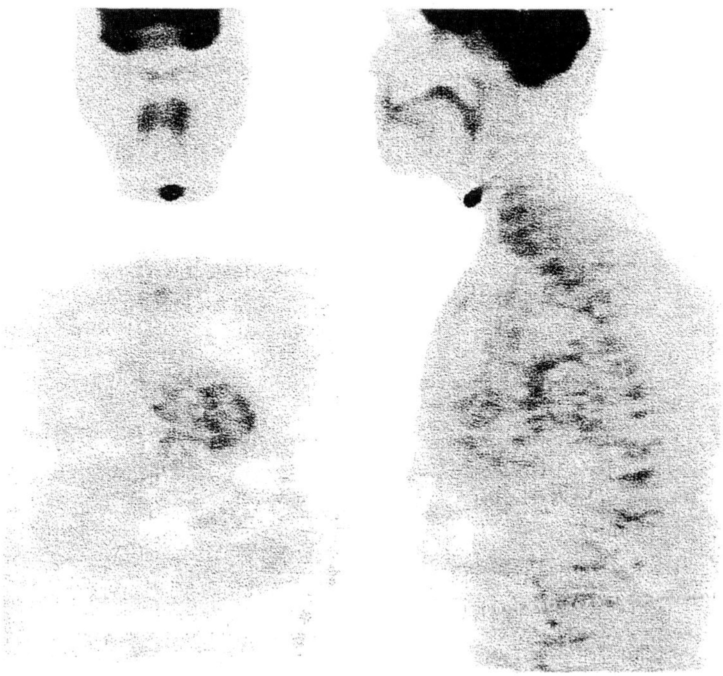

FIGURE 1.—Coronal (**left**) and sagittal (**right**) views acquired with PET. Increased FDG uptake just left of midline in the anterior neck (*arrows*) is shown. (Courtesy of Yeretsian RA, Blodgett TM, Branstetter BF IV, et al: Teflon-induced granuloma: A false-positive finding with PET resolved with combined PET and CT. *AJNR Am J Neuroradiol* 24:1164-1166, 2003. Copyright by American Society of Neuroradiology.)

CT imaging may allow precise diagnosis and prevention of unnecessary interventions.

► I do not often include case reports in the YEAR BOOK since they are generally of rather limited value. I have included this one because of several points. First of all, the occurrence of FDG activity on PET imaging in the area of the vocal chord is not an uncommon finding. This is usually symmetrical uptake. It can be identified often as benign muscular activity. In this particular individual, the uptake is at the site of a previously injected vocal chord. The question that arises is whether or not the combined PET/CT accomplished what the authors' suggest.

The patient was known to have had a Teflon injection because of laryngeal nerve injury and therefore uptake in that area would not be surprising. Given the history and the finding, it certainly would be suspected that this might be the cause of the uptake. The area of increased uptake clearly was at the site of the injection, as shown on the CT, but the case remains perplexing because the thyroglobulin was increasing with no known cause. So then has this patient proven to be a false-positive resolved with PET/CT or is it possibly a false-negative because of PET/CT? I would be more comfortable if a biopsy had been taken of the vocal chord at the time of the fiberoptic laryngoscopy.

M. D. Blaufox, MD, PhD

Evaluation of Dosimetry of Radioiodine Therapy in Benign and Malignant Thyroid Disorders by Means of Iodine-124 and PET

Eschmann SM, Reischl G, Bilger K, et al (Univ of Tübingen, Germany)

Eur J Nucl Med 29:760-767, 2002 10–4

Background.—In the use of radioiodine therapy for thyroid cancer, difficulties in dosing can arise. Target volumes may be inaccurate because of small lesions that are difficult to outline with ultrasound or other imaging modalities, and because calculating radioiodine uptake can vary in the absence of any attenuation or scatter correction. The use of PET with ^{124}I permits high spatial resolution images that can be corrected for scatter and attenuation, so that tissue radioactivity can be accurately quantified. ^{124}I was considered unsuitable for PET imaging because only about 22% of its disintegrations are positrons, but phantom measurements revealed that it had utility for tumorlike objects against relatively low background activity. Patients having radioiodine therapy for thyrotoxicosis or thyroid cancer participated in an evaluation of the suitability of ^{124}I and PET to assess dosimetry.

Methods.—Phantom scans were performed to evaluate the accuracy of PET. An EEC phantom was used, having 6 spheres of different diameters filled with 3 to 30 MBq of ^{124}I. The PET data obtained 1 to 13 days after simultaneous administration of an oral therapeutic dose of ^{131}I and a diagnostic dose of ^{124}I were used to calculate patient dosimetry. The results were compared with findings from intratherapeutic probe measurements and clinical outcome.

Results.—Phantom studies found an inaccuracy of the measured activity concentration of 10%. For ^{124}I, the inaccuracy of volumetry was 20% when the sphere diameters exceeded 13 mm, and 50% for spheres whose diameter was 10 mm. No effect was found in the probe measurements of ^{131}I when ^{124}I was applied. For nodular goiter studies, the mean uptake and effective half-life of the whole thyroid gland showed good correlation between the data obtained with ^{124}I and with ^{131}I. However, significant differences in specific uptake were found between the two during regional analysis of autonomous nodules and normal tissue, with radiation doses to autonomous nodules varying from 177 to 633 Gy, and those of perinodular tissue from 47 to 126 Gy. Effective half-life values did not show these variations. For patients with thyroid cancer, thyroid remnants received doses of 350 to 1420 Gy, and tumor metastases received 70 to 170 Gy.

Conclusions.—Dosimetry with ^{124}I is feasible, with the combination of ^{124}I and PET permitting the accurate calculation of radiation doses as well as the acceptable estimation of tumor or tissue volumes. Good correlation was noted between probe measurements of thyroid uptake and PET in patients with benign thyroid disease. The dosimetry for thyroid nodules and normal thyroid tissue was successfully differentiated by using ^{124}I PET. The absolute quantification that can be achieved can be especially useful in dosimetric evaluations for patients with thyroid cancer to establish dose-response curves, for analyzing the stunning phenomenon, or to evaluate the effects of pharmacologic interventions before radioiodine therapy is undertaken.

► The role of PET in thyroid disease has great potential and will be expanding. It is unfortunate that even though the Medicare system in the United States approved the use of PET for head and neck tumors, originally it specifically excluded thyroid. This was a mistake that has now been corrected with a limited approval in patients with increased thyroglobulin and with negative whole body ^{131} scans. There is no question that a significant subpopulation of patients with thyroid disease will benefit from PET imaging. Recent efforts to use ^{124}I offer even greater promise than FDG. This certainly provides a very reliable quantitative technique for estimating dosing for patients with recurrent disease. Without question, ^{124}I has a role in both benign and malignant diseases utilizing PET, as the authors conclude. I find it exciting that it has the promise of providing us with a rational approach to choosing therapeutic doses.

M. D. Blaufox, MD, PhD

Combined Positron Emission Tomography/Computed Tomography Imaging of Recurrent Thyroid Cancer

Zimmer LA, McCook B, Meltzer C, et al (Univ of Pittsburgh, Pa)
Otolaryngol Head Neck Surg 128:178-184, 2003 10–5

Introduction.—Patients who have elevated serum thyroglobulin levels and negative ^{131}I scans are a small, yet significant group of patients with recurrent thyroid cancer. CT permits high-resolution, cross-sectional anatomical imaging. There are several limitations in the use of this modality for recurrent thyroid cancer. ^{18}FDG PET is valuable in patients with differentiated thyroid cancer with increased serum thyroglobulin levels and negative ^{131}I scans. The limited spatial resolution and lack of anatomical detail with PET make it difficult for precise anatomical localization of tumor. A prototype of combined PET/CT imaging was used to localize recurrent disease in patients with thyroid cancer.

Methods.—Eight patients with suspected recurrent thyroid cancer with elevated serum thyroglobulin or calcitonin levels underwent combined PET/CT imaging using a proton-type device. All 8 patients previously underwent total thyroidectomy and ^{131}I ablation for thyroid carcinoma. Negative ^{131}I scan results were observed in patients with papillary carcinoma.

Results.—Four (50%) patients had recurrent disease in the head and neck. Eleven lesions were detected in these 4 patients. Three patients (8 lesions) underwent surgical removal of disease. All 3 patients had pathologic verification of recurrence; 6 (75%) lesions were positive.

Conclusion.—Combined PET/CT imaging is useful in the diagnosis and anatomical localization of recurrent thyroid cancer.

► CT has a limited, if any, role in evaluation of thyroid cancer. Although this study shows the value of PET, it does not make clear how CT really contributed to the diagnosis. Detailed anatomical localization in thyroid cancer is of minor value since the patients are going to be treated with radioactive iodine in almost all situations. There may be a small subset of patients in whom there is an isolated lesion that is going to be approached surgically and in whom further anatomical information is helpful. But other than this relatively rare indication, it is difficult to understand what value combined PET/CT has over the currently accepted indication of using for PET in patients with rising thyroglobulin and negative ^{131}I scans.

M. D. Blaufox, MD, PhD

Comparison of Methods for Thyroid Volume Estimation in Patients With Graves' Disease

van Isselt JW, de Klerk JMH, van Rijk PP, et al (Univ Med Ctr Utrecht, The Netherlands)

Eur J Nucl Med Mol Imaging 30:525-531, 2003 10–6

Background.—The volume of the thyroid is an important consideration when choosing the radioiodine dosage for patients with Graves' hyperthyroidism. The accuracy of each of 3 methods for determining thyroid volume—planar scintigraphy (PS), SPECT, and US—was compared with that of MRI in patients with Grave's disease.

Methods.—The study included 25 patients (3 men, 22 women; mean age, 42.2 years) with Graves' disease who were referred for radioiodine therapy. All patients underwent MRI, PS, SPECT, and US to determine thyroid volume. During MRI, thyroid segmentation was performed manually using gadolinium-enhanced, T1-weighted images, and thyroid volume was measured by a summation-of-areas technique. PS images underwent filtering and thresholding (Fig 1), and thyroid volume was calculated using a standard surface formula. The SPECT images were iteratively reconstructed and filtered, and a threshold method was applied before thyroid volume was determined by an automatic segmentation algorithm. For US images, thyroid volume was measured using an ellipsoid volume model for multiple 2-dimensional measurements.

Results.—The mean thyroid volume calculated by MRI was 25.0 mL (range, 7.0-56.3 mL). PS measurements correlated poorly with MRI measurements (r^2 = 0.61), and PS calculations had considerable bias (−4.00). The mean relative difference between PS and MRI values was 33.2%. In contrast, SPECT volumes correlated well with those of MRI (r^2 = 0.84) with little bias (1.83). The mean relative difference between SPECT and MRI values was 2.3%. US volumes had the best correlation with MRI values (r^2 = 0.97), but bias with US was high (6.8) because of underestimation. The mean relative difference between US and MRI values were about equal.

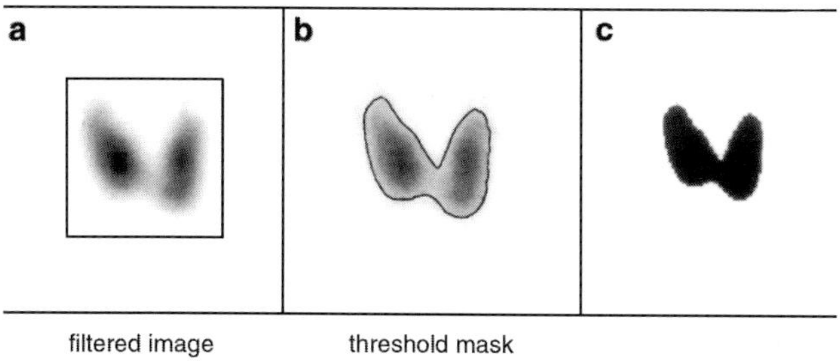

FIGURE 1.—Planar scintigraphy of the thyroid in patient No. 6. **a**, Box ROI around the thyroid; **b**, automatic contour detection with a 30% threshold; **c**, image after segmentation. *Abbreviation: ROI*, Region of interest. (Courtesy of van Isselt JW, de Klerk JMH, van Rijk PP, et al: Comparison of methods for thyroid volume estimation in patients with Graves' disease. *Eur J Nucl Med Mol Imaging* 30:525-531, 2003.)

Conclusion.—SPECT is more accurate than PS for measuring thyroid volume in patients with Graves' disease. US is the most accurate of these 3 modalities, but only if a correction is made for underestimation.

▶ It is interesting to see how various approaches to measuring thyroid volume correlate. It would have been interesting also if the authors had investigated a simple physical examination of the thyroid to see how well that would do against the more sophisticated imaging techniques. Although it certainly is nice to know the volume of the thyroid relatively accurately, the wide variability in dosimetry approaches to treatment still leaves us with no generally accepted and reproducible method for the treatment of Graves' disease.

M. D. Blaufox, MD, PhD

A Retrospective Review of the Effectiveness of Recombinant Human TSH as a Preparation for Radioiodine Thyroid Remnant Ablation

Robbins RJ, Larson SM, Sinha N, et al (Mem Sloan-Kettering Cancer Ctr, New York)

J Nucl Med 43:1482-1488, 2002 10–7

Background.—After a total or near-total thyroidectomy for differentiated thyroid carcinoma, radioiodine remnant ablation (RRA) is generally undertaken to destroy normal thyroid remnants and any microscopic deposits of thyroid carcinoma, thereby reducing the number of local recurrences and improving overall survival. Studies of the efficacy of RRA have been based on treatments given after thyroid hormone withdrawal (THW). Another option is to perform RRA after preparation with recombinant human thyroid-stimulating hormone (rhTSH). The 2 methods were compared when some clinicians chose to follow the traditional THW preparation and others selected the method using rhTSH. The rates of successful remnant ablation were assessed, with the expectation that no differences would be noted.

Methods.—Eighty-seven patients' records were reviewed retrospectively, with the treatment option chosen by the individual physician providing care. Forty-two patients had RRA after THW, and 45 had RRA after rhTSH preparation.

Results.—Patients in the rhTSH group were statistically older than those in the THW group and were also more likely to have an N0 status at initial diagnosis. Patients having THW had significantly lower free thyroxine (T_4) levels and elevated serum TSH levels before ablation, which reflects their withdrawal from thyroid hormone, whereas patients having rhTSH had normal free T_4 levels and a slightly elevated baseline TSH level. The initial diagnostic scan for the rhTSH group used a slightly but significantly higher amount of ^{131}I than was used for the THW group. After RRA, complete ablation was achieved in 80.9% of the THW group and 84.4% of the rhTSH group. A partial response was achieved in 16.7% of the THW group and 15.6% of the rhTSH group.

Conclusions.—No significant difference in outcome developed between the 2 groups of patients evaluated. Thus, THW and rhTSH offer equally effective methods of preparing for RRA. Further evaluation should be undertaken to confirm these findings. If confirmed, the choice of preparation for RRA (THW vs rhTSH) would be made on the basis of the patient's quality of life and the "cost" of hypothyroidism versus the cost of rhTSH, and not on the likelihood of a complete ablation, which appears to be similar for these 2 preparation methods.

► One of the undesirable aspects from the patient's point of view of the preparation for thyroid remnant ablation is the withdrawal of thyroid hormone supplement and the onset of hypothyroidism. Most patients are unhappy with the adverse effect, although relatively brief, that hypothyroidism has on their lifestyle. The use of rhTSH preparation for radioiodine thyroid remnant ablation has many attractive features, both for the physician and the patient. This retrospective study, which points out some of the limitations of such a study, nevertheless suggests that the use of rhTSH is an effective means of preparing patients for remnant ablation. Although definitive data are not yet available, many physicians are beginning to routinely use this technique. It would certainly be worthwhile to have a prospective study completed before this becomes the norm so that there can be a sound scientific basis for this approach. One of the problems we encounter in clinical medicine is that therapeutic approaches are sometimes followed without adequate scientific evidence, and in some situations we find that we have been doing things wrong even though everybody thought we were doing them right. Painful as it is, there is no way to avoid the need of laying a firm scientific foundation for any therapeutic approach.

M. D. Blaufox, MD, PhD

Differentiation Between Healthy Thyroid Remnants and Tumor Tissue After Radioiodine Therapy in Patients With Differentiated Thyroid Carcinoma Using In Vitro Phosphorus-31 Magnetic Resonance Spectroscopy

Moka D, Dietlein M, Raffelt K, et al (Univ of Cologne, Köln, Germany)

Am J Med 112:634-641, 2002 10–8

Background.—The growth and spread of many tumors are triggered by changes in cell membrane metabolism, which can lead to systemic alterations in levels of phospholipids. We sought to determine whether plasma levels of several phospholipids could differentiate between healthy remnants of thyroid tissue and residual tumor tissue or metastases in patients with thyroid carcinoma.

Methods.—We measured plasma phospholipid levels by phosphorus-31 magnetic resonance spectroscopy (^{31}P-MRS) in blood samples from 30 patients with thyroid cancer who had been rendered hypothyroid in preparation for diagnostic or therapeutic administration of iodine-131. All patients had undergone total thyroidectomy. Iodine-131 whole-body scintigraphy and measurements of thyroglobulin values during up to 3 years of follow-up were used to distinguish patients in remission from those with only healthy thyroid remnants and those with tumor tissue or metastases.

Results.—Mean (±SD) levels of sphingomyelin (0.33 ± 0.06 mmol/L vs. 0.46 ± 0.03 mmol/L, P <0.0001) and phosphatidylcholine (1.34 ± 0.19 mmol/L vs. 2.15 ± 0.33 mmol/L, P <0.0001) were significantly lower in patients with metastatic thyroid cancer (n = 8) than in patients (n = 12) who were in remission. Patients with only remnants of thyroid tissue (n = 10) also had significantly lower phospholipid levels than did patients in remission, but significantly greater levels that did patients with tumor tissue or metastases.

Conclusion.—These preliminary results suggest that ^{31}P-MRS may be useful in helping to differentiate the presence of tumor tissue, remnants of thyroid tissue not requiring further treatment, and remission in patients with thyroid cancer.

▶ I am not sure that there is a real need to differentiate normal thyroid tissue from cancer in patients with recurrent thyroid carcinoma. Since most of these patients undergo thyroid ablation and since the location of residual thyroid tissue is very characteristic, this should not really be a difficult clinical problem. It is interesting that this in vitro test has some correlation with the presence or absence of normal thyroid tissue and thyroid metastases, but measurements of thyroglobulin and thyroid scanning have proven very reliable and valuable in following these patients. Furthermore, the lack of a more definitive confirmation of the observations is of some concern.

M. D. Blaufox, MD, PhD

Parathyroid Surgery: Separating Promise From Reality

Perrier ND, Ituarte PHG, Morita E, et al (Univ of California, San Francisco; Surgical Service of Veterans Affairs, San Francisco)

J Clin Endocrinol Metab 87:1024-1029, 2002 10–9

Introduction.—There is considerable controversy regarding whether focal, unilateral, or bilateral neck exploration should be used in patients with primary sporadic hyperparathyroidism (HPT) because of improved preoperative localization tests and intraoperative parathyroid (IOPTH) assay. Seventy-one patients undergoing parathyroid (PTH) surgery between October 1998 and June 1999 were prospectively monitored to determine the use of independent and combined imaging and biochemical techniques.

Methods.—Patients underwent preoperative sestamibi scans, intraoperative γ-probe examinations, and IOPTH monitoring. Accuracy was considered completion of resection if the surgeon depended solely on these imaging and biochemical studies. Adenoma localization by sestamibi scanning was correct in 95% of 59 patients with solitary adenomas. It was correct in 25% of 14 patients with multiple adenomas. Sestamibi scanning incorrectly identified a single hot spot in 64% of patients with secondary and tertiary disease. The probe was not useful in locating other glands after a single gland was removed in patients with hyperplasia. Intraoperative PTH was accurate in 78% of patients with primary disease and 45% of patients who had non-primary disease.

Conclusion.—A minimal approach may be useful in a select group of patients with no familial primary HPT, secondary or tertiary disease, coexisting thyroid pathology, or an equivocal sestamibi scan. Only patients with a positive single hot spot on sestamibi scan should be considered for a minimally invasive procedure. This means only 64% of patients with hyperparathyroidism are candidates for a minimally invasive approach. Findings of a combination of a solitary hot spot on sestamibi scan and a drop in IOPTH allow the surgeon to make the correct decision concerning the need to convert to a bilateral approach in 93% of selected patients.

▶ The use of the gamma probe is rapidly expanding to the point where its routine use in HPT is approaching the clinical state of practice. This article is useful in defining those patients in whom this approach is most likely to be of help. Certainly keeping parathyroid surgery minimally invasive is a great benefit to the patient, provided there is proper selection of those in whom there is a low likelihood of leaving behind any abnormal tissue.

M. D. Blaufox, MD, PhD

Limitations of Technetium 99m Sestamibi Scintigraphic Localization for Primary Hyperparathyroidism Associated With Multiglandular Disease

Katz SC, Wang GJ, Kramer EL, et al (New York Univ)

Am Surg 69:170-175, 2003 10–10

Introduction.—Successful surgical treatment of primary hyperparathyroidism necessitates the localization and excision of the parathyroid tissue responsible for excessive parathyroid hormone secretion while assuring that patients have adequate endogenous parathyroid hormone production to maintain eucalcemia. In the selection of patients with primary hyperparathyroidism for unilateral parathyroidectomy, the surgeon must be able to diagnose multiglandular disease either preoperatively or intraoperatively. A retrospective review was performed of 123 patients who underwent surgical treatment for primary hyperparathyroidism to ascertain the feasibility of selecting patients for minimally invasive surgery based on preoperative imaging.

Methods.—All patients were treated by a single surgeon between January 1993 and January 2000. All 123 patients underwent ^{99m}Tc-sestamibi scan and 119 underwent high-resolution cervical US. One patient in whom ^{99m}Tc-sestamibi revealed increased uptake in the mediastinum also underwent a CT scan.

Results.—Surgery was successful in all 123 patients. Excision of the abnormal parathyroid tissue resulted in persistent postoperative eucalcemia. Four parathyroid glands were detected during surgery in all except 2 patients. One hundred eight (87.8%) patients had solitary adenomas; 15 (12.2%) had disease of 2 or more glands. Seventeen (13.8%) patients had enlarged glands in ectopic sites. One patient underwent a limited thoracotomy in lieu of neck exploration after ^{99m}Tc-sestamibi and CT scanning showed a mediastinal adenoma. The sensitivity and specificity of the ^{99m}Tc-sestamibi scan was superior to high-resolution US in patients with solitary adenomas and those with multiglandular disease.

Conclusion.—Unilateral exploration based exclusively of preoperative imaging may not identify a significant number of patients with bilateral multiglandular disease.

► It is interesting that these authors report a rather low sensitivity for sestamibi in patients with hyperparathyroidism and multiglandular disease. It certainly is well accepted that in parathyroid hyperplasia and other multiglandular disease, there is a relatively low sensitivity of the test. In describing the patient population, the authors do not explain how they excluded the possible presence of secondary hyperparathyroidism. This could be a confounding factor, and it would be interesting to have a little more data in that regard.

Some authors have suggested that since the risk of bilateral disease is relatively small, it is justified to remove the identified adenoma so that surgery is rapid with low risk. Patients who continue to have signs of disease could be re-operated. A preferable approach is to remove the identified adenoma and to have serum parathyroid hormone levels available at the time of surgery. Since these drop rapidly, the exploration could be extended in those cases where a cure is not resultant.

M. D. Blaufox, MD, PhD

^{99m}Tc-tetrofosmin or ^{99m}Tc-sestamibi for Double-Phase Parathyroid Scintigraphy?

Fröberg AC, Valkema R, Bonjer HJ, et al (Erasmus Med Ctr, Rotterdam, The Netherlands)

Eur J Nucl Med 30:193-196, 2003 10–11

Introduction.—The use of preoperative imaging in patients with hyperparathyroidism remains controversial. Yet, the need for localization of parathyroid adenomas before re-operation is widely accepted. Trials comparing ^{99m}Tc-tetrofosmin and ^{99m}Tc-sestamibi in a double-phase protocol have reported conflicting findings. The sensitivity of double-phase ^{99m}Tc-sestamibi and double-phase ^{99m}Tc-tetrofosmin for localization of parathyroid adenomas were compared with the use of both visual and quantitative analysis.

Methods.—Twelve patients (mean age, 56.3 years) with suspected hyperparathyroidism referred for scintigraphy were evaluated. Patients underwent ^{99m}Tc-sestamibi scintigraphy. One month later, scintigraphy was repeated with ^{99m}Tc-tetrofosmin. Visual interpretation was made without knowledge of the lesion-to-thyroid (L/T) ratios; the L/T ratios were determined on all images for quantification.

Results.—Nine patients underwent surgery. Eight parathyroid adenomas or hyperplastic glands were histologically verified in 7 patients; 1 patient had a histologically verified parathyroid carcinoma. All of these patients had positive ^{99m}Tc-sestamibi scintigram results; only 2 ^{99m}Tc-tetrofosmin scintigrams were positive. There was a significant increase in the lesion-to-thyroid ratio from 10 minutes to 90 minutes and 150 minutes post infusion which was not observed on scintigraphy with ^{99m}Tc-tetrofosmin.

Conclusion.—^{99m}Tc-tetrofosmin is not a good alternative to ^{99m}Tc-sestamibi in a double-phase parathyroid scintigraphy protocol due to the lack of time in the L/T ratio in most patients.

► Although there is no question that parathyroid disease can be identified with tetrofosmin, the majority of investigators prefer sestamibi. In this small study, there seems to be an unequivocal advantage of sestamibi over tetrofosmin. It is unfortunate that throughout the article the authors lump parathyroid adenomas and hyperplastic glands together without clearly specifying how many glands had adenomas and how many were hyperplastic. This is probably dictatated by the very small size of the series.

However, it is important to make a distinction between hyperplasia and adenomas because of the very significant difference in sensitivity of the parathyroid scan in these 2 diseases. It would be surprising if the authors' results of having positive sestamibi scans in all of the patients who were operated and had histologically confirmed disease occurred in a significant number of patients with hyperplasia. Part of this 100% sensitivity for sestamibi can be attributed to the fact that in 3 patients in whom the scan was negative or equivocal, there was no surgical exploration.

M. D. Blaufox, MD, PhD

Clinical Outcomes and Fiscal Consequences of Bilateral Neck Exploration for Primary Idiopathic Hyperparathyroidism Without Preoperative Radionuclide Imaging or Minimally Invasive Techniques

Schell SR, Dudley NE (Univ of Florida, Gainesville; Malcolm Randall Veterans Affairs Med Ctr, Gainesville, Fla; Univ of Oxford, England)

Surgery 133:32-39, 2003 10–12

Background.—Excellent results have been obtained in the treatment of patients with primary hyperparathyroidism without using preoperative localizing studies, yet more and more patients are routinely being referred for preoperative radionuclide localization studies before undergoing a primary operation. This approach has been touted as the quickest, most successful, and least costly way of treating primary idiopathic hyperparathyroidism, but the basis for these claims is unproved. The treatment outcomes achieved in patients who underwent standard parathyroid surgery without preoperative localization studies were compared with the results reported in the literature for patients who had been selected to undergo preoperative radionuclide imaging before minimally invasive parathyroid surgery.

Methods.—A prospective gathering of information from 688 patients having their first neck exploration for hyperparathyroidism included diagnostic, treatment, and outcome data. No preoperative localization studies were used; the identification of all parathyroid glands was facilitated by the use of methylene blue intraoperatively. The results in terms of outcomes and costs were compared with reports by centers that advocate the use of scan-directed minimally invasive parathyroid surgery.

Results.—None of the patients died. No patients had injuries to the recurrent laryngeal nerves, and there were no cases of postoperative hemorrhage, infection, or persistent symptomatic hypocalcemia. Fewer than 2% of the patients had a keloid or dystrophic scar at the incision site. A total of 2520 of 2752 glands were identified without using preoperative studies. For 78.7% of the patients, single gland adenomas were noted; 8 of 542 patients had an adenoma in a supernumerary parathyroid gland. Double adenomas were located in 22 patients, and multigland hyperplasia was found in 98 patients. Ten patients had parathyroid carcinoma that was diagnosed and treated at the primary operation. For 97.7% of patients, cure was achieved. The average cost per patient was $1243 for patients with multigland disease, hyperplasia, or malignancy requiring a 48-hour hospital stay; the mean cost for patients with a single adenoma was $1107. If the stay was shortened to 24 hours, the estimated cost decreased to $767 per patient with a single adenoma. The cost for scan-directed approaches averaged $1123 per patient with a single adenoma; adding the cost of failed imaging increased the average to $1263 per patient.

Conclusions.—The cost for scan-directed surgery was higher than that for surgery without preoperative localization scans in patients with primary idiopathic hyperparathyroidism. The use of scanning is not supported by the outcomes or the costs incurred for this intervention.

► This article is truly an example of comparing apples and oranges. The authors suggest that their treatment outcome is less expensive and equally successful with that of institutions that practice scan-directed surgery. The problem is, however, that the 688 patients who were "prospectively" collected are, in fact, representative of a retrospective analysis of cases performed over a 32-year period. Undoubtedly, surgical technique and costs have varied greatly during this time but are analyzed in a current context. Rather than compare their own experience with both techniques, the authors are comparing and contrasting their experience with that reported in the literature. Clearly, there are differences in skill and costs from institution to institution. When these skills and costs are compared not only between institutions but between countries, the general applicability of the findings is subject to serious question. However, with that said, the article is provocative and challenges the currently held concept that nuclear imaging has an important role to play in the surgical treatment of hyperparathyroidism. Although I do not agree with the authors' conclusions and some of their methodology, I recommend the paper as an expression of an important contrasting point of view.

M. D. Blaufox, MD, PhD

The False Negative Technetium-99m-Sestamibi Scan in Patients With Primary Hyperparathyroidism: Correlation With Clinical Factors and Operative Findings

Merlino JI, Ko K, Minotti A, et al (Case Western Reserve Univ, Cleveland, Ohio)

Am Surg 69:225-230, 2003 10–13

Background.—Technetium-99m (^{99m}Tc) sestamibi scintigraphy is often used before initial neck exploration in patients with primary hyperparathyroidism. However, its high false-negative rate in this application, is of concern. To determine possible explanations for these false-negative findings, the clinical factors that correlate with a false-negative ^{99m}Tc sestamibi scan were investigated.

Methods.—The study included 89 patients (16 men, 73 women; mean age, 56 years) with primary hyperparathyroidism who underwent parathyroidectomy during an 11-year period. Of these patients, 76 had a single adenoma, and 13 had multiglandular disease. All patients underwent preoperative ^{99m}Tc scintigraphy. The results of scintigraphy were correlated with clinical, operative, and pathologic findings.

Results.—Of the 89 patients, 68 (76%) had a true-positive scan, 20 (22%) had a false-negative scan, and 1 (1%) had a false-positive scan. The overall sensitivity of ^{99m}Tc sestamibi scanning was 77%, with a positive predictive value (PPV) of 99%. Sensitivity increased to 84% when only adenomas were included (PPV remained at 99%). All 4 patients with parathyroid hyperplasia (100%) and 4 (44%) of 9 patients with double adenomas had a false-negative scan. Patients with a normal preoperative calcium level were also significantly more likely to have a false-negative scan than those with abnormal levels. A true-positive scan was significantly more common for patients with a single adenoma than for patients with multiglandular disease (83% vs 38%; odds ratio, 7.754). Larger adenomas were also more likely to have a true-positive scan than were smaller adenomas. True-positive scans were also significantly more common among patients with an inferior rather than a superior adenoma (90% vs 59%; odds ratio, 6.261).

Conclusion.—About 20% of patients with primary hyperparathyroidism who undergo preoperative ^{99m}Tc sestamibi scintigraphy will have a false-negative result. Although its PPV is high, this approach is less accurate for detecting abnormal parathyroid tissues in patients with small adenomas, multiglandular disease, superior adenomas, or normal preoperative calcium levels. These characteristics should prompt the surgeon to perform bilateral exploration.

▶ Although the technetium-99m sestamibi scan has assumed a major role in the diagnosis and treatment of primary hyperparathyroidism, it continues to be the subject of a very large literature. The fact that so much continues to be written about it probably represents the existence of a number of unresolved issues. A very important issue is an understanding of the particular factors that lead to false/negative scans in patients. The factors that these authors have identified are those that most of us would intuitively have expected to be a source of problems. An exception, perhaps, is the difficulty with superior adenomas. The data are slightly confounded, including 4 patients with hyperplasia, but, in this large series, that does not represent a major problem. In the discussion, the authors present the sensitivity using only adenomas, which better reflects the most accurate aspect of the scan. It would be worthwhile to see some additional studies of the sensitivity and specificity of patients with primary hyperparathyroidism whose lesions are in the upper pole to confirm this surprising finding.

M. D. Blaufox, MD, PhD

Preoperative Parathyroid Localization: Correlating False-Negative Technetium 99m Sestamibi Scans With Parathyroid Disease

Westreich RW, Brandwein M, Mechanick JI, et al (Mount Sinai Hosp, New York)

Laryngoscope 113:567-572, 2003 10–14

Introduction.—The recent emphasis on minimally invasive directed parathyroid surgery has increased the surgeon's dependence on preoperative parathyroid localization. ^{99m}Tc sestamibi scanning is usually considered the gold standard for preoperative localization; sensitivities of 75% to 100% and specificities of 75% to 90% have been reported. In all reported series, there is a subset of patients for whom preoperative localization is either equivocal or negative. A subset of patients from a parathyroid database with false-negative sestamibi scans were evaluated to elucidate characteristics that could affect testing.

Methods.—Twenty patients with negative preoperative scan results and verified parathyroid disease were compared with 22 consecutive patients with positive scan results and confirmed parathyroid disease. Medical records were examined retrospectively for data concerning clinicopathologic and radiologic findings. Variables correlated were as follows: age; gender; concomitant thyroid disease (Hashimoto's thyroiditis, papillary thyroid carcinoma, thyroid adenoma); preoperative parathyroid hormone values; location and number of enlarged parathyroid glands; parathyroid weight; and the relative proportion of chief cells, clear cells, oxyphil cells, and adipose tissue.

Results.—Patients with preoperative false-negative scans were more likely to have an enlarged parathyroid with a high proportion of clear cells ($P = .01$). A trend was observed ($P = .1$) that correlated increased parathyroid fat content and false-negative scans. Positive preoperative scan results were more likely to be linked with a higher percentage of oxyphil cells ($P = .02$). Univariate analysis for other variables, along with logistic regression analysis, did not reach statistical significance.

Conclusion.—This is the largest clinicopathologic review of false-negative sestamibi scans to date. ^{99m}Tc uptake is associated with parathyroid oxyphil cell content. False-negative scans can occur with parathyroid glands containing predominately clear cells.

► An important step toward improving the sensitivity of any diagnostic test is the acquisition of an understanding of the reasons for false-negative examinations. In many situations once that is understood, the problems can be corrected. This article very nicely reviews false-negative tests in parathyroid disease. Unfortunately, the finding that a high proportion of clear cells leads to a negative scan, as well as possibly increased parathyroid fat, is somewhat disappointing since these are factors which are not easily corrected. However, it is valuable to have an explanation for the false-negative tests so that we can have a better understanding of the limitations of the exam. Hopefully, at some point an agent will become available that is concentrated by the clear cell. If so, in patients in whom there is a very strong suspicion of a parathyroid adenoma and in whom the sestamibi scan is negative, a second procedure could be considered.

M. D. Blaufox, MD, PhD

Ultrasonography for Preoperative Localization of Enlarged Parathyroid Glands in Primary Hyperparathyroidism: Comparison With ^{99m}Technetium Sestamibi Scintigraphy

Haber RS, Kim CK, Inabnet WB (Mount Sinai School of Medicine, New York)

Clin Endocrinol (Oxf) 57:241-249, 2002 10–15

Background.—The identification and excision of enlarged parathyroid glands are essential in the successful surgical management of primary hyperparathyroidism. Preoperative parathyroid imaging techniques have permitted the use of surgical approaches that are less invasive than bilateral neck exploration. The results achieved with ultrasonography in localizing enlarged parathyroid glands in 120 consecutive patients with primary hyperparathyroidism were reported, as were correlations with surgical findings in 86 patients referred for surgery. A comparison was made with the results obtained with ^{99m}technetium sestamibi scintigraphy in 99 patients.

Methods.—All 94 women and 26 men (mean age, 60 years) had elevated serum calcium and intact parathyroid hormone levels determined by immunoassay; none had previous parathyroid surgery or secondary hyperparathyroidism. A single observer performed high-resolution ultrasonography; both early and delayed (2-hour) views were obtained with ^{99m}technetium sestamibi scintigraphy. Correlations were made with simultaneous thyroidal ^{123}I uptake in the majority of patients.

Results.—For 92 of the 120 unselected patients referred for imaging, ultrasonography localized enlarged parathyroid glands, and all but one were solitary. One or more abnormal parathyroid glands were removed in 86 of the 88 patients; no abnormal parathyroid glands were found at surgery in the other 2 cases. Surgery resulted in an apparent cure in 82 cases. Ninety-three percent of the adenomas were solitary, with lower parathyroid glands involved more often than upper glands. Ultrasonography allowed correct prediction of the surgical findings in 74% of cases, with 17% having negative examinations, 6% having adenomas predicted at the wrong site, and

2% having putative solitary enlarged glands identified when multigland disease was present. Of the 86 patients in whom enlarged parathyroid glands were found at surgery, ultrasonography was accurate in 83% of cases; the positive predictive value was 90%. Sestamibi scintigraphy was applied in 99 patients, localizing putative abnormal parathyroid glands in 87 cases (88%). Comparing scintigraphic findings and surgical results, sestamibi imaging was correct in 61 of 74 cases (82%), yielded negative examinations in 8% of cases, made a false-positive prediction of a solitary adenoma at the wrong site in 1%, made a false-positive prediction of a putative second adenoma in 5%, and predicted a putative solitary adenoma in patients with hyperplasia in 3%. The positive predictive value for sestamibi scintigraphy was 90%. Comparing the 2 methods, it was less likely that ultrasonography would produce a positive test result (80%) than sestamibi imaging (92%). For eutopic solitary adenomas, the likelihood of a correct positive test result was essentially the same regardless of imaging method. The likelihood of obtaining useful added information by combining the 2 tests was low (Table 5).

Conclusions.—As parathyroid imaging techniques, ultrasonography and sestamibi scintigraphy produced relatively comparable results. The advantages of ultrasonography include low cost, convenience, no radiation exposure, the ability to define anatomic details precisely, and the ability to detect concomitant thyroid nodules and carcinoma. The advantages of sestamibi scintigraphy include a slightly increased likelihood of obtaining a positive test result and better sensitivity in detecting ectopic parathyroid adenomas.

TABLE 5.—Results of Combined Ultrasonographic and Sestamibi Parathyroid Imaging Results in 99 Unselected Patients With Primary Hyperparathyroidism

(A) Sestamibi imaging results in patients with positive *vs.* negative ultrasonography

	Sestamibi imaging result			
	Positive, concordant with ultrasonography	Negative	Positive, discordant for location *vs.* ultrasonography	Positive, ultrasonography negative
Ultrasonography positive ($n = 73$)	53	10	10	—
Ultrasonography negative ($n = 26$)	—	2	—	24

(B) Ultrasonography results in patients with positive *vs.* negative sestamibi imaging

	Ultrasonography imaging result			
	Positive, concordant with sestamibi	Negative	Positive, discordant for location *vs.* sestamibi	Positive, sestamibi negative
Sestamibi positive ($n = 87$)	53	24	10	—
Sestamibi negative ($n = 12$)	—	2	—	10

Note: Values shown represent the number of patients with the indicated imaging results.

(Courtesy of Haber RS, Kim CK, Inabnet WB: Ultrasonography for preoperative localization of enlarged parathyroid glands in primary hyperparathyroidism: Comparison with ^{99m}technetium sestamibi scintigraphy. *Clin Endocrinol (Oxf)* 57:241-249, 2002. Reprinted by permission of Blackwell Publishing.)

► Although these authors suggest that ultrasonography may have a role in preoperative localization of parathyroid adenomas, there is not much to really support this suggestion. Sestamibi scintigraphy has a significantly higher sensitivity than ultrasonography and has been generally accepted as the most effective approach to preoperative localization. The concept of doing 2 tests does not seem justified in view of the small number of additional cases in which the localization might be obtained. This is especially true since mibi scintigraphy was more sensitive for ectopic parathyroid adenomas where the problem of localization is particularly difficult. Although it is helpful for the surgeon to know on which side the adenoma is likely located to minimize operative time, the failure to accurately localize the adenoma in the neck is not a severe problem. On the other hand, ectopic parathyroids are extremely difficult to approach surgically and in that situation, the scan becomes invaluable. If ultrasound is not of great help in this particular situation, there seems to be little justification for including it in the diagnostic algorithm.

M. D. Blaufox, MD, PhD

Intraoperative Gamma Probe Detection of Insulinoma in an Elderly Patient With Pancreatic Cystic Lesions

Rosière A, Ernst YJ, Roelants V, et al (Université Catholique de Louvain, Yvoir, Belgium)

Clin Endocrinol (Oxf) 57:547-549, 2002 10–16

Introduction.—Insulinoma is a rare endocrine tumor that can be erroneously attributed to cerebrovascular disease in the elderly due to predominant neurogenic symptoms. Reported was an elderly patient in whom a diagnosis of insulinoma was difficult because of morphological changes of the pancreas that occur with age.

Case Report.—Woman, 81, was seen for recurrent episodes of confusion, abnormal behavior, and possible nocturnal hypoglycemia. She had been admitted 1 month earlier to another hospital and diagnosed with cerebral vascular accident. During the first night after admission, she had grand mall seizures provoked by a reduction in plasma glucose to 1.5 mmol/L. Her plasma insulin and C-peptide levels were 80.4 pmol/L and 0.6 pmol/mL, respectively. A pancreatic CT scan, MRI, and arteriography results were normal. On ^{111}In-DTPA-octreotide scintigraphy, a hotspot was observed in the pancreatic tail (Fig 1). Intraoperative pancreatic US and palpation were noncontributory as a result of multiple pancreatic cysts and nodular lesions. A gamma-detecting probe localized a small tumor that was labelled preoperatively with ^{111}In-DTPA-octreotide. Intraoperative insulin measurements in portal venous blood verified the successful removal of a well-encapsulated insulinoma that was 6 mm in diameter. Her insulin levels dropped to 60.3 pmol/L (glycemia, 7.8 mmol/

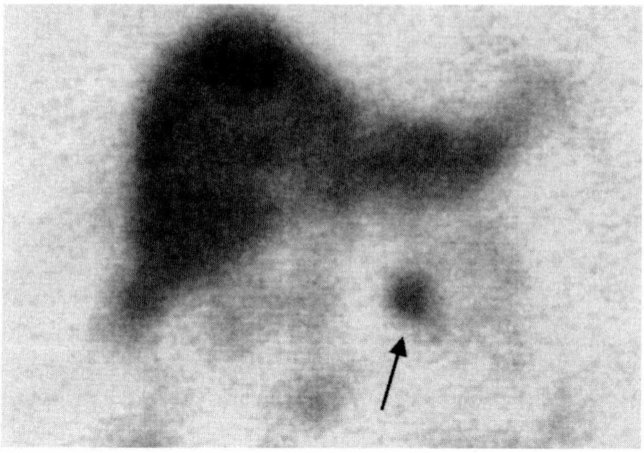

FIGURE 1.—^{111}In-DTPA-octreotide scintigraphy (coronal slice) showing a hotspot (*arrow*) in the tail of the pancreas. (Courtesy of Rosière A, Ernst YJ, Roelants V, et al: Intraoperative gamma probe detection of insulinoma in an elderly patient with pancreatic cystic lesions. *Clin Endocrinol (Oxf)* 57:547-549, 2002. Reprinted by permission of Blackwell Publishing.)

L). Ten days after surgery, the patient was discharged with normal glucose profiles. At 1-month follow-up, she had recovered fully.

Conclusion.—Pancreatic cystic lesions increase with age, making the intraoperative localization of insulinoma challenging. Intraoperative gamma probe detection of the tumor labelled with ^{111}In-DTPA-octreotide may be a useful surgical tool.

▶ This case report supports the very wide potential utility of the intraoperative gamma probe. A new device that has recently appeared, it is essentially a very small, solid-state gamma camera that provides images as a localizing technique rather than counts. Although it will not be as easy to manipulate as the probe, it provides one more approach to the intraoperative localization of lesions that may be difficult to find by other means.

M. D. Blaufox, MD, PhD

Insulin Stimulates Liver Glucose Uptake in Humans: An ^{18}F-FDG PET Study

Iozzo P, Geisler F, Oikonen V, et al (Univ of Turku, Finland; CNR (Natl Research Council), Pisa, Italy; Technical Univ of Munich; et al)

J Nucl Med 44:682-689, 2003 10–17

Background.—The liver is vital to glucose hemostasis, yet our understanding of hepatic glucose uptake is incomplete because of the liver's inaccessibility to direct measurements. Thus, 3 different methods—^{18}F-FDG PET, graphic analysis, and 3-compartment modeling—were used to determine the effect of insulin on hepatic glucose uptake in subjects with varying degrees of insulin sensitivity (IS).

Methods.—The study included 31 men as follows: 8 young athletes (high IS), 16 healthy but sedentary adults (normal IS), and 7 older adults with mild coronary artery disease (low IS). All of the high IS subjects and 9 of the normal IS subjects underwent euglycemic clamping; the other 8 normal IS subjects underwent fasting glucose studies. The low IS subjects underwent both studies, on separate days. All subjects underwent whole-body ^{18}F-FDG PET to determine glucose uptake by the liver. Data were also analyzed using a 3-compartment model to estimate ^{18}F-FDG plasma and tissue levels and ^{18}F-FDG-6-phosphate tissue levels. A graphical analysis was also done.

Results.—Whole-body insulin-mediated glucose uptake increased significantly as IS increased; uptakes in the low, normal, and high IS group were 24, 35, and 65 μmol/min per kg, respectively. During hyperinsulinemia, hepatic glucose influx increased significantly (from 1.5 to 2.3 μmol/min per 100 mL), and glucose phosphorylation rates also increased significantly (from 0.36 to 0.55/min $\times$ 10^{-2}); the increases in all 3 groups were similar. However, the glucose phosphorylation-to-dephosphorylation ratio decreased significantly in the low IS group compared with that of the other 2 groups. The glucose phosphorylation-to-dephosphorylation ratio correlated significantly with whole-body insulin-mediated glucose disposal (r = .045). A significant and inverse relationship was noted between glucose influx rates and fasting plasma free fatty acid levels. Both the 3-compartment model and the graphical analysis accurately described the data, although graphical analysis tended to underestimate glucose influx rates during fasting.

Conclusion.—Euglycemic hyperinsulinemia increases glucose uptake in the liver. Low IS is characterized by a reduced glucose phosphorylation-to-dephosphorylation ratio. ^{18}F-FDG PET provides valuable information about hepatic glucose uptake, and both 3-compartment modeling and graphical analysis are useful complementary or alternative approaches to investigating glucose metabolism in the liver.

► Hepatic glucose production and glycogen storage are certainly critical components of the treatment and diagnosis of patients with diabetes. This study, again, shows the great power of PET, which makes it possible to study the role of insulin and liver glucose uptake directly in humans. A possible practical clinical consideration is that in institutions where insulin is used to lower plasma glucose in patients with hyperglycemia at the time of PET study, a possible additional problem to increased muscle uptake may also be an increased hepatic uptake.

M. D. Blaufox, MD, PhD

PET Imaging of Somatostatin Receptors: Design, Synthesis and Preclinical Evaluation of a Novel ^{18}F-Labelled, Carbohydrated Analogue of Octreotide

Wester HJ, Schottelius M, Scheidhauer K, et al (Technische Universität Munčhen, Germany; Univ of Berne, Switzerland)

Eur J Nucl Med 30:117-122, 2003 10–18

Background.—Strategies for somatostatin receptor (sst)–targeted imaging and therapeutic intervention have been intensively investigated for the past 2 decades. The sst ligand ^{111}In-DTPA-octreotide has been approved for routine clinical scintigraphy of sst-expressing tumors, and ^{99m}Tc-depreotide has been approved for the evaluation of lung carcinoma. In recent years, there has been growing interest in sst scintigraphy with PET. The goal of this study was the design, synthesis, and preclinical evaluation of a carbohydrated ^{18}F-labeled ligand for use in sst PET imaging

Methods.—The affinity profile of ^{18}F-FP-Gluc-TOCA was assessed in cells expressing sst1-sst5. Pretreatment experiments in mice and in rats were used to demonstrate the specificity of tumor uptake in vivo. In addition, an ^{18}F-FP-Gluc-TOCA PET study was performed in a patient with a metastatic carcinoid of the liver with unknown primary.

Results.—The tracer cleared rapidly via renal excretion in the mice, showing low uptake in the liver and intestine and high tumor uptake. Tumor-to-nontumor ratios at 60 minutes p.i. reached 25 for blood, 19 for liver, 7 for intestine, 1.6 for kidney, and 56 for muscle. A similar pattern of biodistribution was seen in pancreatic tumor-bearing rats. The tumor uptake in rats was reduced to 36% and 18% of control at 30 and 60 minutes, respectively, by co-injection of 500 µg Tyr^{3}-octreotide, which showed sst-specific uptake. In the ^{18}F-FP-Gluc-TOCA-PET study of a patient with a metastatic carcinoid of the liver, the tracer showed superior pharmacokinetic properties in regard to rapid urinary excretion and low uptake in the liver, kidney, and spleen. Multiple liver lesions and previously unknown focal uptake of the abdomen were clearly visible.

Conclusion.—^{18}F-FP-Gluc-TOCA is a promising tracer for use in PET imaging of sst-positive tumors and warrants further investigation.

▶ Although ^{18}F-FDG is an extremely versatile radiopharmaceutical, it presents us with the usual problem that we face in nuclear medicine of nonspecific uptake of our imaging agents. The next decade should see a significant number of new agents introduced which are more specific and will expand the use of PET and improve on its sensitivity and specificity, especially in nonneoplastic diseases. Many of the agents currently being considered are labeled with carbon-11 which suffers from the disadvantage of its short half life, making it less practical for widespread application. The introduction of ^{18}F-labeled compounds is far more desirable. This is a significant contribution since octreotide has already been shown to be of value in a wide variety of diseases associated with increased somatastin receptor, and its label with ^{18}F allows for better imaging characteristics.

M. D. Blaufox, MD, PhD

Clinical Value of Somatostatin Receptor Imaging in Patients With Suspected Head and Neck Paragangliomas

Schmidt M, Fischer E, Dietlein M, et al (Universität zu Köln, Germany)

Eur J Nucl Med 29:1571-1580, 2002 10–19

Background.—Paragangliomas or glomus tumors of the head and neck are rare, usually benign neuroendocrine tumors that can cause cranial nerve dysfunction. These tumors express somatostatin, and thus somatostatin receptor scintigraphy (SRS) might help in their localization. The clinical value of SRS in patients with head and neck paragangliomas was examined.

Methods.—The subjects were 19 patients (3 males and 16 females 11-78 years of age) with known or suspected paragangliomas of the head and neck, based on CT or MRI. Each patient was injected IV with 140-220 MBq ^{111}In-octreotide, then 4-6 and 24 hours thereafter underwent [^{111}In-DTPA-D-Phe^{1}]-octreotide scintigraphy. Whole-body and planar images were examined to determine qualitative tracer uptake. Results of SRS were compared with those of CT and MRI, histologic examination, and clinical follow-up.

Results.—Results of SRS were positive in 9 patients, including 3 with previously undiagnosed paragangliomas and 6 with recurrent disease. Tracer uptake was intense in 6 of these 9 patients (Fig 1), moderate in 1 patient, and faint in 2 patients. All 9 of these results were true-positive. SRS correctly ruled out paragangliomas in 9 patients, including 2 patients with ectasia of the bulbus venae jugularis, 2 with a strong family history of paragangliomas, 1 with chronic hyperplastic otitis externa, 1 with granuloma tissue and an organized hematoma, 1 with an acoustic neuroma, 1 with an asymmetric internal carotid artery, and 1 with a jugular vein thrombus. SRS results were false-negative in 1 case, that of a 47-year-old man with recurrent paraganglioma tissue who had previously undergone surgery and postoperative radiotherapy; MRI results were also negative in this case.

Conclusion.—SRS provides important diagnostic information for detecting paragangliomas of the head and neck. SRS can provide information earlier than can CT or MRI, which can be useful in planning treatment. However, because many tumors express somatostatin, SRS is not specific for paraganglioma tissue.

► Anyone who has dealt with patients with tumors of the head and neck is thoroughly aware of the great difficulties of interpreting MRI and CT in this area of very complex anatomy. The advantage of nuclear imaging agents is that the abnormal focus stands out as a hot spot and is relatively easily identified. The combination of nuclear imaging with some form of co-registration with MRI or CT helps to localize these lesions very well. We often, in retrospect, once we have localized a lesion with PET imaging, can go back and see what is

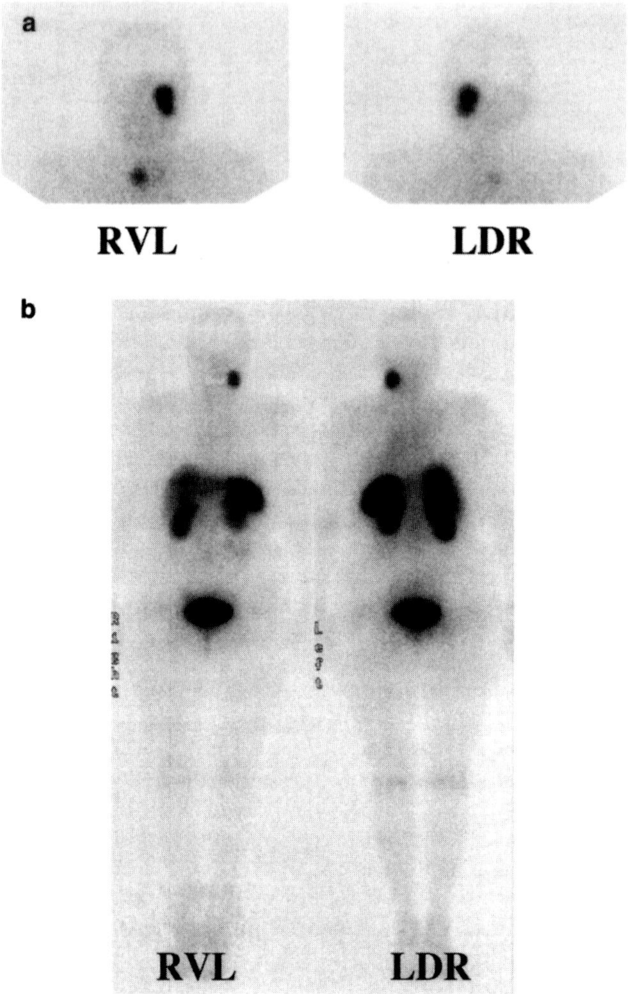

FIGURE 1.—**a**, A 78-year-old woman with a histologically proven recurrent left jugulotympanic paraganglioma. **b**, A 76-year-old woman with a left glomus caroticum tumor which had been known for about 6 1/2 years. *Abbreviations: RVL*, Right ventral left (anterior view); *LDR*, left dorsal right (posterior view). (Courtesy of Schmidt M, Fischer E, Dietlein M, et al. Clinical value of somatostatin receptor imaging in patients with suspected head and neck paragangliomas. *Eur J Nucl Med* 29:1571-1580, 2002. Copyright, Springer-Verlag.)

present on the CT, although the findings are relatively subtle. The uptake of somatostatin by paragangliomas of the head and neck is an encouraging approach to diagnosis of lesions in this area. Although the tumor is very rare, it is still very encouraging to have a very good diagnostic test.

M. D. Blaufox, MD, PhD

Safe and Effective Inhibition of Renal Uptake of Radiolabelled Octreotide by a Combination of Lysine and Arginine

Rolleman EJ, Valkema R, de Jong M, et al (Erasmus Med Centre, Rotterdam, The Netherlands)

Eur J Nucl Med 30:9-15, 2003 10–20

Background.—Scintigraphy with [^{111}In-DTPA^0]octreotide is the method of choice for detecting and staging somatostatin receptor–positive lesions, including neuroendocrine tumors, breast cancer, and small-cell lung cancer. Peptide receptor radionuclide therapy (PRRT) also uses radiolabeled octreotide and other somatostatin analogues, but the high renal uptake of the radiolabeled compounds can produce renal radiation toxicity, limiting the usefulness of PRRT. The uptake of low molecular weight proteins can be inhibited by cationic compounds such as amino acids, so current PRRT protocols use amino acids to reduce renal uptake, which also reduces the dose of radiation to the kidney by approximately 40%. The various amino acid solutions used were evaluated for their effectiveness in reducing renal uptake of radioactivity in PRRT and for the side effects produced.

Methods.—The 26 patients with end-stage neuroendocrine tumors received either diagnostic (220 MBq) or therapeutic (7-10 GBq) doses of [^{111}In-DTPA^0]octreotide with at least one dose not accompanied by an amino acid co-infusion. The amino acid solutions used included a commercially available amino acid solution (AA), lysine preparations, or a combination of lysine and arginine (LysArg). Saline/glucose infusions were given to evaluate the effect of volume administration alone.

Results.—Saline/glucose solutions did not alter the renal uptake of [^{111}In-DTPA^0]octreotide or uptake by the spleen, liver, or tumors. A 20% inhibition was produced with the use of AA or 25 or 50 g of lysine. An inhibition of about 44% was achieved by using a co-infusion of 75 g of lysine, whereas 25 g of lysine plus 25 g of arginine produced a 33% inhibition. Serum potassium levels rose significantly when patients were given 75 g of lysine and LysArg, reaching toxic levels in 3 of 6 patients receiving the 75-g dose of lysine. No alterations in the serum levels of sodium, phosphate, or chloride occurred. Vomiting was the principal side effect of the amino acid infusions, especially those receiving AA; vomiting also occurred in 6% of patients who received no amino acid infusion.

Conclusions.—Renal radioactivity was best inhibited with the use of 75 g of lysine, but this was accompanied by severe hyperkalemia and proved unsuitable for clinical use. The degree of vomiting with AA was profound. LysArg produced the second best results, with no serious hyperkalemia and no vomiting. Thus, infusion of 25 g of lysine plus 25 g of arginine was both effective and safe for patients having PRRT.

► Renal uptake of many imaging compounds presents a problem both in diagnosis and in therapy. Renal uptake may cause problems in interpretation, especially when some of the radionuclide is in the ureter and can be mistaken for the "hot spot." Renal excretion can either reduce the effective radiation dose given in therapy for some conditions or may be a problem because of undesirable radiation to the kidney and bladder. Amino acids have been used extensively in efforts to deal with this problem. The authors report that LysArg reduces renal radioactivity in patients being treated with radiolabeled octreotide and that it results in no significant on serious side effects. However, these agents do cause significant elevations of serum potassium levels, and the experience reported here is relatively limited, with only 11 patients receiving the LysArg combination and with 1 patient reaching a serum potassium level of 6.0 mmol/L. This work suggests that LysArg can inhibit renal radioactivity in PRRT, but further work is needed to clarify its role and support its safety.

M. D. Blaufox, MD, PhD

SPECT Semiquantitative Analysis of Adrenocortical ^{131}I-6β-Iodomethyl-Norcholesterol Uptake to Discriminate Subclinical and Preclinical Functioning Adrenal Incidentaloma

La Cava G, Imperiale A, Olianti C, et al (Univ of Florence, Italy)

J Nucl Med 44:1057-1064, 2003 10–21

Background.—The functional assessment of benign adrenal masses is an important concern because several late clinical consequences may be expected in patients with borderline preclinical functional increase. The terms "subclinical Cushing's syndrome" (SC-CS) and "preclinical Cushing's syndrome" (PC-CS) have often been used synonymously; however, the PC-CS patients are at risk for development of an overt Cushing's syndrome (CS). The purpose of this study was to determine the clinical reliability of a proposed ^{131}I-6β-iodomethyl-norcholesterol (^{131}I-NP-59) uptake semiquantitative evaluation method for the characterization of adrenocortical masses in a selected population of patient with disease clinically classified as subclinical and preclinical Cushing's syndrome according to Reincke's definition.

Methods.—A total of 47 patients with incidentally discovered unilateral adrenal masses were examined with abdominal SPECT after IV injection of ^{131}I-NP-59 at 24, 48, 72, and, in some cases, 96 hours after tracer injection (Fig 1). A standard elliptical region of interest was manually drawn and connected with the adrenals and liver, avoiding the gallbladder region. The adrenal region of interest integral count, which was determined by summing the 24-, 48-, and 72-hour counting values, was normalized by the hepatic integral count. The adrenal percentage of relative uptake (UPT%) was then computed.

Results.—Discriminant analysis was performed on 3 variables—UPT%, adrenocorticotropic hormone serum concentration, and CT mass dimension—to determine the variable, or combination of variables, that best discriminated between the SC-CS and PC-CS groups. Univariate analysis showed that, compared with both ACTH and CT mass dimension, the UPT% variable was the most significant discriminating variable between the SC-CS and PC-CS groups, with overall accuracy, sensitivity, and specificity equal to 90%, 91%, and 89%, respectively. Stepwise discriminant analysis

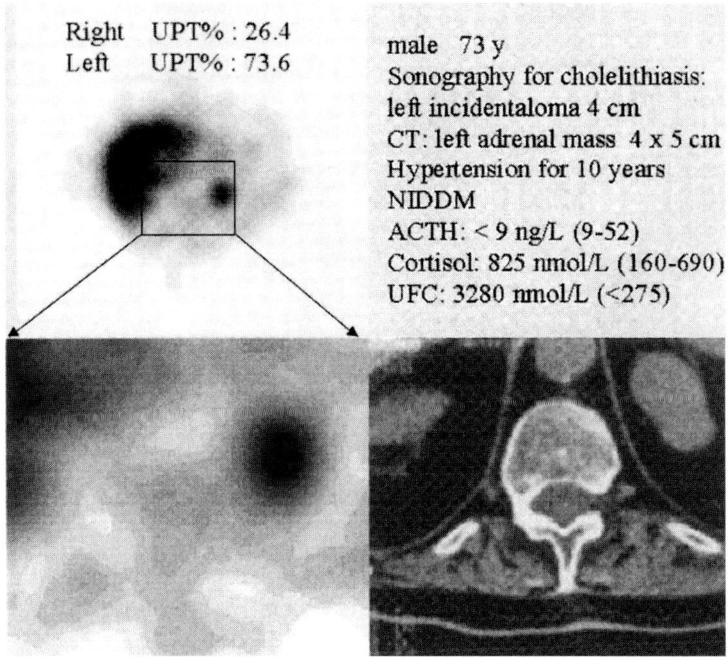

FIGURE 1.—Typical adrenal incidentaloma SPECT study at 72 hours after ^{131}I-NP-59 injection in patient classified, according to Reincke (Reincke M: Subclinical Cushing's syndrome. *Endocrinol Metab Clin North Am* 29:43-56, 2000), as preclinical Cushing's syndrome. Scintigraphic study shows typical example of concordant pattern: increased radiotracer uptake on side of lesion demonstrated on CT scan (4 × 5 cm left corticoadrenal adenoma). *Abbreviations: NIDDM*, Non–insulin-dependent diabetes mellitus; *ACTH*, adrenocorticotropic hormone; *UFC*, urinary freecortisol. (Reprinted by permission of the Society of Nuclear Medicine from La Cava G, Imperiale A, Olianti C, et al: SPECT semiquantitative analysis of adrenocortical ^{131}I-6β-iodomethyl-norcholesterol uptake to discriminate subclinical and preclinical functioning adrenal incidentaloma. *J Nucl Med* 44:1057-1064, 2003.)

of all 3 variables yielded a classification matrix that correctly classified all 9 patients in the SC-CS group and 18 of 22 patients in the PC-CS group, with 100% positive and 69% negative predictive values and an overall accuracy, sensitivity, and specificity of 87%, 82%, and 100%, respectively.

Conclusion.—The indication from these initial findings is that the use of the semiquantitative method proposed in this report in association with both laboratory screening for cortisol production and CT mass dimension measurement can increase the clinical diagnostic accuracy of PC-CS. This technique could be used to follow adrenal mass function whenever hormonal or clinical features suggest adrenocortical hyperfunction.

► Early disease is always difficult to find. Any methodology that helps us make a diagnosis before obvious clinical symptomatology has appeared is certainly welcome. The authors' suggestion that a semiquantitative analysis of adrenocortical imaging with SPECT can accomplish this is attractive. It is remarkable how with the inherent quantitative capability of nuclear medicine technology, we actually have so few truly useful quantitative procedures. Our closest approach to quantitation always seems to end up being a semiquantitative one. As the authors point out, incidental detection of adrenal masses is not uncommon with the high number of imaging procedures currently performed. This problem extends to PET as well, where it also is not uncommon to be faced with a dilemma of whether or not an adrenal is imaged is of clinical significance.

M. D. Blaufox, MD, PhD

11 Renal

Introduction

Although productivity in renal nuclear medicine has fallen during the last several years, it is interesting to note that the range of articles published has a considerably broader perspective. Of course, there are the usual articles on clearance, some of which have been included in this YEAR BOOK. However, we now have a number of articles devoted to evaluation of significant parenchymal damage, including one that I have included on the use of PET to evaluate renal blood flow in the face of severely decreased renal function. A very important development in the renal area is the emergence of competing radiographic techniques. For instance, an article is included here that reviews the use of ultrasound in the grading of renal cortical damage in the presence of obstruction. MR renography is even put forth as a possible alternative to radionuclide renography using gadopentetate dimeglumine. Although I am not convinced of the value of this approach as an alternative to conventional renography, it is an interesting technique to consider. Another MR article abstracted here suggests that this technique may even be superior to conventional radionuclide techniques.

An abstract on color Doppler of the testis is included, and there is no question of the impact of this radiographic technique on nuclear medicine. In our institution, we have seen a decrease in the utilization of testicular scanning from as much as 1 or 2 scans per week to virtually zero. This is a result of most patients with testicular disease being referred for ultrasound.

Another unfulfilled promise in nuclear medicine is its application in penile disease. Although some promising studies were published several years ago, the technique was rapidly supplanted by the use of ultrasound. A novel although uncommon application of penile scintigraphy is abstracted here in a study that suggests that it may be of value in differentiating the stable and unstable phases of Peyronie's disease. All together, although progress in nuclear medicine study of renal disease has slowed, the field still is active and hopefully over the next several years, newer and more innovative techniques will be introduced, in particular the use of PET imaging.

M. Donald Blaufox, MD, PhD

Indexing Glomerular Filtration Rate to Suit Children

Bird NJ, Henderson BL, Lui D, et al (Addenbrooke's Hosp, Cambridge, England; Harley Street Clinic, London; Middlesex Hosp, London)
J Nucl Med 44:1037-1043, 2003 11–1

Background.—Glomerular filtration rate (GFR) is usually indexed to body surface area (BSA) to allow comparison of persons of differing size. However, this application of BSA has been criticized, not only in relation to GFR but also in relation to other hemodynamic variables. This approach is not suitable for children because they have a relatively high BSA simply because of their small size. A variable for which there is good evidence for indexing GFR in children is total body water; however, it is not practical to obtain this measurement every time GFR is measured. An investigation was conducted to identify an appropriate, simple whole-body variable based on height and weight suitable for indexing GFR that would be simultaneously appropriate for both children and adults.

FIGURE 1

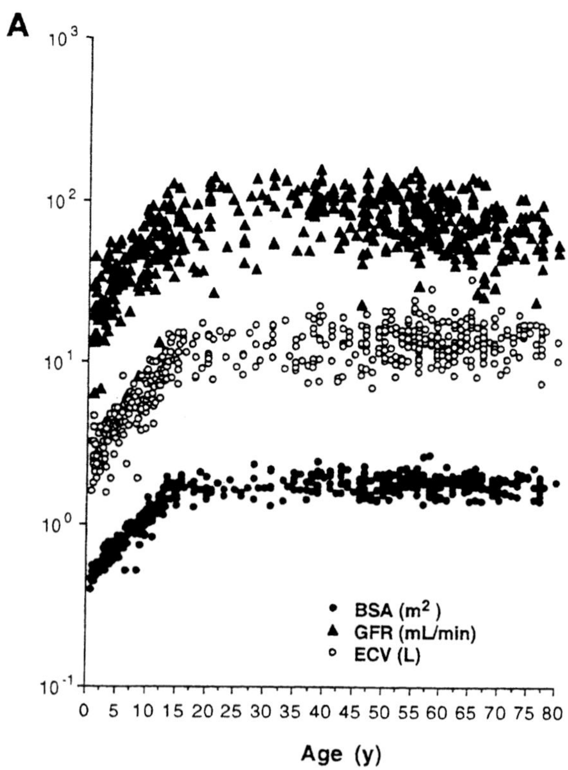

(*Continued*)

Methods.—An analysis was conducted of a database of 532 routine clinical GFR measurements, each based on 3 venous blood samples obtained between 2 and 4 hours after injection of ^{51}Cr-ethylenediaminetetraacetic acid. The purpose of the analysis was to determine the GFR and, using only the half-time of the slope of the clearance curve, the quotient GFR to extracellular fluid volume (ECV). BSA was determined from the Haycock formula, which is based on height and weight raised to indexes to give units of area. An equation analogous to Haycock's was formulated in which the indexes of height and weight were varied to provide an iterative best fit to ECV instead of BSA.

Results.—The GFR, ECV, and BSA were found to increase as functions of age until about age 13 years, corresponding to a BSA of about 1.35 m^2, which was taken as the cutoff point between children and adults (Fig 1). As humans grow, the ratio of height to effective radius changes as a nonlinear function of surface area; thus, humans must change shape as they grow. A new equation was proposed: ECV = $weight^{0.6469} \times height^{0.7236} \times 0.02154$.

ECV corresponding to a BSA of 1.73 m^2 (whether measured or estimated from the new equation) was 12.9 L. GFR indexed to this new equation cor-

FIGURE 1 (cont.)

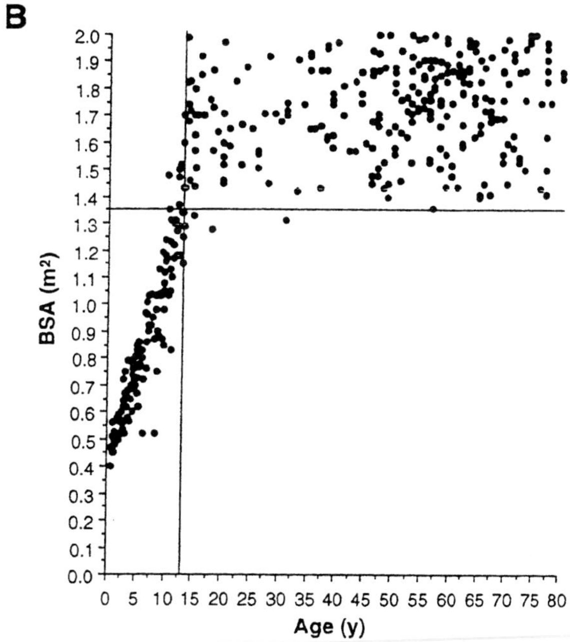

FIGURE 1.—A, Increase in glomerular filtration rate (*GFR*), measured extracellular fluid volume (*ECV*), and body surface area (*BSA*) as function of age. All increase broadly exponentially until about age 13 years, when they all stop increasing fairly abruptly. B, Population with BSA above cutoff value of 1.35 m^2 (*horizontal line*) includes only 5 (of 131) children (less than13 years of age; *vertical line*), and population below cutoff value of 1.35 m^2 includes only 3 (of 401) adults. (Reprinted by permission of the Society of Nuclear Medicine from Bird NJ, Henderson BL, Lui D, et al: Indexing glomerular filtration rate to suit children. *J Nucl Med* 44:1037-1043, 2003.)

related more closely with GFR indexed to ECV than did GFR indexed to BSA and, along with GFR/ECV, showed a greater decline as a function of age than did GFR/BSA.

Conclusion.—When GFR is required in absolute units rather than as a rate of turnover of extracellular volume, the rate is appropriately indexed to indexes of height and weight as defined by the new equation presented in this report. This procedure will avoid disadvantages to children from indexing to body surface area and can reveal higher values of filtration function in children than have previously been reported.

► This study is directed at an extremely difficult problem in children. The measurement of renal function is hard to characterize because of the relationship of renal function to body size and changes that occur with age. Serum creatinine and creatinine clearance are particularly unreliable in children because of the rapid changes in muscle mass. This study uses a very large number of patients to derive a new approach indexed to height and weight and keyed to ECV rather than BSA. Hopefully, other centers will be able to apply these results and determine their reliability. The issue of concern is, of course, the fact that equations drawn upon specific populations sometimes fail when used more generally.

M. D. Blaufox, MD, PhD

Comparison of Relative Renal Function by Renal Scintigraphy and Lateralized Creatinine Clearance in Children With Bilateral Vesicoureteral Reflux

Mindrup SR, Cooper CS, Hodroff MA, et al (Univ of Iowa, Iowa City)
Urology 61:816-819, 2003 11–2

Objectives.—To evaluate the relative renal function on preoperative and postoperative renal scintigraphy with lateralized creatinine clearance. Multiple factors affect renal blood flow and glomerular filtration that alter the relative renal function calculated by renal scintigraphy. The relative renal function according to renal scintigraphy in children with bilateral vesicoureteral reflux has not been compared with lateralized creatinine clearance.

Methods.—We retrospectively reviewed the charts of 45 children treated surgically for bilateral vesicoureteral reflux. The average age at time of reimplantation was 5.3 years. Bilateral ureteral catheters were placed intraoperatively. Lateralized creatinine clearance was measured with 24-hour urine collections postoperatively from each catheter. Bladder catheterization was not performed during the renal scans.

Results.—Thirty-six of 45 children had preoperative 1 to 3-minute relative renal function assessed by scintigraphy, 28 had a postoperative assessment, and 24 had both. Preoperative relative renal function ranged between 51% and 94% (mean 61.3%) in the higher functioning kidney. Postoperative renal function ranged from 47% to 90% (mean 60.5%) in the higher functioning kidney. A strong correlation existed between preoperative relative renal function and lateralized creatinine clearance ($P < 0.0001$). Similarly, a significant correlation existed between the postoperative assessment and lateralized creatinine clearance ($P < 0.0003$). No significant difference occurred between the preoperative and postoperative 1 to 3-minute relative renal function ($P = 0.3552$).

Conclusions.—The 1 to 3-minute relative renal function determined by renal scintigraphy accurately reflects the relative renal function determined by lateralized creatinine clearance. Bladder catheterization does not appear necessary for accurate determination of relative renal function by renal scan even in the presence of bilateral reflux.

► It is interesting to see a comparison with individual function measured by nuclear medicine techniques and individual creatinine clearance. These measurements are particularly difficult to obtain at this time because of the trend away from invasive measurements of differential renal function. The authors have a reasonably large series from which to make their assessment. The results are quite surprising since the agents used were glucoheptonate and dimercaptosuccinic acid. It is generally accepted practice not to measure relative renal function with these agents until about 1 to 2 hours after the injection when the radioactivity is localized in the cortex, and there is maximum target to background ratio. These results would be difficult to validate since few centers would have the data or patient population to carry out such a study. Therefore, if we accept this as presented, there would be strong support to consider using the 1- to 3-minute uptake of these agents for relative renal function, which, certainly, greatly simplifies the measurement. It might be interesting to obtain some studies comparing the 1- to 3-minute uptake with the 1- or 2-hour uptake.

M. D. Blaufox, MD, PhD

Radionuclide Voiding Patterns in Children With Vesicoureteral Reflux

Vlajković M, Ilić S, Bogićević M, et al (Clinical Ctr Nis, Yugoslavia; Clinical Ctr Serbia, Belgrade, Yugoslavia)

Eur J Nucl Med Mol Imaging 30:532-537, 2003 11–3

Background.—Many children with primary vesicoureteral reflux (VUR) also have voiding dysfunction. The efficacy of indirect radionuclide cystography (IRNC) to identify these children was determined.

Methods.—The study included 74 neurologically intact children (14 boys, 60 girls), 2 to 14 years old with VUR as confirmed by contrast micturating cystourethrography. All patients underwent IRNC with ^{99m}Tc DTPA. An IV injection of 37 MBq per 10-kg body weight DTPA was given, then voiding urodynamics were examined in the posterior view with acquisition of 90 frames every 2 seconds.

Results.—As many as 64 of these patients with primary VUR (86%) had symptoms of urinary tract dysfunction. IRNC identified 3 groups of patients with VUR: 27 patients with normal urodynamic results, 43 patients with de-

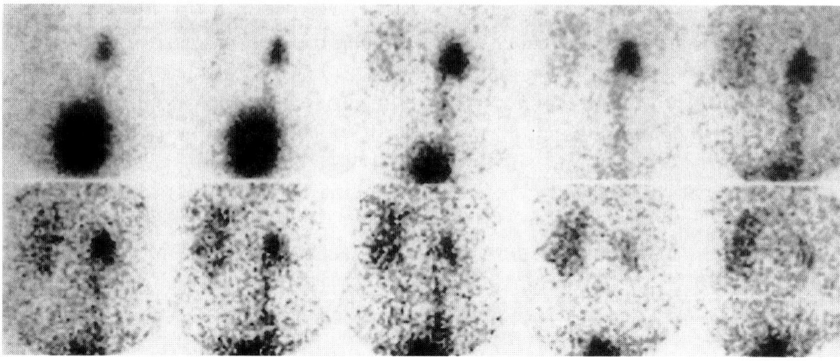

FIGURE 1.—Characteristic indirect radionuclide cystography findings during and after micturition in a child with vesicoureteral reflux and detrusor hyperreflexia, also illustrating the mechanism for refilling the bladder. (Courtesy of Vlajković M, Ilić S, Bogićević M, et al: Radionuclide voiding patterns in children with vesicoureteral reflux. *Eur J Nucl Med Mol Imaging* 30:532-537, 2003.)

trusor hyperreflexia (Fig 1), and 4 patients with detrusor-sphincter dyssynergia. Logistic regression analysis identified functional bladder capacity (FBC), peak flow rate (PFR), and ejection fraction (EF) as significant independent predictors of a voiding disorder. Patients whose FBC was < 82% or > 134% had a 4-fold higher risk of having a voiding disorder. Patients whose PFR was < 11 mL/s or > 31 mL/s had a 15-fold higher risk of a voiding disorder. Patients whose EF was < 89% had almost a 16-fold higher risk of a voiding disorder. These 3 variables could characterize each of the 3 groups described previously. Patients with a normal voiding pattern had normal FBC with near-normal PFR and EF. Patients with bladder instability had markedly lower FBC, PFR, and EF. Patients with detrusor-sphincter dyssynergia had higher bladder volume, near-normal PFR, and slightly lower or near-normal EF. If voiding dysfunction were defined as abnormalities in at least 2 of these 3 variables, IRNC would be true-positive in 38 (80.9%) of 47 patients and true-negative in 21 (77.8%) of 27 patients.

Conclusion.—Most of these children with primary VUR had symptoms of urinary tract dysfunction. IRNC could identify 3 voiding patterns that correlated with the presence or absence of voiding dysfunction in children with VUR. IRNC had high sensitivity and specificity and should be considered a first-line test for identifying children with VUR who have abnormal voiding patterns.

► It is important to be aware of the possible association between bladder dysfunction and vesicoureteral reflux. This study shows that a very significant number of children may have problems that need to be addressed besides the reflux itself. Unfortunately, the authors do not mention whether the urine cultures were done at the time of the study. A possible confounding factor in this investigation would be the concurrent presence of urinary tract infection. Regardless of whether infection was present or not, this article properly brings to our attention factors that should be considered in the evaluation of any patient with vesicoureteral reflux.

M. D. Blaufox, MD, PhD

Renal Parenchymal Damage in Sibling Vesicoureteric Reflux
Cascio S, Yoneda A, Chertin B, et al (Our Lady's Hosp for Sick Children, Dublin)
Acta Paediatr 92:17-20, 2003 11–4

Background.—The siblings of children with vesicoureteric reflux (VUR) are at increased risk of having reflux and associated renal parenchymal damage. However, questions remain about whether renal damage occurring in asymptomatic siblings results from congenital renal dysplasia or acquired pyelonephritis. Rates of renal damage were assessed in siblings of children with VUR, including those with and without a history of UTI.

Methods.—The analysis included 226 siblings from 107 families of VUR patients, studied during an 11-year period. These siblings were identified as having VUR on contrast voiding cystourethrography. This examination was performed for documented urinary tract infection (UTI) in 64 siblings and for screening purposes in 55 asymptomatic siblings. The incidence of renal parenchymal damage, assessed by dimercaptosuccinic acid (DMSA) scanning, was compared for siblings with and without a history of UTI.

Results.—Renal nephropathy was detected in 26% of renal refluxing units (RRUs) of siblings with a history of UTI versus 7% of RRUs in the asymptomatic siblings. The rate of mild renal damage was higher in the siblings with documented UTI: 21% of RRUs, compared with just 2% of RRUs in the asymptomatic siblings. In contrast, the rate of moderate to severe renal damage was similar between groups: 5% and 4% of RRUs, respectively.

Conclusions.—Among the siblings of children with VUR, those with a history of documented UTI have a higher rate of mild renal parenchymal damage than asymptomatic siblings studied for screening purposes only. However, moderate to severe renal scarring affects similar proportions of these 2 groups of siblings. Further study is needed to assess the effectiveness of screening to prevent renal damage in asymptomatic siblings of VUR patients.

▶ This article represents one more example of the great potential value of technetium DMSA scans in patients with known or suspected renal disease. There is no other way that these data could have been acquired.

M. D. Blaufox, MD, PhD

Objective Evidence of a High Prevalence of Renal Damage in Women With Type 2 Diabetes by Technetium-99m DMSA Renal Cortex Scan Findings

Wu H-C, Huang W-S, Lin C-C, et al (China Med College, Taichung, Taiwan; Tri-Service Gen Hosp, Taipei, Taiwan)

Urology 61:50-54, 2003 11–5

Objectives.—To compare control women with men and women with type 2 diabetes mellitus (DM) for the prevalence and type of renal damage due to urinary tract infections (UTIs) using technetium-99m dimercapto-succinic acid (^{99m}Tc DMSA) renal scanning. Women with DM have UTIs more often than do women without DM. It is unknown, however, what the prevalence and type of renal damage due to UTI are in these women.

Methods.—Three groups of patients: 28 control women without type 2 DM and a history of UTIs, 25 male patients with type 2 DM but without a history of UTIs, and 103 female patients with type 2 DM underwent ^{99m}Tc DMSA renal scan (Fig 2). The 103 women with type 2 DM were separated into three groups: 36 women without a history of UTIs, 34 patients with a history of cystitis only, and 33 with a history of pyelonephritis.

Results.—All the control women and male patients with type 2 DM without a history of UTIs had normal ^{99m}Tc DMSA renal scan findings. However, 39.8% of women with type 2 DM had abnormal ^{99m}Tc DMSA renal scan findings. Women with type 2 DM without a history of UTI had a significantly lower prevalence of abnormal renal scan findings than did those with a history of cystitis only or pyelonephritis. In addition, the prevalence of abnormal renal scan findings was significantly higher in women with type 2 DM with pyelonephritis than in those with a history of cystitis only. Renal scars on ^{99m}Tc DMSA renal scans were found in women with type 2 DM and a history of pyelonephritis (Table 3).

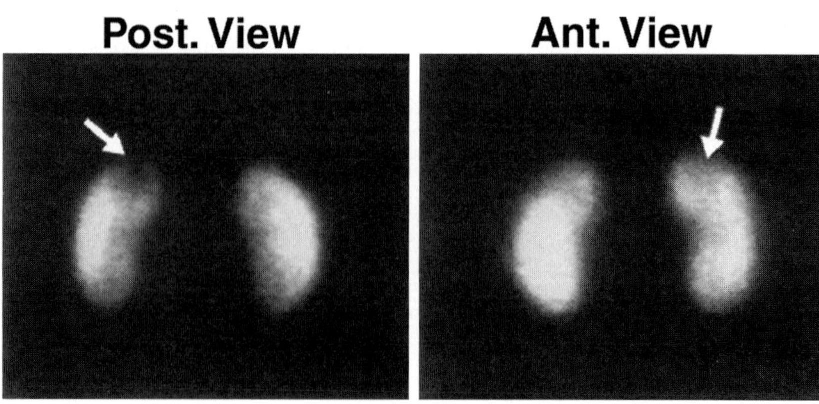

FIGURE 2.—^{99m}Tc DMSA renal scan revealing normal contour, decreased activity in the lateral and medial aspects of upper pole in left kidney (*arrow*), and no volume loss. *Abbreviations: Post.*, Posterior; *Amt.*, anterior. (Reprinted from Wu H-C, Huang W-S, Lin C-C, et al: Objective evidence of a high prevalence of renal damage in women with type 2 diabetes by technetium-99m DMSA renal cortex scan findings. *Urology* 61:50-54. Copyright 2003, with permission from Elsevier Science.)

TABLE 2.—Renal Scan Findings Among Female Controls, Male Patients With Diabetes Mellitus, and Female Patients With Diabetes Mellitus

Renal Scan Findings	Female Controls (n)	Type 2 DM Male Patients (n)	Type 2 DM Female Patients (n)		
			Without UTI	Cystitis	Pyelonephritis
Normal	28	25	35	21	6
Inflammation	0	0	1	13	14
Scar	0	0	0	0	13

Abbreviations: DM, Diabetes mellitus; *UTI*, urinary tract infection.

(Reprinted from Wu H-C, Huang W-S, Lin C-C, et al: Objective evidence of a high prevalence of renal damage in women with type 2 diabetes by technetium-99m DMSA renal cortex scan findings. *Urology* 61:50-54. Copyright 2003, with permission from Elsevier Science.)

Conclusions.—Compared with control women and men with type 2 DM, women with type 2 DM, especially if they had a history of UTIs, had a significantly higher prevalence of abnormal ^{99m}Tc DMSA renal scan findings.

► The problem of renal disease in patients with type 2 diabetes mellitus cannot be stressed enough. Diabetes, and especially in those patients with hypertension, has become a primary cause of renal failure and the eventual need for dialysis in patients with renal disease in this country. It is critically important to develop techniques to determine the potential onset of renal disease so that effective therapies can be initiated. One of the routinely used methodologies is the measurement of microalbuminuria.

It is interesting to note in this study that although the urinary protein excretion was above normal and at a level where one would begin to be concerned about potential renal damage, there was no significant difference in excretion between those patients with diabetes who had normal scans, inflammation, or scarring. Therefore, it appears that the DMSA scan provides an additional bit of information about the possibility of renal disease and may potentially help to find these people earlier. If these studies are corroborated, they can prove to be a very important approach to the evaluation of the patient with diabetes.

M. D. Blaufox, MD, PhD

Dynamic Renal Blood Flow Measurement by Positron Emission Tomography in Patients With CRF

Juillard L, Janier MF, Fouque D, et al (Hôpital Edouard Herriot, Lyon, France; Université Claude Bernard, Lyon, France; Hôpital Cardiologique, Bron, France; et al)

Am J Kidney Dis 40:947-954, 2002 11–6

Background.—Renal blood flow (RBF) is a vital ingredient in kidney function, so its measurement yields an important insight into renal physiology. However, RBF measurements are difficult to obtain noninvasively in humans. Among the noninvasive methods used to measure single-kidney

RBF are electron beam CT, renograms, and possibly MRI; conventional para-3-hippurate (PAH) clearance only estimates RBF and is inaccurate with more severe chronic renal failure (CRF). PET allows dynamic regional blood flow measurements and was evaluated for its ability to detect acute changes in RBF in patients with CRF.

Methods.—Eight men with hypertension and moderate CRF underwent PET-RBF using oxygen 15–labeled water ($H_2{}^{15}O$) before and 5, 40, 80, and 120 minutes after a 10-mg IV injection of quinaprilat was administered. Before the quinaprilat injection and 20, 60, 100, and 140 minutes thereafter, PAH was used to measure the effective renal plasma flow (ERPF) and glomerular filtration rate (GFR), and inulin clearance was determined.

Results.—All patients were able to undergo PET successfully. At baseline, the mean PET-RBF was 221 mL/min/100 g; the values 5, 40, 80, and 120 minutes after quinaprilat injection increased 15.4%, 25.9%, 18.9%, and 22.9%, respectively. For ERPF, the mean baseline value was 225 mL/min/1.73 m^2; no significant changes occurred after quinaprilat injection. No significant changes were noted for PAH-ERPF or GFR; a slight decrease in GFR plus an increase in ERPF led to a significant decline in the filtration fraction 100 and 140 minutes after quinaprilat administration. A high correlation was noted between PET-RBF and PAH-ERPF values (Fig 4). Facial flush developed a few minutes after quinaprilat injection in 5 patients, but no other adverse effects were noted. A significant decline was noted in diastolic blood pressure and mean arterial pressure after patients received the quinaprilat; heart rate was not significantly affected. A significant decrease in serum angiotensin-converting enzyme activity was seen 40, 80, and 120 minutes after

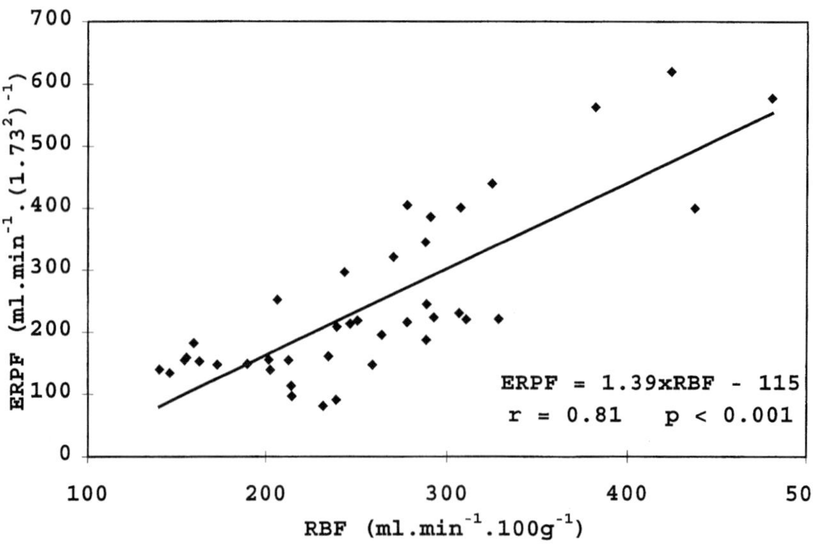

FIGURE 4.—Correlation ($r = 0.81$; $P \leq .001$) between PET-RBF and PAH-ERPF. *Abbreviations*: *RBF*, Renal blood flow; *PAH*, para-aminohippuric acid; *ERPF*, effective renal plasma flow. (Courtesy of Juillard L, Janier MF, Fouque D, et al: Dynamic renal blood flow measurement by positron emission tomography in patients with CRF. *Am J Kidney Dis* 40:947-954, 2002. Copyright National Kidney Foundation.)

the injection of quinaprilat. No significant changes in serum potassium or creatinine levels occurred.

Conclusions.—PET was able to detect and monitor RBF dynamically in patients with CRF. A significant increase in PET-RBF was noted after a single IV injection of an angiotensin-converting enzyme inhibitor. PET proved to be both reliable and sensitive for determining RBF, possibly more sensitive than PAH clearance for detecting acute changes in RBF in humans.

► It is encouraging that we are beginning to see more applications of the use of PET in a variety of renal diseases. Most importantly, this is beginning to make the transition from the laboratory animal to applications in humans. However, it is unfortunate that at the present time, most of the PET imaging agents are compounds that require the immediate proximity of a cyclotron. Studies measuring RBF with PET and ^{15}O-labeled water go back to the early 1960s when Mike Terpogossian was experimenting in this area. He provided very interesting physiologic data, but because of the need for the immediate proximity of a cyclotron, it did not prove practical. Although the authors are still dependent on a short-lived positron emitter, it is quite interesting that they were able to show the potential use of this approach in patients with CRF. It is interesting that in these patients, there was a significant increase in blood flow after the administration of quinaprilat. One might tend to question this significant vasodilatory effect in patients with intrinsic renal disease; however, the findings are corroborated by the changes in PAH clearance. We are desperately in need of an agent that can be used with PET to estimate RBF that employs a readily available positron emmiter with a sufficient half-life to be practical for clinical use. In the meantime, more studies like this are needed to help us better understand the basic physiology of renal disease in humans and to provide techniques for evaluation of therapeutic interventions.

M. D. Blaufox, MD, PhD

Ultrasound Grade of Hydronephrosis and Severity of Renal Cortical Damage on ^{99m}Technetium Dimercaptosuccinic Acid Renal Scan in Infants With Unilateral Hydronephrosis During Followup and After Pyeloplasty

Konda R, Sakai K, Ota S, et al (Tohoku Univ, Sendai, Japan)

J Urol 167:2159-2163, 2002 11–7

Background.—In infants with urinary tract dilatation, there may or may not be active obstruction, and the condition may improve or resolve spontaneously. Therefore, the principal indication for surgery, especially when the patient has asymptomatic hydronephrosis that was detected prenatally, is the function in the obstructed kidney. Among the methods to detect renal function are ultrasonography and ^{99m}technetium (Tc) dimercaptosuccinic acid (DMSA) renal scans. Tubulointerstitial injury is a primary lesion of the obstructed kidney, and such renal damage is more likely to be revealed by detecting tubular dysfunction than by measuring glomerular filtration rate and renal plasma flow. Surgery would be indicated in patients with hydronephrosis who are shown to have tubulointerstitial injury. DMSA renal scans and ultrasonography were performed in infants with unilateral hydronephrosis during follow-up and after pyeloplasty to evaluate whether ultrasound hydronephrosis grade is reflective of the severity of the renal cortical damage, and to monitor the recovery of function in the obstructed kidneys once surgery was accomplished.

Methods.—Eighty boys and 19 girls had unilateral hydronephrosis detected before 1 year of age, with 76% of these detected prenatally. The Society for Fetal Urology (SFU) grading system was used to grade the ultrasound images. The DMSA renal scan assessed the severity of renal cortical damage, with absolute function of the right and left kidneys estimated by DMSA uptake and calculation of the relative DMSA uptake (Fig 1).

Results.—No cortical damage was detected on DMSA scans for kidneys with grade 1 or 2 hydronephrosis. However, cortical damage was detected in 10 of 19 kidneys with grade 3 hydronephrosis, and 49 of 50 kidneys with grade 4 disease. Moderate or mild damage was present on the DMSA renal scans for 10 kidneys with grade 3 hydronephrosis and 33 kidneys with grade 4 disease. Sixteen kidneys with grade 4 hydronephrosis had severe cortical damage. The 2- and 24-hour relative uptakes of DMSA were strongly and significantly correlated. Relative DMSA uptake decreased significantly as the hydronephrosis grade increased. There were no significant differences in relative DMSA uptake among grades 1 to 3 hydronephrosis (Fig 2), but relative DMSA uptake in grade 4 cases was significantly lower than in grades 1 to 3. In 40 patients, pyeloplasty was performed because of renal damage detected on the DMSA renal scan. The relative DMSA uptake was 39.9% and

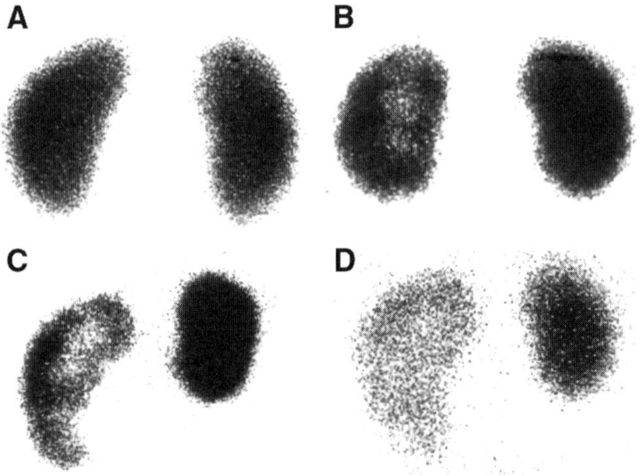

FIGURE 1.—Representative cases classified by DMSA renal scan with obstructed kidney at **left. A,** Normal—no cortical damage. **B,** Mild—focal renal cortical damage in central area. **C,** Moderate—more general renal cortical damage with greater renal length but some areas of normal cortex. **D,** Severe—global cortical damage. (Courtesy of Konda R, Sakai K, Ota S, et al: Ultrasound grade of hydronephrosis and severity of renal cortical damage on ^{99m}technetium dimercaptosuccinic acid renal scan in infants with unilateral hydronephrosis during followup and after pyeloplasty. *J Urol* 167:2159-2163, 2002.)

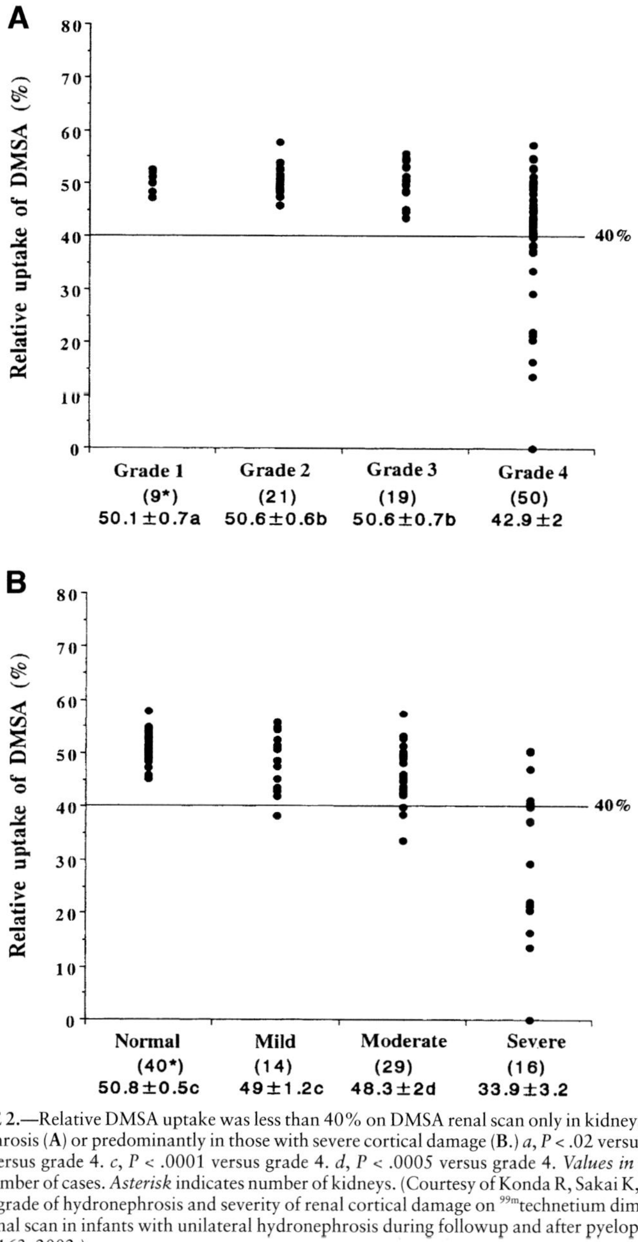

FIGURE 2.—Relative DMSA uptake was less than 40% on DMSA renal scan only in kidneys with grade 4 hydronephrosis (**A**) or predominantly in those with severe cortical damage (**B**.) *a*, $P < .02$ versus grade 4. *b*, $P < .0005$ versus grade 4. *c*, $P < .0001$ versus grade 4. *d*, $P < .0005$ versus grade 4. *Values in parentheses* represent number of cases. *Asterisk* indicates number of kidneys. (Courtesy of Konda R, Sakai K, Ota S, et al: Ultrasound grade of hydronephrosis and severity of renal cortical damage on ^{99m}technetium dimercaptosuccinic acid renal scan in infants with unilateral hydronephrosis during followup and after pyeloplasty. *J Urol* 167:2159-2163, 2002.)

SFU grade was 3 or 4, with moderate or severe renal damage noted in all but one case. When 36 of these 40 patients were evaluated up to 2 years after the surgical procedure, the mean cortical damage score and mean relative DMSA uptake had improved significantly.

Conclusions.—The SFU hydronephrosis grade based on ultrasonographic findings proved to correlate well with the severity of the cortical damage or decline in renal differential function detected with DMSA renal scans. A higher risk for a significant decline in renal function accompanies grade 4 hydronephrosis. DMSA renal scans proved useful in determining surgical indications and monitoring changes in renal function after surgery.

► This study shows very nicely the utility of DMSA scanning in children with unilateral hydronephrosis. The authors present clear evidence that the scan was of great value in guiding the decision for surgery and in the follow-up of these children. It is important to note that this study originates from a department of urology, so that here we are being informed by the user of the value of one of our services.

M. D. Blaufox, MD, PhD

Role of Radioisotope Renal Scans in the Choice of Nephrectomy Side in Live Kidney Donors

Shokeir AA, Gad HM, El-Diasty T (Mansoura Univ, Egypt)

J Urol 170:373-376, 2003 11–8

Objective.—Living donors are a major source of kidneys for transplantation. Previously, the choice of which kidney to use has been based on morphologic findings of imaging studies. The use of radioisotope renal scanning for preoperative evaluation of potential live kidney donors was reported.

Methods.—During a 21-month period, radioisotope renal scanning was performed in 300 consecutive live kidney donation candidates. The renal scan was added to standard laboratory and imaging tests, with selective measurement of glomerular filtration rate (GFR) for each kidney. Based on experience with the initial 100 donors, the technique was standardized, and the normal GFR difference between kidneys resulting from technical and normal physiologic factors was quantified. In the remaining 200 donors who served as the study group, a GFR difference exceeding the normal mean was considered to represent a significant disparity in function between kidneys.

Results.—In the initial 100 potential donors, the mean GFR was similar between the 2 kidneys: 57.7 mL/min for the left and 58.09 mL/min for the right. The average disparity in clearance was 6.12 mL/min, with a range of 0 to 14.25 mL/min. The average disparity accounted for 5.31% of the total GFR, as measured by renography.

For the 200 potential donors in the study group, the 2 kidneys were classified as having comparable GFRs in 58% of cases. Thus, in 42% of donors, renal scanning showed a disparity in function: the left kidney had better function in 24.5% of donors, and the right kidney had better function in 17.5% of donors. The lower-functioning kidney was selected for nephrectomy, even if anatomic factors (eg, multiple renal arteries) suggested otherwise. When kidney function was comparable, selection was based on anatomic factors.

Conclusions.—More than 40% of living renal donor candidates show a disparity between function of the 2 kidneys on preoperative radioisotope renal scanning. The findings suggest that a GFR difference of more than 6 mL/min is significant. In this situation, the lesser functioning kidney should be taken for donation. Radioisotope scans to measure split kidney function should be included in the evaluation of potential living kidney donors.

▶ Although I believe that all institutions using live kidney donors test to determine whether total renal function in the donor is normal, I am not aware of any data on how many of these institutions routinely look at individual renal function. The authors' suggestion that in patients in whom there is a greater than normal difference in renal function between the 2 sides, the side with the lesser function should be chosen as the donor kidney, is certainly worth some consideration. However, I am not sure that this choice should be made irrespective of the anatomic findings. Live kidney donation puts the donor at risk, and in patients who have no evidence of kidney disease, even though it would be preferable to remove the kidney with lesser function, there is no reason to think that leaving that kidney and taking the other kidney would cause any harm to the donor. If that is true, then anatomic conditions cannot be ignored. If the anatomy of the kidney is such that there is an increased risk to the donor or an increased risk of failure from taking one particular kidney, this may override the observed difference in function.

M. D. Blaufox, MD, PhD

MR Renography Using a Dynamic Gradient-Echo Sequence and Low-Dose Gadopentetate Dimeglumine as an Alternative to Radionuclide Renography

Ten HS, Ang ES, Wong WC, et al (Changi Gen Hosp, Singapore; Singapore Gen Hosp; et al)

AJR 181:441-450, 2003 11–9

Introduction.—Renal function and urinary obstruction can be assessed by performing MRI with gadolinium-based tracers. However, the inability to produce renographic curve and dynamic serial images like those created on radionuclide renography makes it difficult to evaluate split renal function and urinary excretion. An approach to acquiring MR signal intensity-time renographic curves and dynamic serial images was reported.

Methods.—The analysis included 21 studies from 19 patients in whom both radionuclide studies and MR renography were performed no more than 3 months apart. Two of the studies were unusable because of technical errors in MR renographic acquisitions. A dynamic, 2-dimensional spoiled gradient-echo fast low-angle shot T1-weighed sequence with a conventional 1.5 T MRI unit was used to obtain serial MR renograms. Imaging was performed by using low-dose IV furosemide and gadopentetate dimeglumine, 0.025 mmol/kg. With the use of data on intensity-time curves in regions of interest over the renal parenchyma and whole kidney, split renal function

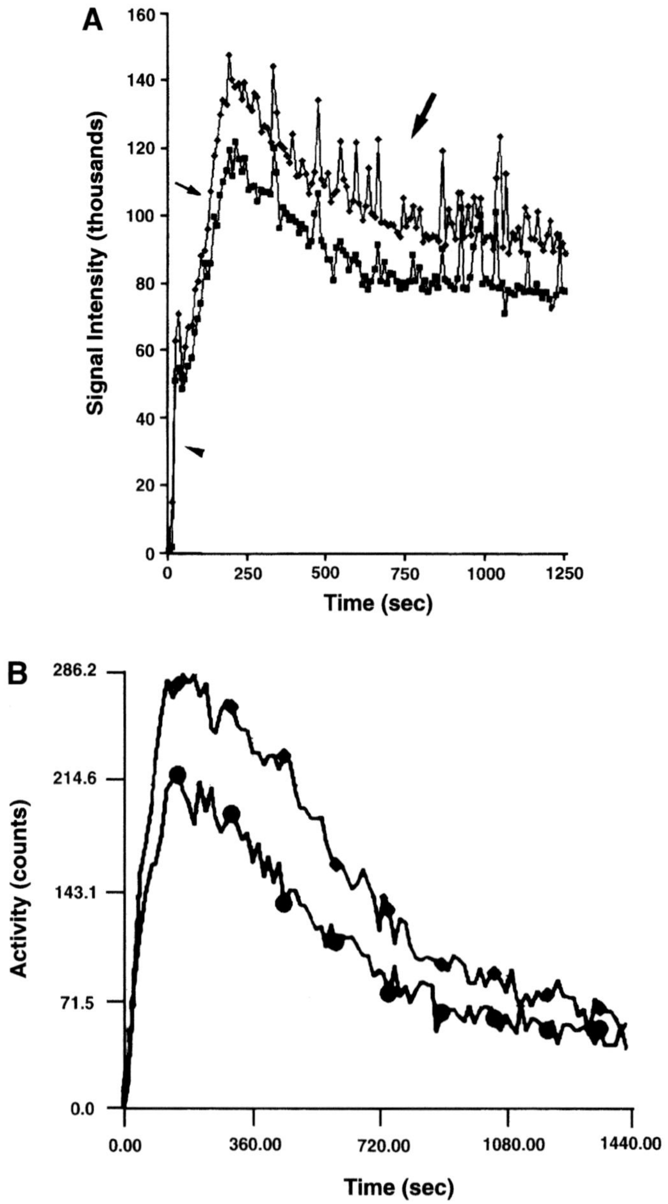

FIGURE 2.—45-year-old woman with hematuria from urinary tract infection. Graph of MR renogram (**A**) reveals similar curve pattern to graph of radionuclide renogram (**B**). Graph of MR renogram (**A**) shows characteristic curve pattern consisting of three segments corresponding to vascular (*arrowhead*), parenchymal (*thin arrow*), and excretory (*thick arrow*) phases. Parenchymal phase is initiated by minimal signal drop at end of initial vascular peak (peak-trough pattern). Split renal function between the right (*diamonds*) and left (*squares*, **A**; *circles*, **B**) kidneys acquired with radionuclide renography (**B**) and MR renography (**A**) also shows good agreement; values of 56%, 44% and 55%, and 45%, respectively, were obtained. (Courtesy of Ten HS, Ang ES, Wong WC, et al: MR renography using a dynamic gradient-echo sequence and low-dose gadopentetate dimeglumine as an alternative to radionuclide renography. *AJR* 181:441-450, 2003. Reprinted with permission from the *American Journal of Roentgenology*.)

and urinary excretion were assessed. The findings were compared with those of radionuclide renography.

Results.—The MR renographic findings for volume-corrected split renal function were strongly correlated with the results of radionuclide renography ($r = 0.97$). Weighted kappa statistics showed good agreement between 2 observers in terms of the excretory curve patterns resulting from MR versus radionuclide renography (Fig 2).

Conclusions.—MR renography performed by means of a low-dose gadopentetate dimeglumine technique yields intensity-time curves and serial dynamic images similar to those of radionuclide renograms. It permits assessment of split renal function and urinary excretion. Significant limitations remain to be overcome, but the MR renography technique offers much better visualization of the kidneys and urinary outflow tract than radionuclide renography, and may permit MR urography and MR angiography to be performed in a single examination.

► As radiographic techniques continue to be refined, we are seeing more and more capability for doing dynamic and time-related studies. Although there is still considerable room for improvement, there is no question that some of the data which previously could only be obtained with nuclear medicine techniques, can now be obtained by alternate radiographic methods. A major difference, of course, is that the MR is using a glomerular filtration rate (GFR)-excreted agent, while in nuclear medicine we have available to us many alternative agents to examine different aspects of renal function. However, for the nephrologists, the GFR is generally the measurement upon which clinical decisions are made. It is unfortunate that the authors chose to use technetium-99m MAG3 for the isotopic study for comparison. I would have liked to have seen a comparison of DTPA renography with gadolinium renography. That way we would be comparing the 2 procedures based on the GFR, and we could have had a better feeling for whether or not there is the same information in the 2 studies as the investigators suggest. Given a gadolinium renogram and a technetium DTPA renogram, the curves if they are indeed the same, should be basically superimposable, and the difference in the divided function should not be statistically significant between the 2 studies. It would be nice to see those data sometime in the future.

M. D. Blaufox, MD, PhD

MR Imaging of Kidneys: Functional Evaluation Using F-15 Perfusion Imaging

Grattan-Smith JD, Perez-Bayfield MR, Jones RA, et al (Emory Univ, Atlanta, Ga)

Pediatr Radiol 33:293-304, 2003 11–10

Background.—The widespread use of maternal sonography and the recognition of urologic abnormalities in the workup of febrile urinary tract infections in children have resulted in an increase in the diagnosis of both antenatal and postnatal hydronephrosis. An accurate determination of obstruction is needed to determine whether surgical intervention is required, and children with hydronephrosis are typically evaluated with a combination of diuretic renal scintigraphy, US, and voiding cystourethrography. However, there is no gold standard for the assessment of obstruction. This study evaluated the utility of dynamic contrast-enhanced MR urography in the investigation of children with hydronephrosis to define urinary anatomy, calculate differential real function, and assess urinary tract obstruction.

Methods.—Forty children with unilateral hydronephrosis underwent dynamic contrast-enhanced MRI. The study group included 14 girls and 26 boys ranging in age from 1 month to 14 years (mean age, 1.4 years). Information from traditional imaging modalities was compared with the information obtained from the single MR study.

Results.—Anatomical imaging with MR urography was found to be superior to other modalities. When surgery versus nonsurgery was used as the decision point, MR urography had a sensitivity of 100%, specificity of 71%, positive predictive value of 86%, negative predictive value of 100%, and diagnostic efficiency of 90%. For renal scintigraphy, the sensitivity was 96%, the specificity was 56%, the positive predictive value was 76%, the negative predictive value was 90%, and the diagnostic efficiency was 79%.

Conclusion.—These findings show that dynamic contrast-enhanced MR urography provides superior information when compared with US and diuretic renal scintigraphy. In addition, the data are obtained in a single study without the use of ionizing radiation. MR urography will likely replace renal scintigraphy in the evaluation of hydronephrosis in children.

▶ This study represents one more example of how conventional radiologic imaging such as MR and CT is beginning to impact on nuclear medicine. This is a result of increasing sophistication of the technology and increasing capability to perform functional-type studies. The authors' suggest that their technique using F-15 perfusion imaging is more sensitive and specific than the nuclear medicine technique and has the advantage that it avoids ionizing radiation. Whether their suggestion that MR urography will replace renal scintigraphy in the evaluation of hydronephrosis in children is correct remains to be seen.

Questions to be raised are whether subsequent studies can duplicate the authors' results, what is the cost efficacy of an MR study versus a nuclear study, and what is the relative risk considering the very low radiation dose from a renal scintigram. However, regardless of what the answers to these questions turn out to be, we must acknowledge that nuclear medicine is being challenged by other techniques which can, to some extent, provide similar functional information. Renal nuclear medicine has been rather static during the last several years, and if we are going to compete with these techniques, we have to move forward and improve our own.

M. D. Blaufox, MD, PhD

Color Doppler Sonography and Scintigraphy of the Testis: A Prospective, Comparative Analysis in Children With Acute Scrotal Pain

Nussbaum Blask AR, Bulas D, Shalaby-Rana E, et al (George Washington Univ, Washington, DC)

Pediatr Emerg Care 18:67-71, 2002 11–11

Background.—In adults, testicular torsion and nonsurgical causes of acute scrotal pain can be differentiated with the use of testicular color Doppler sonography, which has essentially replaced scintigraphy as the method of choice. For the pediatric population, color Doppler sonography has produced good results, but false-negative examinations have been reported, caused by intermittent torsion, lesser degrees of torsion, lack of blood flow detection in a normal testis, or decreased but present blood flow in a testis with torsion. Testicular color Doppler sonography was compared with testicular scintigraphy for the ability to distinguish between surgical and nonsurgical testicular conditions.

Methods.—The 46 children evaluated ranged in age from 1 day to 18 years (median age, 11 years). All were evaluated by both scintigraphy and color Doppler sonography by 2 radiologic teams blinded to the results of the other modality. The radiologic diagnosis was reported as surgical, nonsurgical, or indeterminate and was compared with the patient's surgical or clinical diagnosis.

Results.—Twelve patients had surgically proved testicular torsion, one had testicular torsion based on the development of late testicular atrophy, and one had either undiagnosed torsion or postinflammatory infarction that produced late testicular atrophy. Thirty-two patients had nonsurgical diagnoses. Sonography was accurate in diagnosing 11 of the 14 surgical conditions and 31 of the 32 nonsurgical conditions, whereas scintigraphy accurately identified 11 of the surgical conditions and 29 of the nonsurgical conditions. There was intermediate or good agreement between the 2 modalities. No false-positive results were obtained on sonography, and there were only 3 false-negative examinations, for a sensitivity of 78.6%, a specificity of 96.9%, and an accuracy of 91.3%. In 34 of 44 boys, the asymptomatic testis demonstrated color flow. On scintigraphy, 2 false-positive examinations and 2 false-negative examinations occurred, for a sensitivity of 78.6%, a specificity of 90.6%, and an accuracy of 87.0%.

Conclusions.—Pediatric patients with acute scrotal pain can be imaged with either testicular color Doppler sonography or scintigraphy, with similar sensitivity. Sonography is possible even when flow is hard to detect in the testes of prepubertal asymptomatic boys. A few false-negative results are obtained with each modality.

► It is interesting that the authors report a similar sensitivity and specificity for color Doppler sonography and scintigraphy in the diagnosis of testicular torsion. Regardless of the relative value of the 2 tests, it appears that most institutions have switched to color Doppler as the procedure of choice. We rarely perform scrotal scintigraphy at this time, whereas several years ago it was a relatively common emergency nuclear medicine procedure. The only statement that the authors make that I would take issue with is their suggestion that the 2 studies may provide complementary information. Our policy has always been that emergency surgical treatment should never be delayed for a diagnostic study. Our philosophy has been that it is better to operate on a testicle that turns out not to have torsion, than to risk losing testicular function unnecessarily by an avoidable delay. Therefore, when a study is requested, if we cannot perform it immediately, we advise the surgeon to take the patient directly to the operating room if she thinks that is indicated. The suggestion of interposing a second test will introduce additional delays and therefore reduce the likelihood of viability in those patients who actually have torsion. I believe that a policy should be established where one or the other test is the test of choice and that test should be performed, or whichever test is more readily accessible should be performed.

M. D. Blaufox, MD, PhD

Penile Scintigraphy With ^{99m}Tc-Human Immunoglobulin G: A Novel Method for Distinguishing the Unstable and Stable Phases of Peyronie's Disease

Erdogru T, Boz A, Köksal T, et al (Akdeniz Univ, Antalya, Turkey)
BJU Internatl 90:703-706, 2002 11–12

Background.—Peyronie's disease (PD) is a connective tissue disorder of the penis in which there is fibrous inelastic scar tissue formation in the tunica albuginea of the corpora cavernosa and adjacent erectile tissue. There are 2 phases in PD: an unstable phase, also termed the inflammatory/acute phase, and a stable phase, called the fibrotic/chronic phase. The surgical management of PD must be accomplished during the stable phase, but it can be difficult to determine when the disease transitions from the unstable to the stable phase. Deformity and pain on erection are characteristic of the unstable phase, which can last 12 to 18 months; dense fibrosis on the plaque side and stable deformity mark the stable phase. A technique using human IgG labeled with ^{99m}Tc (^{99m}Tc-IgG) is used in scintigraphy to locate inflammatory lesions and may help distinguish the 2 phases of PD. The value of penile scintigraphy with ^{99m}Tc-IgG in differentiating the 2 phases of PD was evaluated.

Methods.—Twenty-five patients with PD (mean age, 56 years) and 7 without PD were assessed by means of a detailed sexual history, serum chemistry panel, color Doppler ultrasonography during simultaneous intracavernosal injection of papaverine (50 mg) and stimulation, and ^{99m}Tc-IgG scintigraphy. Measurements of nocturnal penile tumescence, dynamic infusion cavernosometry, cavernosonography, and cavernosal artery systolic occlusion pressure were obtained as needed. Images were obtained 30 minutes, and 1, 2, 3, and 4 hours after administration of 370 MBq of ^{99m}Tc-IgG. A positive scan was defined as having focal accumulation of radiopharmaceutical consistent with PD plaque formation.

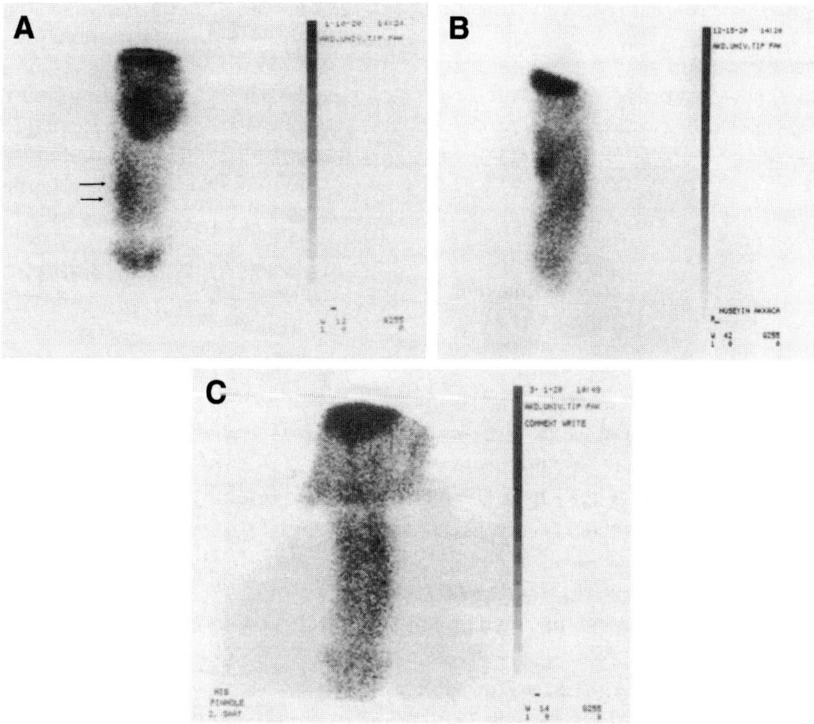

FIGURE 1.—**A**, Increased accumulation of radionuclide activity at the same location as a painful palpable plaque (5 months). **B**, Increased nuclear activity on the **right side** of the mid-penis, consistent with the painful, palpable nodule at 8 months after the onset of Peyronie's disease (PD). **C**, Complete resolution of activity 1 year after the onset of PD. (Courtesy of Erdogru T, Boz A, Köksal T, et al: Penile scintigraphy with ^{99m}Tc-human immunoglobulin G: A novel method for distinguishing the unstable and stable phases of Peyronie's disease. *BJU Internatl* 90:703-706, 2002. Reprinted by permission of Blackwell Publishing.)

Results.—Fourteen patients were in the stable phase and 11 in the unstable phase, with a mean interval from onset of PD until appearance at the clinic of 21 months (range, 2-120 months). Localized ^{99m}Tc-IgG activity was noted in 10 patients in the unstable phase (Fig 1); the other patient had a palpable nodule on the right side of the radix penis. Two patients had complete resolution of the activity after 1 year. Twelve patients with stable PD had no change in ^{99m}Tc-IgG activity over the course of 1 year, and two had more activity on the plaque side. The control group showed no local increase in activity.

Conclusions.—Significantly more ^{99m}Tc-IgG activity was found in 10 patients who had palpable nodules on the same side. The plaques all occurred in the midshaft of the penis. After 1 year, 2 patients had total resolution of activity on the plaque side. Thus, the differentiation of the 2 phases of PD was successfully accomplished with penile ^{99m}Tc-IgG imaging.

▶ The role of penile scintigraphy has been greatly diminished by improved ultrasound techniques and the ready availability of Doppler. One of the major areas that was observed early for a possible role of nuclear medicine was in patients with problems of impotence. Although the radionuclide techniques have provided some information about the basic physiology in this situation, they have not proven particularly important in general clinical management. Although PD is a relatively uncommon condition, the investigators were able to accumulate 25 patients in a relatively short period. Their suggestion that there is a role for nuclear imaging in PD seems well substantiated, and this appears to be an area where nuclear penile imaging can continue to be of some help to urologists.

M. D. Blaufox, MD, PhD

12 Vascular

Introduction

During the past several years, the major articles in the vascular section have been devoted to the lymphatics and evaluation of lymphedema. As in previous years, we do have a couple of studies devoted to that subject that I have included in this section. However, I am delighted that I have been able to add a few more studies suggesting a broader application of nuclear medicine in vascular imaging. Arguably, the article on thyroid angiography could have been in the thyroid section but I chose to put it here to try to provide a little further emphasis on the potential of angiography for nuclear medicine techniques. Included in this section are approaches to perfusion, vascular imaging, left to right shunts, and even the role of PET in the evaluation of hemangiomas. This represents a very great broadening of the indications for vascular related studies in nuclear medicine and perhaps represents a resurgence of interest in this area. I had suggested to the publishers a couple of years ago that we should omit the section on vascular disease from the YEAR BOOK because of the lack of productivity. This year we see a resurgence of interest in this area and if this keeps up for another year to two, I think I will have been proven wrong and the publishers were quite right in overruling my suggestion and deciding to maintain this section for an indefinite period of time.

M. Donald Blaufox, MD, PhD

A Comparison of Radionuclide Thyroid Angiography, ^{99m}Tc-MIBI Scintigraphy and Power Doppler Ultrasonography in the Differential Diagnosis of Solitary Cold Thyroid Nodules

Demirel K, Kapucu Ö, Yücel C, et al (Gazi Univ, Ankara, Turkey)

Eur J Nucl Med Mol Imaging 30:642-650, 2003 12–1

Background.—Thyroid nodules are a common occurrence, with an incidence of at least 4% to 7% in the general population. However, the rate of malignancy is relatively low, as only 5% of thyroid nodules are malignant. After exclusions of hypothyroidism and hyperthyroidism by measurement of thyroid-stimulating hormone level, fine-needle aspiration biopsy (FNAB) is the first and most important diagnostic procedure for the evaluation of a thyroid nodule. FNAB is safe, easily performed, has no complications, and is cost effective.

However, FNAB is not suitable for differentiation of follicular adenoma from follicular carcinoma. The purpose of this study was to determined the comparative diagnostic value of radionuclide thyroid angiography (RTA), ^{99m}Tc-methoxyisobutylisonitrile (^{99m}Tc-MIBI) scintigraphy, and power Doppler US (PDUS) in the differentiation of benign and malignant thyroid nodules.

Methods.—Forty-three patients were prospectively studied. Perfusion in the nodules in RTA was compared with perfusion in the surrounding thyroid tissue and classified as avascular (0), hypovascular (1), isovascular (2), or hypervascular (3). Uptake of ^{99m}Tc-MIBI in the nodules compared with that in the surrounding thyroid tissue was scored for both early and delayed images as cold (0), decreased (1), equal (2), or increased (3). PDUS patterns were classified as nodule vascularization patterns.

Results.—Histologic examination revealed thyroid carcinoma in 9 patients and benign conditions in 34 patients. Sensitivity, specificity, and accuracy were 89%, 100%, and 97%, respectively, for RTA; 100%, 76%, and 81%, respectively, for PDUS; and 67%, 91%, and 86%, respectively, for ^{99m}Tc-MIBI (when nodules with increased uptake in both the early and the delayed images and a positive retention index were considered as malignant).

Conclusion.—RTA, ^{99m}Tc-MIBI scintigraphy, and PDUS may all aid in the preoperative assessment of solitary and cold thyroid nodules. However, this study found RTA to be the most accurate and specific method for the differentiation of malignant from benign thyroid nodules.

► The differential diagnosis of thyroid nodules has always been and continues to be a difficult problem. The authors suggest that ^{99m}Tc-MIBI scintigraphy and PDUS may provide some additional information in characterizing benign thyroid nodules. Their finding that RTA yielded the best differential is certainly an interesting finding. Given the complex nature of the diagnostic approach that they have described, their statement in the Discussion that "The optimum diagnostic and therapeutic strategy for patients with a solitary thyroid nodule is still a matter of debate" is probably still the operative phrase.

M. D. Blaufox, MD, PhD

Gallium-67 SPECT Scintigraphy May Be Useful in Diagnosis of Temporal Arteritis

Reitblat T, Ben-Horin CL, Reitblat A (Ben-Gurion Univ, Ashkelon, Israel)
Ann Rheum Dis 62:257-260, 2003 12–2

Background.—For patients with the typical symptoms of temporal arteritis and a positive biopsy, the diagnosis is rather straightforward. However, about half of patients with temporal arteritis have a negative biopsy, and other diagnostic tools are needed in these cases. The utility of quantitative gallium-67 citrate (^{67}Ga SPECT) in the diagnosis of temporal arteritis was determined.

Methods.—The study included 9 patients with temporal arteritis (5 men, 4 women; mean age, 70.1 years) and 6 patients undergoing ^{67}Ga SPECT to evaluate febrile disease (control group). Five of the 6 patients with temporal arteritis who underwent biopsy had negative results. All subjects were injected with IV 8 to 10 mCi ^{67}Ga, then underwent SPECT 48 hours later. The ^{67}Ga uptake ratio in both temporal areas was measured on transaxial and coronary slices.

Results.—Compared with the control subjects, each patient with temporal arteritis had increased ^{67}Ga uptake in both temporal areas (Fig 2). The ^{67}Ga uptake ratio in the coronary view was 1.47 compared with 1.11 in the

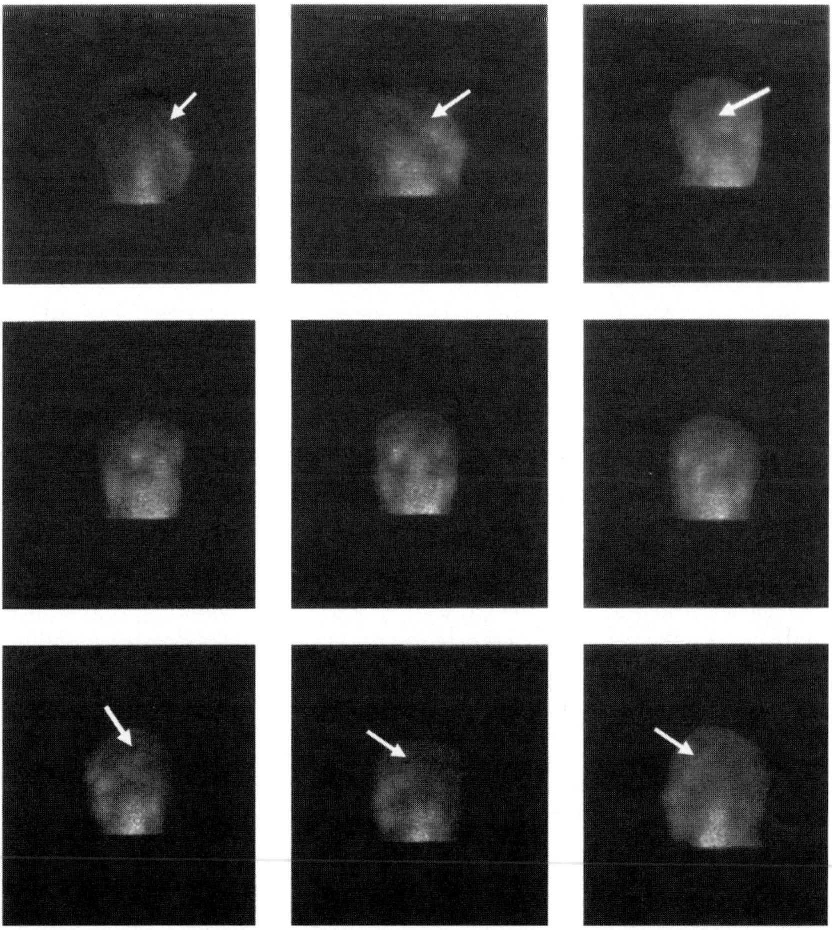

FIGURE 2.—Three-dimensional volume cine pictures show increased ^{67}Ga uptake in the temporal regions (*arrows*). (Courtesy of Reitblat T, Ben-Horin CL, Reitblat A: Gallium-67 SPECT scintigraphy may be useful in diagnosis of temporal arteritis. *Ann Rheum Dis* 62:257-260, 2003. Reproduced by permission of the BMJ Publishing Group.)

control group, and that in the transaxial view was 1.31 compared with 1.04 in the control group. Prednisone pretreatment in 8 patients did not affect these findings.

Conclusion.—^{67}Ga SPECT of the skull may be a useful noninvasive tool for diagnosing temporal arteritis.

▶ This small study suggests that gallium-67 may aid in the diagnosis of temporal arteritis. As the authors themselves point out, the diagnosis of temporal arteritis in most patients is relatively straightforward. The study suffers from the fact that the control group was not composed of patients who were possibly suffering from temporal arteritis but rather simply normal controls. The problem that really needs to be addressed is whether gallium can be useful for patients who are thought to have temporal arteritis but for whom it is not clear. Perhaps we will see more from these authors as they explore the problem further.

M. D. Blaufox, MD, PhD

Scintigraphic Diagnosis of a Right to Left Shunt in End-Stage Lung Disease

Graves MW, Kiratli PO, Mozley D, et al (Univ of Pennsylvania)

Respir Med 97:549-554, 2003 12–3

Purpose.—The presence of a right to left shunt influences the surgical approach to lung transplantation in patients with end-stage pulmonary disease. The purposes of this study included comparing contemporaneous lung scintigraphy with cardiac catheterization in the detection of intracardiac shunts in patients with end-stage lung disease and the point prevalence of right to left shunting was determined in patients with several different types of end-stage lung disease

Methods.—Hundred and twenty six patients with end-stage lung disease who were candidates for lung transplantation underwent perfusion images of the lungs with Tc-99m-labeled macro-aggregated albumin (MAA). Planar scans of the brain and the kidneys were performed contemporaneously. Statistical analyses included correlation of the clinical, laboratory and scintigraphic variables. Group means were compared with the students *t*-test (two-tailed *P*-value).

Results.—There were 21 patients with primary pulmonary hypertension (PPH), 72 with emphysematous lung disease (COPD), 22 with pulmonary fibrotic disease (PF), and 11 with congenital heart disease (CHD) leading to pulmonary hypertension. Only 13 patients (10.3%) were found to have a right to left shunt. Of these, 4 had PPH, 2 had PF, and 7 had CHD. No shunts were found in patients with emphysema. All the positive studies had abnormally increased activity in both the brain and the kidneys. However, there were 25 cases with renal activity, and none of these patients had brain activity or clinical evidence of a shunt. Increased pulmonary artery pressure was associated with scintigraphic presence of a shunt. There were no cases of a right to left shunt with a mean pulmonary artery pressure less than 50 mmHg. In the subset of patients with a pulmonary pressure greater than 50 mmHg, approximately 40% of the patients had a right to a left shunt. There were no measurable differences in the spirometry results, right ventricular ejection fraction (RVEF) or left ventricular ejection fraction (LVEF) in the subgroup of patients with PPH and right to left shunt in comparison with patients with PPH but without a right to left shunt.

Conclusions.—The findings indicate that images of the brain, but not the kidneys, are an effective way to diagnose extrapulmonary right to left shunts in patients with end-stage pulmonary disease. The problem of a right to left shunt is uncommon in patients with emphysematous lung disease and relatively common in patients with primary pulmonary hypertension.

► The authors suggest that brain imaging is important in evaluating a possible left to right shunt in end stage lung disease. They suggest that this may be somewhat more reliable than renal imaging since free pertechnetate is excreted by the kidney, and renal uptake does not always reflect a shunt. However, no data are given about the quality control of technetium-99m macro-aggregated albumin that was used. Quality assurance and care that there is a minimal amount of free pertechnetate is important in any study of this type. The data raise the question of whether the radiopharmaceutical used might have had an unusual amount of free pertechnetate, since prior studies using the kidney as a guide for shunt have proven very reliable. If the authors would confirm that the material they used contained the same amount of free pertechnetate as is encountered in most radiopharmaceutical preparations, their point would be quite important.

M. D. Blaufox, MD, PhD

Evaluation of Hemangioma by Positron Emission Tomography: Role in a Multimodality Approach

Hatayama K, Watanabe H, Ahmed AR, et al (Gunma Univ, Maebashi, Japan)
J Comput Assist Tomogr 27:70-77, 2003 12–4

Background.—Many imaging methods have been used to diagnose hemangioma and to distinguish these tumors from other soft tissue tumors. The utility of PET in identifying malignant hemangioma was compared to that of CT, MRI, and digital subtraction angiography (DSA).

Methods.—The medical records of 16 patients (4 males and 12 females, ages 12-61 years) with histopathologically proven hemangioma of the extremities were reviewed. Preoperatively, all 16 patients underwent MRI, all 16 underwent PET with FDG, 14 underwent DSA, 12 underwent PET with fluorine-18 alpha-methyltyrosine (FMT), and 11 underwent CT. Findings with each of these imaging studies were compared.

Results.—All hemangiomas imaged with FDG-PET or FMT-PET revealed areas of increased tumor uptake. Standardized uptake values (SUVs) for FDG-PET ranged from 0.7 to 0.67, and SUVs for FMT-PET ranged from

0.14 to 1.00. In all cases, these SUVs indicated a benign tumor. FDG-PET SUVs did not correlate significantly with tumor size, but FMT-PET SUVs did ($r = 0.664$). CT detected 9 of the 11 tumors imaged but missed 2 tumors with FDG-PET SUVs of 0.8 and 1.1. Furthermore, CT showed calcifications in 2 tumors with an FDG-PET SUV of 0.7 and 0.73. MRI also detected all 16 tumors, and its signal characteristics were relatively consistent. DSA identified 12 of 14 tumors. In particular, pooling and cotton-wool staining on DSA correlated significantly with more intense FDG accumulation during PET.

Conclusion.—FDG-PET and FMT-PET may be the most reliable methods for distinguishing benign hemangiomas from other soft tissue tumors. FDG-PET results correlate with blood pooling, and FMT-PET results correlate with tumor size. CT results suggest that FDG may have less accumulation in hemangiomas with phleboliths. DSA results suggest that ischemia due to localized blood retention may accelerate anaerobic glycolysis, which would explain the higher FDG uptake in areas of blood retention.

► The authors suggest that FDG-PET may play a useful role in differentiating the benign hemangioma from malignant tumors. The study included only patients with histopathologically documented hemangiomas. In order to be sure that this conclusion is warranted, it would be necessary to conduct a comparison of FDG uptake utilizing the authors' technology in patients with malignant as well as benign tumors. Although the authors have clearly shown the FDG uptake is relatively low in patients with hemangioma, they do not provide us with sufficient information about the FDG uptake that could occur in malignant lesions that could be confused with hemangioma. Further study of this provocative question is warranted. Certainly, the authors' optimistic conclusion seems likely to be vindicated.

M. D. Blaufox, MD, PhD

Dynamic Lymph Flow Imaging in Patients With Oedema of the Lower Limb for Evaluation of the Functional Outcome After Autologous Lymph Vessel Transplantation: An 8-Year Follow-up Study

Weiss M, Baumeister RGH, Hahn K (Ludwig-Maximilians-Univ of Munich)

Eur J Nucl Med 30:202-206, 2003 12–5

Introduction.—The physiologic transport of radiotracers occurs during lymphoscintigraphy and permits evaluation of the function of the lymphatic system of the lower limbs. The functional outcome of microsurgical intervention on lymph drainage was assessed via lymphoscintigraphy after autologous lymph vessel transplantation.

Methods.—Eight patients with primary or secondary lymphedema of the lower limb were evaluated before and for 8 years after autologous lymph vessel transplantation. ^{99m}Tc-labelled nanocolloid was subcutaneously injected into the first interdigital space of the affected limb and sequential images were obtained up to 6 hours post injection. A numerical transport index was established for semiquantitative assessment by assigning scores of up to

9 on each of these criteria: lymphatic transport kinetics, distribution pattern of the radiopharmaceutical, time to appearance of lymph nodes, visualization of lymph nodes, and visualization of lymph vessels/grafts. Ti values below 10 were defined as normal.

Results.—For all 8 patients, lymphatic function significantly ($P \leq .01$) improved after microsurgical treatment. Permanent function of vessel grafts was indicated by persistently low Ti values throughout the observation period, impressively demonstrating the success of this complex microsurgical approach. Two of 8 patients with scintigraphic visualization of the vessel graft had a markedly better postoperative outcome, compared with those without visualization of the vessel graft.

Conclusion.—Lymph vessel transplantation significantly enhanced lymph drainage in patients with primary or secondary lymphedema of the lower limb. Lymphoscintigraphy is useful in planning microsurgical treatment and in monitoring postoperative outcome.

► Another example of the simplicity and utility of lymphoscintigraphy. The images are particularly impressive.

M. D. Blaufox, MD, PhD

Post-Therapeutic Lymphedema: Scintigraphy Before and After Autologous Lymph Vessel Transplantation: 8 Years of Long-term Follow-up

Weiss M, Baumeister RGH, Hahn K (Ludwig-Maximilians Univ of Munich)

Clin Nucl Med 27:788-792, 2002 12–6

Background.—Evaluation of the function of the lymphatic system can be accomplished noninvasively with lymphoscintigraphy. The outcome in terms of lymph drainage after microsurgical intervention for patients with secondary lymphedema was monitored using lymphoscintigraphy, adhering to visual and semiquantitative criteria.

Methods.—The 12 patients evaluated ranged in age from 32 to 73 years (mean age, 56 years), and all had secondary lymphedema of an upper extremity. A baseline scintigraphic study was conducted, with follow-up extending for 8 years after the microsurgical procedure.

Results.—Lymphatic function improved significantly in 11 of the 12 patients after the autologous lymph vessel transplantation. Drainage of the radiopharmaceutical was facilitated, and the transport index declined markedly from preoperative values. Before lymph vessel transplantation, the radiopharmaceutical was distributed diffusely, with lymph nodes only recognized with difficulty and lymph vessels undetectable (Fig 1). After treatment, there was partially diffuse drainage, with both the axillary lymph nodes and the vessel graft clearly visualized on scintigraphy.

Conclusions.—Significantly improved lymph drainage was achieved with lymph vessel transplantation in these patients with secondary lymphedema. Assessment of this status was provided by lymphoscintigraphy and an eval-

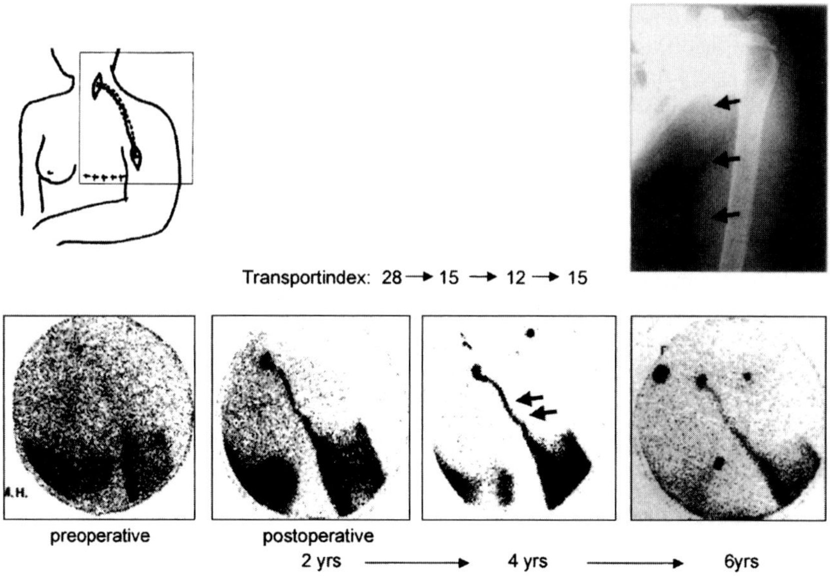

FIGURE 1.—Secondary lymphedema of the left arm. (Courtesy of Weiss M, Baumeister RGH, Hahn K: Post-therapeutic lymphedema: Scintigraphy before and after autologous lymph vessel transplantation: 8 years of long-term follow-up. *Clin Nucl Med* 27(11):788-792, 2002.)

uation by the transport index. This method was easy to perform, produced reliable results, proved to be safe, and is readily available for this use.

► The use of ^{99m}Tc-labeled nanocolloid presents a remarkably simple technique for evaluation of lymph flow after subcutaneous injection. The authors present a very simple technique for evaluating lymph flow before and after therapy in patients with secondary lymphedema of an upper extremity. The use of a "transport index" is a neat method for objectively demonstrating the degree of the obstruction and the effect of therapy on its relief. It is worthy of comment here that there is no substitute for applying some quantitative technique to the evaluation of a kinetic situation. Although the evaluation of serial images of any organ can provide the interpreter with a qualitative assessment of changes with time, it is fraught with considerable error. The apparent concentration of radioactivity is greatly affected by a variety of physical factors, not the least of which is the processing of the study. The introduction of some quantitative technique, whether it be an index or a curve of the changing concentration, greatly facilitates the correct and reliable interpretation of a kinetic study. The authors have wisely included such an approach in this interesting report.

M. D. Blaufox, MD, PhD

13 Central Nervous System

Introduction

Although imaging of the brain is a relatively small portion of the studies performed in a nuclear medicine laboratory, it continues to be an important part of radionuclide imaging. Studies for determination of brain death are still performed in many nuclear medicine departments, and more data confirming the cost effectiveness of the studies are presented in a following abstract. The evaluation of the patient with medically refractory seizure disorder continues to be problematic, and both PET and SPECT imaging have a role in this evaluation. New techniques for evaluating ictal and inter-ictal studies are being developed and are discussed in the abstracts.

Radionuclide imaging is likely to have an increasingly important role in the differential diagnosis of the causes of dementia. Medicare presently is considering the coverage of FDG-PET imaging for the identification of Alheizmer's disease. If that indication is approved by Medicare, a marked increased utilization of FDG-PET imaging of the brain will be seen.

R. Edward Coleman, MD

Outcomes of Patients Referred for Confirmation of Brain Death by 99mTc-Exametazime Scintigraphy

Harding JW, Chatterton BE (Royal Adelaide Hosp, South Australia)

Intensive Care Med 29:539-543, 2003 13–1

Background.—The guidelines of the Australian and New Zealand Intensive Care Society (ANTICS) regarding the diagnosis of brain death emphasize that the diagnosis is primarily clinical and relies on the establishment of a causative mechanism, exclusion of potentially reversible "mimics," and the clinical triad of coma, absent brainstorm reflexes, and apnea. Confirmatory tests are necessary when these preconditions are not met or when the examination is incomplete, and the utility of 99mTc-labeled exametazime scintigraphy is widely recognized in these circumstances. Clinical outcomes in patients referred for confirmation of brain death by 99mTc-labeled exametazime scintigraphy were reviewed, and any tangible benefit that was identified was assessed.

Methods.—This retrospective case note review was conducted in the ICU and nuclear medicine department of a tertiary-level acute care hospital. A total of 66 consecutive patients in whom a clinical diagnosis of brain death could not be established underwent 99mTc-labeled exametazime scintigraphy from February 1993 to March 2002. Case notes for 56 of these patients were available for review.

Results.—Brain death was confirmed in 77% of these patients on the basis of absent supratentorial and infratentorial uptake. In patients in whom brain death was not confirmed, a normal scan was seen in 30%, with the remainder showing patchy reduced infratentorial or supratentorial uptake. All of the patients with scintigraphic appearance of brain death subsequently died. Among the patients in whom brain death could not be confirmed, 11 of 13 patients died soon afterward. Two patients with normal brain scintigraphy regained consciousness and survived for an extended period. When brain death was not confirmed by scintigraphy, the time to certification of death was longer (44.7 hours vs 7 hours), and organ donation was less common, even when a subsequent clinical diagnosis was established.

Conclusions.—The indication from these findings is that the prognosis for patients with suspected brain death remains poor, regardless of the findings on 99mTc-labeled exametazime scintigraphy but that the results of the scan do affect the time to withdrawal of therapy or organ donation. Thus, 99mTc-labeled exametazime scintigraphy in these cases provides a significant cost benefit; in addition, an occasional long-term survivor is seen.

► Very rarely do we see any perfusion in patients with suspected brain death who are referred to us for evaluation of cerebral perfusion. We perform only approximately 1 brain death study per month, so we do not have a large experience. The discussion of the findings and outcomes in patients who do have some cerebral perfusion is most interesting.

R. E. Coleman, MD

Postictal Psychosis in Temporal Lobe Epilepsy

Leutmezer F, Podreka I, Asenbaum S, et al (Abteilung der Krankenanstalt Rudolfstiftung, Vienna; Max Planck Institut für Neurologische Forschung, Köln, Germany)

Epilepsia 44:582-590, 2003 13–2

Background.—Postictal psychosis (PIP) accounts for about 25% of psychoses in epilepsy. The psychopathology of PIP is often polymorphic, and the most frequently reported symptoms are abnormal mood, paranoid delusions, and fluctuating impairment of consciousness and orientation. Its course is usually benign, with remission of psychotic symptoms over several days, often without the need for neuroleptic treatment. However, in rare cases, chronic psychoses may develop from recurrent or even a single episode of PIP. A possible relationship between PIP and certain types of epilepsy has often been stressed but has not been elucidated. Five patients with temporal lobe epilepsy (TLE) in whom psychotic symptoms developed during video-EEG monitoring are reported.

Methods.—All 5 patients in this report were evaluated for suspected focal epilepsy and underwent intensive video-EEG monitoring for the purpose of surgical treatment of their refractory epilepsy. The patients were studied with hexamethylpropyleneamine-oxime SPECT (HMPAO-SPECT) during and after the psychotic event.

Results.—In comparison with the interictal state, all of the SPECT scans obtained during PIP manifest bifrontal and bitemporal hyperfusion patterns. Some of the SPECT studies also showed unilateral left lateral frontal hyperperfusion. These cortical blood-flow patterns appeared to be distinct from patterns obtained during complex partial seizures.

Conclusions.—It would appear from these findings that postictal psychoses in patients with temporal lobe epilepsy are associated with hyperactivation of both temporal and frontal lobe structures. This hyperperfusion may be a reflection of ongoing (subcortical) discharges or may simply be a manifestation of dysregulation of cerebral blood flow.

► If a laboratory does many imaging studies in patients with suspected temporal lobe epilepsy, postictal psychosis is likely to be seen. SPECT brain perfusion studies in the postictal state demonstrate hyperactivation of the temporal and frontal lobe structures. The significance of this interesting finding is yet to be determined.

R. E. Coleman, MD

Neocortical Temporal FDG-PET Hypometabolism Correlates With Temporal Lobe Atrophy in Hippocampal Sclerosis Associated With Microscopic Cortical Dysplasia

Diehl B, LaPresto E, Najm I, et al (Cleveland Clinic Found, Ohio)

Epilepsia 44:559-564, 2003 13–3

Background.—Atrophy of the hippocampal formation and regional FDG-PET hypometabolism have been associated with medically intractable temporal lobe epilepsy caused by hippocampal sclerosis (HS), with or without cortical dysplasia (CD). However, the relationship between areas of functional and structural abnormalities has not been well documented. The association between FDG-PET metabolism and temporal lobe and hippocampal atrophy in patients with histologically proved isolated HS and HS related to CD was investigated.

Methods.—En bloc resection of the mesial and anterolateral neocortical structures was performed on 23 patients. Ten had isolated HS, and 13 had HS associated with microscopic CD. Measurements of temporal lobe and hippocampal volumes were obtained.

Findings.—Significant ipsilateral PET hypometabolism was noted in all 3 regions studied in all patients. The most prominent hypometabolism in patients with isolated HS was found in the anterior and mesial temporal lobe. In patients with HS associated with CD, the most prominent hypometabolism was in the lateral temporal lobe. Temporal lobe and hippocampal volumes on the epileptogenic side were significantly smaller.

In the patients with HS associated with CD but not in those with HS alone, PET asymmetries ipsilateral and contralateral to the epileptogenic zone and temporal lobe volume asymmetries were significantly associated in the anterior and lateral temporal lobes. The 2 groups did not differ significantly in mesial temporal hypometabolism.

Conclusion.—Temporal neocortical microscopic CD with concurrent HS correlates with more prominent lateral temporal metabolic dysfunction compared with isolated HS in temporal lobe atrophy. Further research is needed to verify these data and to correlate PET hypometabolic patterns with outcomes in patients undergoing surgery for HS with or without CD.

► The abnormalities on the FDG-PET scan in patients with temporal lobe epilepsy are larger than the abnormalities noted on MRI and noted at pathology. The association of larger abnormalities on the PET scan with CD is an interesting observation. Furthermore, the demonstration that the abnormality with HS to the medial temporal cortex and the abnormality with CD extend to the lateral temporal cortex may help explain some of the concordancy that we see between PET and other imaging studies, including pathology.

R. E. Coleman, MD

Extratemporal Hypometabolism on FDG PET in Temporal Lobe Epilepsy as a Predictor of Seizure Outcome After Temporal Lobectomy

Choi JY, Kim SJ, Hong SB, et al (Sungkyunkwan Univ, Seoul, Korea)

Eur J Nucl Med Mol Imaging 30:581-587, 2003 13–4

Background.—In the management of patients with medically intractable temporal lobe epilepsy (TLE), the prediction of seizure control is important, and the use of FDG PET has been suggested as providing reliable predictive data after surgical interventions. The presence and severity of temporal lobe hypometabolism have shown an association with the degree of seizure relief achieved after surgery. The presence of extratemporal hypometabolism after surgery in patients with TLE seems to predict poor seizure control but may not be an independent factor in this process. Whether subcortical hypometabolism is also predictive of postoperative seizure outcomes in patients with TLE was investigated, as was the significance of extratemporal hypometabolism in this determination.

Methods.—FDG-PET images were obtained in 47 patients with intractable unilateral mesial TLE over a period of 2 months before they underwent anterior temporal lobectomy; the regional metabolic status was then compared with images obtained after surgery. The follow-up period was a mean of 6.1 years.

Results.—Forty-nine percent of the patients were free of seizures after surgery, 40% were nearly free or had rare seizures, and 11% still had seizures. All patients had temporal cortex hypometabolism, and 18 had hypometabolism limited to the ipsilateral temporal cortex, which is termed type 1 cortical metabolic pattern. For 29 patients, cortical hypometabolism was also present; 11 had extratemporal cortical hypometabolism that only affected the ipsilateral cerebral hemisphere (type 2 cortical metabolic pattern), and 18 had hypometabolism in the contralateral cerebral cortex with or without ipsilateral extratemporal cortical hypometabolism (type 3 cortical metabolic pattern). Seventy-eight percent of those with type 1 patterns were free of seizures after surgery. Type 2 patterns were associated with intermediate postoperative seizure control. All patients for whom surgery did not achieve good control had type 2 or 3 cortical metabolic patterns. Ipsilateral thalamic hypometabolism was noted in 12 patients, and bilateral thalamic hypometabolism was noted in 8. Thirty-five percent of those with thalamic hypometabolism were seizure free after surgery; 59% of 27 patients with normal thalamic metabolism became completely free of seizures after surgery. The cortical metabolic pattern and thalamic metabolism as determined on FDG PET were found to be significant predictive indicators of postoperative seizure control on univariate analysis; however, on multivariate analysis, only the cortical metabolic pattern retained independent predictor status.

Conclusions.—When a patient with TLE had extratemporal cortical hypometabolism outside the seizure focus, the postoperative seizure outcome was generally poorer than when this was absent. Thalamic hypometabolism was also associated with a higher likelihood that seizures would persist; however, the relationship was not independent but was possibly the result of extratemporal or temporal pathologic conditions.

▶ Our group[1] has previously shown that the extent of abnormality in the temporal lobe on PET imaging was a predictor of seizure control after a temporal lobectomy. This study demonstrates that extratemporal cortical hypometabolism results in a poorer outcome related to control of seizures.

R. E. Coleman, MD

Reference

1. Radtke RA, Hanson MW, Hoffman JM, et al: Temporal lobe hypometabolism on PET: Predictor of seizure control after temporal lobectomy. *Neurology* 43:1088-1092, 1993.

Stratifying Differences on Ictal/Interictal Subtraction SPECT Images

Koo CW, Devinsky O, Hari K, et al (New York Univ)
Epilepsia 44:379-386, 2003 13–5

Background.—In patients with refractory partial seizures being considered for surgery, ictal and interictal SPECT is commonly used for localization of epileptogenic foci. However, side-by-side comparison of ictal and interictal SPECT scans shows low sensitivity. When the interictal scans are subtracted from the ictal scans, the result is numerous foci of varying pixel values, found throughout the brain. Toward enhancing the accuracy of subtraction SPECT, the magnitude of differences between the ictal and interictal scans was quantified.

Methods.—The prospective study included 13 patients with refractory partial seizures who underwent registration, normalization, and subtraction of interictal from ictal SPECT scans. The foci on these subtraction images were classified as having 75% to 100% of the maximal pixel value (group 1), or 50% to 75% of the maximum (group 2). Group 1 and 2 foci were localized and correlated with the results of surgery and invasive electroencephalographic (EEG) studies (Fig 1).

Results.—The group 1 foci corresponded well with the ictal scalp EEG findings in 10 of the 13 patients, and with the invasive EEG results in 9 of these 10 cases. The group 1 foci were located bilaterally in 7 patients. The group 1 foci also showed good concordance with the areas of surgical resec-

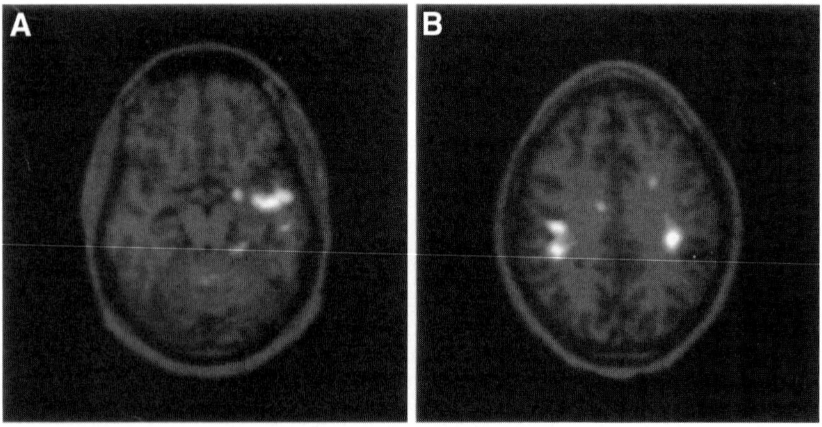

FIGURE 1.—**A**, Group I foci (75%-100% of maximal pixel value). **B**, Group II foci (50%-75% of maximal pixel value) in case 5. Surgical resection of the left temporal lobe was performed and the patient had a seizure-free outcome. Group I foci in this patient were found in the left temporal lobe. We considered this good concordance for both laterality and lobar localization. Conversely, group II foci occurred bilaterally in the frontoparietal lobes; we considered this poor concordance with the surgical resection site because the lobar localization did not match the surgical resection site. Scalp EEG showed bilateral frontocentral foci for the same case. Group I foci showed only left temporal localization and thus was thought to show poor concordance with the scalp EEG. Conversely, group II foci with bilateral frontoparietal localization, overlapping with the central region on scalp EEG, showed good concordance with the group II foci. (Courtesy of Koo CW, Devinsky O, Hari K, et al: Stratifying differences on ictal/interictal subtraction SPECT images. *Epilepsia* 44:379-386, 2003. Reprinted by permission of Blackwell Publishing.)

tion in 10 of 13 patients, 9 of whom also had good concordance with the scalp EEG findings and 8 with the invasive EEG results. Eight of these patients were rendered seizure free by surgery.

In contrast, the group 2 foci correlated well with the ictal scalp EEG findings in 5 of 13 patients, and with the invasive EEG results in 5 of 10. The group 2 foci were distributed in both sides of the brain in 10 patients, all of whom had good results after unilateral surgery. The group 2 foci corresponded to the surgical site in just 6 of 13 patients. These foci were not well correlated with the scalp or invasive EEG findings, but 5 of the patients achieved good postoperative results. Sensitivity in seizure localization was 40% for group 1 foci and 20% for group 2 foci; specificity values were 88% and 79%, respectively.

Conclusions.—As defined in this ictal/interictal subtraction SPECT study, group 1 foci correspond well to seizure foci in patients with refractory partial seizures. In contrast, group 2 foci show a lower level of concordance. These preliminary findings suggest possible gains in specificity and preoperative localization with subtraction SPECT through stratification of ictal/interictal differences.

► I have found that SPECT brain imaging in evaluation of refractory partial seizure disorder is quite difficult to perform and interpret. At our institution, SPECT has not been demonstrated to be particularly useful. The patients who are referred for ictal and interictal SPECT images are those who have not been previously characterized by surface EEG, PET scans, and MRI. We have not used the subtraction methods discussed in this article. We need a better method of evaluating these images than we are now using at our institution.

R. E. Coleman, MD

Alzheimer's Disease: Differences in Technetium-99m HMPAO SPECT Scan Findings Between Early Onset and Late Onset Dementia

Kemp PM, Holmes C, Hoffmann SMA, et al (Southampton Univ, Hampshire, England)

J Neurol Neurosurg Psychiatry 74:715-719, 2003 13–6

Background.—The role of diagnostic imaging procedures in the evaluation of patients with mild Alzheimer disease (AD) remains unclear. With the availability of multicrystal scanners for visualization of the medial temporal lobes, the role of cerebral perfusion imaging in diagnostic evaluation of patients with differing clinical presentations of AD warrants further consideration. The HMPAO SPECT findings of patients with early- and late-onset AD were compared.

Methods.—The retrospective analysis included 2 groups of patients with AD undergoing HMPAO SPECT imaging with the use of a multidetector gamma camera at one British nuclear medicine department. Twenty patients had early-onset AD, presenting before the age of 65 years, and 44 had late-onset AD, presenting after the age of 65. In both groups, disease had been present for a mean of about 2 years; all patients met NINCDS-ADRDA (National Institute of Neurological and Communicative Disorders and Stroke–Alzheimer's Disease and Related Disorders Association) criteria for possible or probable AD. The findings of technetium-99m HMPAO SPECT brain scans were compared visually and by statistical parametric mapping.

Findings.—Analysis of left and right visual perfusion scores suggested that 79% of patients with late-onset AD had greater medial temporal hypoperfusion compared with the posterior association cortices. In contrast, 85% of patients with early-onset AD had greater hypoperfusion to the posterior association cortices, relative to the medial temporal lobe. These differences were supported by statistical parametric mapping and were unaffected by adjustment for severity of disease and duration of illness.

Conclusions.—The findings of HMPAO SPECT brain scanning differ significantly for patients with early- and late-onset AD. In support of the clinical and histopathologic findings, patients with late-onset AD tend to have involvement of the medial temporal lobes associated with clinical memory loss, whereas those with early-onset AD have relatively greater involvement of the posterior cortical association area. These age-related differences may have important implications for the clinical diagnosis of patients with suspected AD, as well as for the interpretation of functional imaging studies.

► The imaging of dementia is being increasingly utilized. Both SPECT brain perfusion imaging and FDG-PET brain metabolic studies are used in evaluating patients with dementia. This article defines some differences in the pattern of abnormality in patients with early onset and late onset of dementia. It would be interesting to know whether similar findings are present on FDG-PET scans.

R. E. Coleman, MD

---

^{99m}Tc-HMPAO and ^{99m}Tc-ECD Perform Differently in Typically Hypoperfused Areas in Alzheimer's Disease

Koulibaly PM, Nobili F, Migneco O, et al (Univ of Nice-Sophia Antipolis, France; Univ of Genoa, Italy)

Eur J Nucl Med Mol Imaging 30:1009-1013, 2003 13–7

Introduction.—Single-photon emission tomography (SPET) of the brain may be performed with ^{99m}Tc-hexamethylpropylene amine oxime (HMPAO) or ^{99m}Tc-*N,N*"-1,2-ethylene diylbis-L-cysteine diethyl ester dihydrochloride (ECD). With their differing pharmacokinetics, the 2 tracers result in significantly different cerebral perfusion findings. The patterns and significance of ^{99m}Tc-HMPAO and ^{99m}Tc-ECD in patients with Alzheimer disease (AD) were compared.

Methods.—The retrospective study included 64 patients with mild to moderate AD: 32 undergoing ^{99m}Tc-HMPAO SPET and 32 undergoing ^{99m}Tc-ECD SPET. The 2 groups were selected with matching for age, sex, and Mini-Mental State Examination scores. Statistical parametric mapping was used to compare the findings of the 2 types of SPET scans.

Results.—A number of different symmetric clusters showed higher uptake ratio values with ^{99m}Tc-ECD than with ^{99m}Tc-HMPAO, including the right and left occipital cuneus, the left occipital and parietal precuneus, and the left superior and middle temporal gyri. Certain smaller clusters—namely, the hippocampus in both sides of the brain—showed higher uptake ratios with HMPAO than with ECD.

Conclusions.—These 2 SPET tracers show differing relative uptake patterns in areas of the brain affected by AD. The clinical impact of the observed discrepancies in ^{99m}Tc-HMPAO and ^{99m}Tc-ECD uptake is unknown and warrants further investigation. The findings also underscore the need for specific normal databases.

▶ I was surprised at the differences demonstrated by these 2 radiopharmaceuticals.

R. E. Coleman, MD

Subject Index

A

Abciximab
effects on microvascular integrity and left ventricular function recovery after primary coronary angioplasty in myocardial infarction, 130
Abdomen
SPET/CT image co-registration with simple and cost-effective tool in, 8
upper, normal organs in, visualized on PET/CT, accuracy of image fusion of, 169
Absorbed fractions
of 6 age-dependent multiregion models of kidney, 31
Acetate
carbon-11, PET with
assessment of forward cardiac output with (in pig), 158
in prostate cancer, 202
Acipimox
administration, feasibility and image quality of dual-isotope SPECT using FDG and Tc-99m tetrofosmin after, 160
ADAM
iodine-123, biodistribution and dosimetry of, 30
Adenoma
parathyroid, double-phase parathyroid scintigraphy with Tc-99m tetrofosmin *vs.* Tc-99m sestamibi for, 248
Adenosine
tracer, as myocardial flow marker (in dog), 44
vs. normal exercise Tc-99m tetrofosmin SPECT, prognostic value of, 144
Adolescence
malignancies during, thyroid neoplasms after therapeutic radiation for, 62
Adrenal
incidentaloma, subclinical and preclinical functioning, SPECT semiquantitative analysis of adrenocortical I-131 6β-iodomethyl-norcholesterol uptake to discriminate, 262
Age
effects on SPECT imaging of stomach, 119
Albumin
technetium-99m macroaggregated, scintigraphic diagnosis of right to left shunt in end-stage lung disease with, 290
Algorithms
OSEM and depth-dependent resolution recovery, for evaluation of global left ventricular function in Tl-201 gated myocardial perfusion SPECT, 161
reconstruction
effect on ROC analysis for assessment of lesion detection performance in 3D PET, 11
ordered subsets, using median root prior and inter-update median filtering, for transmission PET studies, 14
in whole-body PET applications, 12
Allograft
vasculopathy, cardiac, detection with resting echocardiography and quantitative dipyridamole Tc-99m sestamibi SPECT, 133
α-emitting Ra-223
targeting of osseous sites with (in mice), 43
Alteplase
plus heparin *vs.* heparin alone in submassive pulmonary embolism, 81
Alzheimer's disease
early- *vs.* late-onset, Tc-99m HMPAO SPECT findings in, 301
typically hypoperfused areas in, Tc-99m HMPAO *vs.* Tc-99m ECD performance in, 302
Amyloidosis
scintigraphy in, Tc-99m aprotinin, 38
Anatomical
-functional image fusion, benefit in diagnostic work-up of neuroendocrine neoplasms, 172
Androgen
-dependent and androgen-independent prostate cancer, FCH *vs.* FDG PET of, 203
deprivation therapy as initial treatment of metastatic prostate cancer, prognostic value of bone scan after, 218
Aneurysm
ascending aortic, surgical repair, total and partial cardiac sympathetic denervation after, 134

Anger-logic
gadolinium oxyorthosilicate detectors, performance of brain PET camera based on, 18
Angina
pectoris, reversible perfusion abnormalities during dobutamine stress Tc-99m sestamibi SPECT in patients with *vs.* without, late outcome of, 123
vasospastic, myocardial sympathetic denervation, fatty acid metabolism, and left ventricular wall motion in, 132
Angiography
no reflow on, quantitative estimation of myocardial salvage after primary coronary angioplasty in patients with, 140
radionuclide thyroid, *vs.* Tc-99m MIBI scintigraphy and power Doppler ultrasound in differential diagnosis of solitary cold thyroid nodules, 287
Angioplasty
coronary, primary percutaneous transluminal
for myocardial infarction, effects of abciximab on microvascular integrity and left ventricular function recovery after, 130
myocardial salvage in patients with angiographic no reflow after, quantitative estimation of, 140
Annexin A5
in vivo detection of cell death in area at risk in myocardial infarction with, 42
Antibody(ies)
antigranuloctye monoclonal, Fab fragment, Tc-99m, for imaging infection in different clinical settings, 233
labeled, granulocyte scintigraphy with, *vs.* FDG PET and hydromagnetic resonance imaging in assessment of Crohn's disease activity, 232
Anticoagulation
withholding from patients with suspected acute pulmonary embolism and negative CT findings, outcomes after, 88
Antigranulocyte
monoclonal antibody Fab fragment, Tc-99m, for imaging infection in different clinical settings, 233
Anxiety
during isolation and radionuclide therapy, 65
Aortic
aneurysm, ascending, surgical repair, total and partial cardiac sympathetic denervation after, 134
Apcitide
scintigraphy, Tc-99m, in deep vein thrombosis, 99
Apical
hypertrophic cardiomyopathy, SPECT of, 128
Aprotinin
technetium-99m, scintigraphy in amyloidosis with, 38
Arginine
/lysine, inhibition of renal uptake of radiolabeled octreotide by, 261
Arteritis
temporal, gallium-67 SPECT in, 288
Artery
coronary, disease, suspected, attenuation and scatter correction in myocardial SPET in, 154
Arthritic
finger joints, novel *vs.* conventional imaging procedures in, 224
Atomic bomb
survivors
fast neutrons measured in Hiroshima at distances relevant to, 59
lung cancer risk in, joint effects of radiation and smoking on, 56
mortality of, 57
Atrophy
temporal lobe, in hippocampal sclerosis associated with microscopic cortical dysplasia, neocortical temporal FDG-PET hypometabolism correlates with, 297
ATSM
copper, PET for hypoxia in myocardium with (in dog), 46
copper-60, PET for tumor hypoxia in lung cancer with, 97
Attenuation
correction
CT-based, in calculation of semi-quantitative indices of FDG uptake in PET, 16
in myocardial SPET, 154

B

Barostat
comparison with SPECT imaging of stomach, 119

Bicycle
exercise stress in PET for assessment of coronary flow reserve, 163
Biopsy
sentinel node, for breast cancer, sequential dermal-peritumoral radiocolloid injection for, 212
Biventricular
dynamic physical phantom, validation of gated blood pool SPECT cardiac measurements tested using, 22
Bleeding
gastrointestinal
occult, clinical utility of nuclear medicine imaging for detection, 113
scintigraphy, importance of delayed images in, 112
Blood
flow
myocardial (*see* Myocardium, blood flow)
renal, dynamic measurement by PET in CRF, 273
pool
SPECT, gated, cardiac measurements with, validation using biventricular dynamic physical phantom, 11
tomography, gated, *vs.* gated myocardial perfusion tomography for calculation of left ventricular volumes and ejection fraction, 149
BMIPP
iodine-123, scintigraphy of myocardial sympathetic denervation, fatty acid metabolism, and left ventricular wall motion in vasospastic angina with, 132
iodine-125, uptake in stunned myocardium (in mice), 162
Body
mass index, effects on SPECT imaging of stomach, 119
Bomb
atomic (*see* Atomic bomb)
Bone
metastases from breast cancer disguised by osteopoikilosis, 223
scan(s)
hot spots in ribs on, solitary, 215
prognostic value in patients with metastatic prostate cancer treated initially with androgen deprivation therapy, 218
serial, in follow-up of clinically localized low to intermediate grade prostate cancer managed with watchful observation alone, 219
three-phase, *vs.* other imaging modalities in arthritic finger joints, 224
Bowel
disease, active inflammatory, Tc-99m (V) DMSA scintigraphy in, 115
Brain
death confirmation by Tc-99m exametazime scintigraphy, outcome of patients referred for, 295
PET camera based on Anger-logic gadolinium oxyorthosilicate detectors, performance of, 18
tumor
recurrent metastatic, after stereotactic radiosurgery, methionine PET differentiating radiation necrosis from, 197
response to gamma knife radiosurgery, semiquantitative FDG PET in prediction of, 196
Breast
cancer (*see* Cancer, breast)
Breath
tests, carbon-14 urea, in children, no radiation protection reasons for restrictions on, 69
Breathing
oxygen-enriched, effect on myocardial uptake of Tc-99m sestamibi, 137
Bronchial
carcinoid follow-up, somatostatin receptor scintigraphy for, 179

C

Camera
gamma, hand-held
semiconductor-based, performance of, 26
PET, brain, based on Anger-logic gadolinium oxyorthosilicate detectors, performance of, 18
Cancer
breast
biopsy for, sentinel node, sequential dermal-peritumoral radiocolloid injection for, 212
mammary nodes in, internal, lymphoscintigraphic visualization with subtumoral radiocolloid injection, 210
metastatic to bone, disguised by osteopoikilosis, 223
after radiation for pediatric tumors, megavoltage, 69

cervix
advanced, para-aortic lymph node metastasis in, FDG PET after negative CT for, 206
pelvic insufficiency fracture after pelvic irradiation in, 220
recurrent, PET in detection of, 205
colorectal, FLT *vs.* FDG PET in, 190
esophagus
response to induction therapy, and whole body FDG PET, 188
sentinel nodes with Tc-99m colloidal rhenium sulfide in, 209
squamous cell, metastases to regional lymph nodes from, CT *vs.* FDG PET for presurgical detection of, 189
head and neck, squamous cell
locoregional advanced, impact of PET on initial staging and therapy in, 181
recurrent, diagnostic and prognostic value of FDG PET for, 183
tumor aggressiveness and response to intra-arterial chemotherapy and radiotherapy in, FDG PET for prediction of, 182
lung
non-small cell *(see below)*
risk in atomic bomb survivors, joint effects of radiation and smoking on, 56
small cell, prognostic value of FDG PET in, 178
staging with FDG PET/CT, 176
suspected, use of serial questionnaires to evaluate therapeutic efficacy of FDG PET in, 175
lung, non-small cell
cT1 N0 M0, effect of radioisotope sentinel node mapping in, 208
PET in, as predictor of response to chemotherapy, 92
PET in, FDG, 92
staging with PET/CT, 95
treatment of, neoadjuvant, FDG PET as predictor of response to, 177
tumor hypoxia in, Cu-60 ATSM PET of, 97
mortality
of atomic bomb survivors, 57
risk among workers at Mayak Nuclear Complex, 60
prostate
androgen-dependent and androgen-independent, FCH *vs.* FDG PET of, 203
clinically localized low to intermediate grade, managed with watchful observation alone, serial bone scans in follow-up of, 219
metastatic, treated initially with androgen deprivation therapy, prognostic value of bone scan after, 218
PET in, C-11 acetate and FDG, 202
rectal, pelvic recurrence after irradiation for, detection with FDG PET, 191
thyroid
metastases, pulmonary, functioning, effect of radioiodine on prognosis, 185
metastatic, In-111 DTPA-octreotide scintigraphy for, 186
radioiodine therapy in, dosimetry of, evaluation by I-124 PET, 240
recurrent, PET/CT of, 242
risk after thyroid examination with I-131, 63
Carbon-11
acetate PET
assessment of forward cardiac output with (in pig), 158
in prostate cancer, 202
carfenatil PET of cardiac opioid receptors, 34
choline PET in musculoskeletal tumors, 227
glucose *vs.* FDG for quantifying myocardial glucose use with PET (in dog), 45
N-methyl-naltrindole PET of cardiac opioid receptors, 34
pipzA-4 for in vivo evaluation of high-affinity choline uptake system, 39
Carbon-14
urea breath tests in children, no radiation protection reasons for restrictions on, 69
Carcinoid
bronchial, follow-up, somatostatin receptor scintigraphy for, 179
Carcinoma (*see* Cancer)
Cardiac (*see* Heart)
Cardiomyopathy
hypertrophic, apical, SPECT of, 128
ischemic, dobutamine-induced contractile reserve in stunned, hibernating, and scarred myocardium in, 143
Cardiovascular
nuclear medicine, 123

Carfenatil
carbon-11, PET of cardiac opioid receptors with, 34
CCK (*see* Cholecystokinin)
CdZnTe
semiconductor-based gamma camera, hand-held, performance of, 26
Cell(s)
death in area at risk in myocardial infarction, in vivo detection of, 42
exposed to very low x-ray doses, evidence for lack of DNA double-strand break repair in, 71
squamous (*see* Squamous cell)
stem cell transplantation, autologous
with chemotherapy, myeloablative, combined with I-131 MIBG for treatment of neuroblastoma, 194
for lymphoma, aggressive, FDG PET in prediction of clinical outcome, 198
T cell lymphoma, enteropathy-type, FDG PET of, 201
Central nervous system
nuclear medicine, 295
Cervix
cancer (*see* Cancer, cervix)
Chemotherapy
induction, dose-intensive, for high-risk neuroblastoma, MIBG scintigraphy for response to, 193
intra-arterial, in head and neck cancer, FDG PET for response to, 182
in lung cancer, non-small cell, PET as predictor of response to, 92
myeloablative, with autologous stem cell support, combined with I-131 MIBG for treatment of neuroblastoma, 194
neoadjuvant, of non-small cell lung cancer, FDG PET as predictor of response to, 177
Children
breath tests in, carbon-14 urea, no radiation protection reasons for restrictions on, 69
glomerular filtration rate indexed to suit, 266
malignancies in, thyroid neoplasms after therapeutic radiation for, 62
MRI of kidney in, 281
neuroblastoma in, I-131 MIBG in combination with myeloablative chemotherapy with autologous stem cell support for, 194
of patients receiving radioiodine therapy, and radiation dose, 66
scrotal pain in, acute, color Doppler sonography *vs.* scintigraphy of testis in, 283
thyroid cancer risk after thyroid examination with I-131 in, 64
vesicoureteral reflux in (*see* Vesicoureteral, reflux in children)
Cholecystokinin
cholescintigraphy, methodology and normal values using lactose-free fatty meal food supplement, 105
-8, regular *vs.* pharmacy-compounded, gallbladder function obtained with, 106
infusion, IV, *vs.* fatty meal for gallbladder ejection fraction, 103
-33, quantitative cholescintigraphy with, random dose for, and reproducibility of abnormal results, 108
Cholescintigraphy
cholecystokinin, methodology and normal values using lactose-free fatty meal food supplement, 105
quantitative
with CCK-33, random dose for, and reproducibility of abnormal results, 108
evidence of gallbladder function impairment in type 2 diabetes by, 111
Choline
carbon-11, PET with, in musculoskeletal tumors, 227
uptake system, high-affinity, F-18 FA4 and C-11 pipzA-4 for in vivo evaluation of, 39
Chromatid
exchanges, sister, in lymphocytes of nuclear medicine physicians, 67
Clinical
prediction rules, comparison of 2, among patients with suspected pulmonary embolism, 78
Cold
pressor test and endothelial dysfunction in diabetes, 138
Colloid
sulfur, Tc-99m, sequential dermal-peritumoral injection with, for sentinel node biopsy for breast cancer, 212
tin, Tc-99m
injection, subtumoral, lymphoscintigraphic visualization of internal mammary nodes in breast cancer with, 210

sentinel node mapping in cT1 N0 M0 lung cancer with, 208
Colloidal
rhenium sulfide, Tc-99m, sentinel node detection in esophageal carcinoma with, 209
Colorectal
cancer, FLT *vs.* FDG PET in, 190
Compression
ultrasound, venous, in diagnostic strategy for patients with suspected pulmonary embolism, 85
Computed tomography (*see* CT)
Contractile
reserve, dobutamine-induced, in stunned, hibernating, and scarred myocardium in ischemic cardiomyopathy, 143
Contrast
-enhanced MRI *vs.* resting Tl-201 SPECT for myocardial viability early after infarction, 136
Copper
ATSM PET of hypoxia in myocardium (in dog), 46
Copper-60
ATSM PET of tumor hypoxia in lung cancer, 97
Coronary
angioplasty, primary percutaneous transluminal
for myocardial infarction, effects of abciximab on microvascular integrity and left ventricular function recovery after, 130
myocardial salvage in patients with angiographic no reflow after, quantitative estimation of, 140
artery disease, suspected, attenuation and scatter correction in myocardial SPET in, 154
flow (*see* Myocardium, blood flow)
microvascular reactivity, dysregulation in asymptomatic type 2 diabetics, 147
Cortical
dysplasia, microscopic, hippocampal sclerosis associated with, neocortical temporal FDG-PET hypometabolism correlates with temporal lobe atrophy in, 297
Cost
-effective tool, SPET/CT image co-registration in abdomen with, 8
Creatinine
clearance, lateralized, *vs.* renal scintigraphy, relative renal function in children with bilateral vesicoureteral reflux by, 268
CRF
dynamic renal blood flow measurement by PET in, 273
Criticality
accident in Japan, first, analysis of dose distribution for heavily exposed workers in, 53
Crohn's disease
activity, assessment with FDG PET, hydro-MRI, and granulocyte scintigraphy, 232
inactive, Tc-99m interleukin-2 and Tc-99m HMPAO granulocyte scintigraphy in, 115
CT
attenuation correction on PET/CT, respiratory motion artifacts on PET emission images obtained using, 4
-based attenuation correction in calculation of semi-quantitative indices of FDG uptake in PET, 16
findings, negative, and suspected acute pulmonary embolism, outcomes after withholding anticoagulation from patients with, 88
helical, 85
in diagnostic strategy for patients with suspected pulmonary embolism, 85
single-detector, as primary diagnostic test in suspected pulmonary embolism, 87
vs. ventilation/perfusion scan for diagnosis of pulmonary embolism, 79
/PET (*see* PET/CT)
single photon emission (*see* SPECT)
/SPET image co-registration in abdomen with simple and cost-effective tool, 8
spiral *(see* helical *above)*
thin-section reformatted, of solitary hot spots in ribs found on bone scan, 215
in thymic enlargement, 173
vs. FDG PET for presurgical detection of metastasis to regional lymph nodes from esophageal squamous cell carcinoma, 189
Cu
ATSM PET for hypoxia in myocardium (in dog), 46

Cu-60
ATSM PET for tumor hypoxia in lung cancer, 97
Cystic
fibrosis lung, FDG uptake in, 229
lesions, pancreatic, intraoperative gamma probe detection of insulinoma in elderly patient with, 255

D

Death
brain, confirmation by Tc-99m exametazime scintigraphy, outcome of patients referred for, 295
cell, in area at risk in myocardial infarction, in vivo detection of, 42
Delegated Authorization Guidelines
introduction, audit and review of, 71
Denervation
sympathetic
cardiac, total and partial, after surgical repair of ascending aortic aneurysm, 134
myocardial, in vasospastic angina, 132
3'-Deoxy-3'-fluorothymidine
fluorine-18, PET with, *vs.* FDG PET in colorectal cancer, 190
Deoxyglucose
fluorine-18 (*see* FDG)
Depression
during isolation and radionuclide therapy, 65
Depth
-dependent resolution recovery algorithm, for evaluation of global left ventricular function in Tl-201 gated myocardial perfusion SPECT, 161
Dermal
-peritumoral radiocolloid injection, sequential, for sentinel node biopsy for breast cancer, 212
Diabetes mellitus
non-insulin-dependent (*see* type 2 *below*)
type 2
coronary microvascular reactivity dysregulation in asymptomatic patients with, 147
gallbladder function impairment in, evidence by quantitative cholescintigraphy, 111
glucose levels after physiologic meal in, postprandial plasma, effect of altering gastric emptying on, 117
myocardial perfusion in, PET of, 138
renal damage in women with, Tc-99m DMSA renal cortex scan of, 272
Diacetyl-*bis*(N^4-methylthiosemicarbazone)
copper, PET of hypoxia in myocardium with (in dog), 46
copper-60, PET of tumor hypoxia in lung cancer with, 97
Dimercaptosuccinic acid (*see* DMSA)
Dipyridamole
endothelial dysfunction in diabetes and, 138
SPECT, Tc-99m sestamibi, for detection of cardiac allograft vasculopathy, 133
DISIDA
cholescintigraphy, Tc-99m, evidence of gallbladder function impairment in type 2 diabetes by, 111
DMSA
scintigraphy of renal parenchymal damage in sibling vesicoureteric reflux, 271
technetium-99m, scintigraphy with
renal, severity of renal cortical damage in infants with unilateral hydronephrosis during follow-up and after pyeloplasty with, 275
renal cortex, of renal damage in women with type 2 diabetes, 272
(V), Tc-99m, scintigraphy in acute inflammatory bowel disease with, 115
DNA
double-strand break repair in cells exposed to very low x-ray doses, evidence for lack of, 71
Dobutamine
-induced contractile reserve in stunned, hibernating, and scarred myocardium in ischemic cardiomyopathy, 143
ischemia with, repetitive supply-demand, glucose uptake in postischemic and remote myocardium increased by (in pig), 139
stress Tc-99m sestamibi SPECT
prognostic value of, long-term, 127
reversible perfusion abnormalities during, comparison of late outcome in patients with *vs.* without angina having, 123

Doctors (*see* Physicians)
Donors
  live kidney, role of radioisotope renal scans in choice of nephrectomy side in, 278
Doppler
  ultrasound
    color, of testis, in children with acute scrotal pain, 283
    power, *vs.* radionuclide thyroid angiography and Tc-99m MIBI scintigraphy in differential diagnosis of solitary cold thyroid nodules, 287
Dose
  distribution for heavily exposed workers in first criticality accident in Japan, analysis of, 53
Dosimetry, 1
  of ADAM, I-123, 30
  of fluoro-A-85380, F-18, 28
  of FPCIT, F-18, 27
  of radioiodine therapy in benign and malignant thyroid disorders, evaluation by I-124 PET, 240
DTPA
  -octreotide scintigraphy, In-111, for metastatic thyroid cancer, 186
  technetium-99m, voiding patterns in children with vesicoureteral reflux with, 269
Dysplasia
  cortical, microscopic, hippocampal sclerosis associated with, neocortical temporal FDG-PET hypometabolism correlates with temporal lobe atrophy in, 297

E

ECD
  technetium-99m, *vs.* Tc-99m HMPAO, performance in typically hypoperfused areas in Alzheimer's disease, 302
Echocardiography
  resting, with quantitative dipyridamole Tc-99m sestamibi SPECT for detection of cardiac allograft vasculopathy, 133
  3D, *vs.* myocardial perfusion gated SPECT, left ventricular mass measured by, 151
Ejection fraction
  gallbladder, fatty meal *vs.* IV cholecystokinin infusion for, 103
  left ventricular
    calculation with gated myocardial perfusion tomography *vs.* gated blood pool tomography, 149
    using automated quantitative gated SPECT, factors affecting, 165
Elderly
  pancreatic cystic lesions in, intraoperative gamma probe detection of insulinoma in patient with, 255
Electrocardiographic
  changes, exercise-induced, in patients with chronic respiratory diseases, 145
Embolism
  pulmonary (*see* Pulmonary, embolism)
Endocrinology, 235
Endothelial
  dysfunction in diabetes, and dipyridamole and cold pressor test, 138
Enteropathy
  -type T cell lymphoma, FDG PET of, 201
Epilepsy
  temporal lobe
    hypometabolism on FDG PET in, extratemporal, as predictor of seizure outcome after temporal lobectomy, 298
    postictal psychosis in, 296
Esophagus
  cancer (*see* Cancer, esophagus)
  carcinoma (*see* Cancer, esophagus)
Ethanol
  injection, percutaneous, plus radioiodine, *vs.* radioiodine alone in treatment of large toxic thyroid nodules, 37
Exametazime
  scintigraphy, Tc-99m, outcome of patients referred for confirmation of brain death by, 295
Exercise
  -induced electrocardiographic changes in patients with chronic respiratory diseases, 145
  stress, bicycle, in PET for assessment of coronary flow reserve, 163
  training after myocardial infarction improves myocardial perfusion assessed by Tl-201 scintigraphy, 126
  vs. adenosine Tc-99m tetrofosmin SPECT, prognostic value of, 144

Extratemporal
  hypometabolism on FDG PET in temporal lobe epilepsy as predictor of seizure outcome after temporal lobectomy, 298
eZ SCOPE
  performance of, 26

F

FA-4
  fluorine-18, for in vivo evaluation of high-affinity choline uptake system, 39
Fab
  fragment, Tc-99m antigranulocyte monoclonal antibody, for imaging infection in different clinical settings, 233
Fat
  area, supraclavicular, FDG uptake during PET/CT in, 167
Fatty
  acid metabolism in vasospastic angina, 132
  meal
    food supplement, lactose-free, cholescintigraphy using, methodology and normal values for, 105
    vs. IV cholecystokinin infusion for gallbladder ejection fraction, 103
FCH
  PET *vs.* FDG PET of androgen-dependent and androgen-independent prostate cancer, 203
FDG
  F-18
    PET with (*see* PET, FDG)
    uptake in stunned myocardium (in mice), 162
  PEM, initial clinical results, 207
  /Tc-99m tetrofosmin SPECT after acipimox administration, feasibility and image quality of, 160
  uptake
    in lung, cystic fibrosis, 229
    in supraclavicular area fat during PET/CT, 167
    thymic enlargement and, 173
Fibrosis
  cystic, FDG uptake in lung in, 229
Finger
  joints, arthritic, novel *vs.* conventional imaging procedures in, 224
Fiscal
  consequences of bilateral neck exploration for primary idiopathic hyperparathyroidism without preoperative radionuclide imaging or minimally invasive techniques, 249
FLT
  vs. FDG PET in colorectal cancer, 190
Fluorine-18
  3'-deoxy-3'-fluorothymidine PET *vs.* FDG PET in colorectal cancer, 190
  deoxyglucose (*see* FDG)
  FA-4 for in vivo evaluation of high-affinity choline uptake system, 39
  fluoro-A-85380, biodistribution and dosimetry of, 28
  fluorocholine *vs.* FDG for PET of androgen-dependent and androgen-independent prostate cancer, 203
  fluorodeoxyglucose (*see* FDG)
  FPCIT, dosimetry of, 27
  FP-Gluc-TOCA PET imaging, 258
Fluoro-A-85380
  fluorine-18, biodistribution and dosimetry of, 28
Fluorocholine
  fluorine-18, *vs.* F-18 FDG for PET of androgen-dependent and androgen-independent prostate cancer, 203
Fluorodeoxyglucose
  fluorine-18 (*see* FDG)
Food
  supplement, lactose-free fatty meal, cholescintigraphy using, methodology and normal values for, 105
FPCIT
  fluorine-18, dosimetry of, 27
FP-Gluc-TOCA
  fluorine-18, PET imaging with, 258
Fracture
  pelvic insufficiency, after pelvic irradiation in cervix cancer, 220
Fundoplication
  mass index, effects on SPECT imaging of stomach, 119

G

Ga-67 (*see* Gallium-67)
Gadolinium
  oxyorthosilicate detectors, Anger-logic, performance of brain PET camera based on, 18

Gadopentetate
dimeglumine, MR renography using, *vs.* radionuclide renography, 279
Gallbladder
ejection fraction, fatty meal *vs.* IV cholecystokinin infusion for, 103
function
impaired, in type 2 diabetics, evidence by quantitative cholescintigraphy, 111
obtained with regular CCK-8 and pharmacy-compounded CCK-8, 106
Gallium-67
scintigraphy
in paracoccidioidomycosis, for extent of disease, 121
in Wegener's granulomatosis, for disease activity, 230
SPECT in temporal arteritis, 288
Gamma
camera, hand-held semiconductor-based, performance of, 26
knife radiosurgery
brain tumor response to, semiquantitative FDG PET in prediction of, 196
radiation necrosis and recurrent metastatic brain tumor after, methionine PET of, 197
probe detection of insulinoma, intraoperative, in elderly with pancreatic cystic lesions, 255
Gastric
emptying, altering, effect on postprandial plasma glucose levels after physiologic meal in type 2 diabetics, 117
Gastrointestinal
bleeding
occult, clinical utility of nuclear medicine imaging for detection of, 113
scintigraphy, importance of delayed images in, 112
nuclear medicine, 103
Glomerular
filtration rate indexing to suit children, 266
Glucose
carbon-11, *vs.* FDG for quantifying myocardial glucose use with PET (in dog), 45
levels, postprandial plasma, after physiologic meal in type 2 diabetics, effect of altering gastric emptying on, 117
uptake
in liver, insulin stimulates, FDG PET study of, 256
in myocardium, postischemic and remote, repetitive supply-demand ischemia with dobutamine increases (in pig), 139
use on PET as predictor of response to chemotherapy in non-small cell lung cancer, 92
Glycoprotein
IIb/IIIa receptor antagonist scintigraphy, Tc-99m, in deep vein thrombosis, 99
Granulocyte
scintigraphy
with labeled antibodies *vs.* FDG PET and hydromagnetic resonance imaging in assessment of Crohn's disease activity, 232
Tc-99m HMPAO, in inactive Crohn's disease, 115
Granuloma
Teflon-induced, PET/CT of, 238
Granulomatosis
Wegener's, disease activity in, gallium-67 scintigraphic assessment of, 230
Graves' disease
thyroid volume estimation methods in, comparison of, 243
Guidelines
Delegated Authorization, introduction, audit, and review of, 71

H

Hand
-held semiconductor-based gamma camera, performance of, 26
Head and neck
cancer (*see* Cancer, head and neck)
paragangliomas, suspected, clinical value of somatostatin receptor imaging in, 259
Heart
measurements, gated blood pool SPECT, validation using biventricular dynamic physical phantom, 22
opioid receptors, PET imaging of, 34
output, forward, assessment with 1-carbon-11 acetate PET (in pig), 158
sympathetic denervation, total and partial, after surgical repair of ascending aortic aneurysm, 134

transplantation, detection of cardiac allograft vasculopathy with resting echocardiography and dipyridamole Tc-99m sestamibi SPECT after, 133
Hemangioma
PET evaluation of, 291
Hematologic
disorders, splenosis detection in, improved with combined transmission-emission tomography, 120
Heparin
alone or with alteplase in submassive pulmonary embolism, 81
Hepatobiliary
imaging, nuclear, prolonged by opioids given prior to scanning, 109
High Resolution Research Tomograph
single LSO crystal layer, characterization of, 19
Hippocampal
sclerosis, temporal lobe atrophy in, associated with microscopic cortical dysplasia, neocortical temporal FDG-PET hypometabolism correlates with, 297
Histopathologic
response in patient with high-grade sarcoma, FDG PET-guided re-evaluation of, 225
HMPAO
SPECT of postictal psychosis in temporal lobe epilepsy, 297
technetium-99m, *vs.* Tc-99m ECD, performance in typically hypoperfused areas in Alzheimer's disease, 302
Hodgkin's disease
in children, second neoplasms after megavoltage radiation for, 69
Hormone
thyroid-stimulating, recombinant human, as preparation for radioiodine thyroid remnant ablation, 244
Hot spots
in ribs, solitary, on bone scan, 215
Hydromagnetic resonance imaging
vs. FDG PET and granulocyte scintigraphy in assessment of Crohn's disease activity, 232
Hydronephrosis
unilateral, in infants, ultrasound grade of hydronephrosis and severity of renal cortical damage on Tc-99m DMSA renal scan in, during follow-up and after pyeloplasty, 275
Hyperparathyroidism
primary
associated with multiglandular disease, limitations of Tc-99m sestamibi scintigraphic localization for, 247
idiopathic, clinical outcomes and fiscal consequences of bilateral neck exploration without preoperative radionuclide imaging or minimally invasive techniques for, 249
sestamibi scan in, Tc-99m, false negative, 251
Hypertrophic
cardiomyopathy, apical, SPECT of, 128
Hypometabolism
extratemporal, on FDG PET in temporal lobe epilepsy as predictor of seizure outcome after temporal lobectomy, 298
temporal, neocortical, on FDG PET, correlation with temporal lobe atrophy in hippocampal sclerosis associated with microscopic cortical dysplasia, 297
Hypoxia
in myocardium, Cu-ATSM PET of (in dog), 46
tumor, in lung cancer, Cu-60 ATSM PET of, 97

I

Ictal
/interictal subtraction SPECT images, stratifying differences on, 300
Image(s)
delayed, importance in gastrointestinal bleeding scintigraphy, 112
fusion
of abdominal organs, normal upper, visualized with PET/CT, accuracy of, 169
anatomical-functional, benefit in diagnostic work-up of neuroendocrine neoplasms, 172
leukocyte, labeled, pulmonary activity on, 100
quality of dual-isotope SPECT using FDG and Tc-99m tetrofosmin after acipimox administration, 160
SPECT, subtraction, ictal/interictal, stratifying differences on, 300
Imaging
lymph flow, dynamic, after autologous lymph vessel transplantation, 292

magnetic resonance (*see* MRI)
medical, do physicians correctly estimate radiation risks from? 49
nuclear medicine, clinical utility for detection of occult gastrointestinal hemorrhage, 113
procedures, novel *vs.* conventional, in arthritic finger joints, 224
Immunoglobulin
G, technetium-99m human, penile scintigraphy with, for distinguishing unstable and stable phases of Peyronie's disease, 284
Incidentaloma
adrenal, subclinical and preclinical functioning, SPECT semiquantitative analysis of adrenocortical I-131 6β-iodomethyl-norcholesterol uptake to discriminate, 262
Indium-111
DTPA-octreotide scintigraphy for disease detection in metastatic thyroid cancer, 186
leukocyte images, pulmonary activity on, 100
pentetreotide, high-activity, long-term efficacy in treatment of disseminated neuroendocrine tumors, 40
Infant
hydronephrosis in, unilateral, ultrasound grade of hydronephrosis and severity of renal cortical damage on Tc-99m DMSA renal scan in, 275
Infarction
myocardial (*see* Myocardium, infarction)
Infection
imaging in, 229
LeukoScan for, in different clinical settings, 233
Inflammation
imaging in, 229
Inflammatory
bowel disease, active, Tc-99m (V) DMSA scintigraphy in, 115
Instrumentation, 1
PET, and reconstruction algorithms in whole-body applications, 12
Insulin
stimulates liver glucose uptake, FDG PET study of, 256
Insulinoma
gamma probe detection of, intraoperative, in elderly with pancreatic cystic lesions, 255
Interictal
/ictal subtraction SPECT images, stratifying differences on, 300
Interleukin-2
scintigraphy, Tc-99m, in inactive Crohn's disease, 115
Iodine-123
ADAM, biodistribution and dosimetry of, 30
BMIPP scintigraphy of myocardial sympathetic denervation, fatty acid metabolism, and left ventricular wall motion in vasospastic angina, 132
MIBG
imaging for total and partial cardiac sympathetic denervation after surgical repair of ascending aortic aneurysm, 134
scintigraphy of myocardial sympathetic denervation, fatty acid metabolism, and left ventricular wall motion in vasospastic angina, 132
Iodine-124
PET, evaluation of dosimetry of radioiodine therapy in benign and malignant thyroid disorders by, 240
Iodine-125
BMIPP uptake in stunned myocardium (in mice), 162
Iodine-131
6β-iodomethyl-norcholesterol uptake, SPECT semiquantitative analysis to discriminate subclinical and preclinical functioning adrenal incidentaloma, 262
-MIBG combined with myeloablative chemotherapy with autologous stem cell support in neuroblastoma, 194
therapy for functioning pulmonary metastases of thyroid cancer, effect on prognosis, 185
thyroid examination with, thyroid cancer risk after, 63
4-Iodo-L-*meta*-tyrosine
biodistribution and excretion via kidney (in mice), 35
6β-Iodomethyl-norcholesterol
iodine-131, uptake, SPECT semiquantitative analysis to discriminate subclinical and preclinical functioning adrenal incidentaloma, 262

Ischemia
repetitive supply-demand, with dobutamine, glucose uptake in postischemic and remote myocardium increased by (in pig), 139
Ischemic
cardiomyopathy, dobutamine-induced contractile reserve in stunned, hibernating, and scarred myocardium in, 143
Isolation
for radionuclide therapy, depression and anxiety during, 65
Isotope
dual
myocardial perfusion SPECT with, in women with systemic lupus erythematosus, 131
myocardial scintigraphy with, simultaneous, clinical validation of, 150

J

Joint
finger, arthritic, novel *vs.* conventional imaging procedures in, 224

K

Kidney
(*See also* Renal)
donors, live, role of radioisotope renal scans in choice of nephrectomy side in, 278
excretion of 4-iodo-L-*meta*-tyrosine (in mice), 35
models of, 6 age-dependent multiregion, absorbed fractions and radionuclide S values for, 31
MRI of, 281
Knowledge
doctors', of radiation exposure, 51

L

Lactose
-free fatty meal food supplement, cholescintigraphy using, methodology and normal values for, 105
Lesion
detection performance in 3D PET, ROC analysis for assessment of, 11
Leukemia
risk among workers at Mayak Nuclear Complex, 60
Leukocyte
images, labeled, pulmonary activity on, 100
LeukoScan
for imaging infection in different clinical settings, 233
Limb
lower, lymphedema, after autologous lymph vessel transplantation, dynamic lymph flow imaging in, 292
Liver
glucose uptake, insulin stimulates, FDG PET study of, 256
Lobectomy
temporal, seizure outcome after, extratemporal hypometabolism on FDG PET in temporal lobe epilepsy as predictor of, 298
LSO
crystal layer High Resolution Research Tomograph, single, characterization of, 19
Lung
(*See also* Pulmonary)
cancer (*see* Cancer, lung)
cystic fibrosis, FDG uptake in, 229
disease, end-stage, scintigraphic diagnosis of right to left shunt in, 290
perfusion SPECT in diagnosis of pulmonary embolism, 75
scan, observer variability and accuracy of different criteria for interpretation of, 76
Lupus
erythematosus, systemic, in women, SPECT dual isotope myocardial perfusion imaging in, 131
Lutetium
oxyorthosilicate crystal layer High Resolution Research Tomograph, single, characterization of, 19
Lymph
flow imaging, dynamic, after autologous lymph vessel transplantation, 292
node(s)
mammary, internal, in breast cancer, lymphoscintigraphic visualization with subtumoral radiocolloid injection, 210
para-aortic, metastasis in advanced cervical cancer with negative CT findings, FDG PET for, 206
regional, metastases from esophageal squamous cell carcinoma, CT *vs.* FDG PET for presurgical detection of, 189

node(s), sentinel
biopsy, for breast cancer, sequential dermal-peritumoral radiocolloid injection for, 212
detection with Lymphoseek, 212
detection with Tc-99m colloidal rhenium sulfide in esophageal carcinoma, 209
mapping, radioisotope, in cT1 N0 M0 lung cancer, 208
vessel transplantation, autologous, lymphedema after, scintigraphic follow-up, 293
Lymphedema
lower limb, after autologous lymph vessel transplantation, dynamic lymph flow imaging in, 292
after lymph vessel transplantation, autologous, scintigraphic follow-up, 293
Lymphocytes
of physicians, nuclear medicine, sister chromatid exchanges in, 67
Lymphoma
aggressive, clinical outcome after autologous stem cell transplantation, FDG PET for prediction of, 198
T cell, enteropathy-type, FDG PET of, 201
Lymphoscintigraphic
visualization of internal mammary nodes with subtumoral radiocolloid injection in breast cancer, 210
Lymphoseek
for sentinel node detection, 212
Lysine
/arginine, inhibition of renal uptake of radiolabeled octreotide by, 261

M

Magnetic resonance image
/PET fusion in soft tissue sarcoma, 6
Magnetic resonance imaging (*see* MRI)
Magnetic resonance renography
vs. radionuclide renography, 279
Magnetic resonance spectroscopy
phosphorus-31, differentiation between healthy thyroid remnants and tumor tissue after radioiodine therapy for differentiated thyroid carcinoma with, 245
Malignancies
during childhood or adolescence, thyroid neoplasms after therapeutic radiation for, 62
Mammary
nodes, internal, in breast cancer, lymphoscintigraphic visualization with subtumoral radiocolloid injection, 210
Mammography
positron emission, initial clinical results, 207
Mammotomography
with pinhole incomplete circular orbit SPECT, 24
Mayak Nuclear Complex
cancer mortality risk in workers at, 60
Meal
fatty
food supplement, lactose-free, cholescintigraphy using, methodology and normal values for, 105
vs. IV cholecystokinin infusion for gallbladder ejection fraction, 103
physiologic, in type 2 diabetics, effect of altering gastric emptying on postprandial plasma glucose levels after, 117
Medical
imaging, do physicians correctly estimate radiation risks from? 49
Meperidine
prolongs nuclear hepatobiliary imaging when given prior to scanning, 110
MET
PET of recurrent metastatic brain tumor and radiation necrosis after stereotactic radiosurgery, 197
Metabolism
fatty acid, in vasospastic angina, 132
Metaiodobenzylguanidine (*see* MIBG)
Metastases
bone, from breast cancer, disguised by osteopoikilosis, 223
lymph node
para-aortic, in advanced cervical cancer with negative CT findings, FDG PET for, 206
regional, from esophageal squamous cell carcinoma, CT *vs.* FDG PET for presurgical detection of, 189
pulmonary, functioning, of thyroid cancer, radioiodine therapy for, effect on prognosis, 185
Metastatic
brain tumor, recurrent, after stereotactic radiosurgery, methionine PET differentiating radiation necrosis from, 197

prostate cancer treated initially with androgen deprivation therapy, prognostic value of bone scan after, 218
thyroid cancer, In-111 DTPA-octreotide scintigraphy for, 186

Methionine
PET of recurrent metastatic brain tumor and radiation necrosis after stereotactic radiosurgery, 197

Methoxyisobutylisonitrile
technetium-99m, scintigraphy with, *vs.* radionuclide thyroid angiography and power Doppler ultrasound in differential diagnosis of solitary cold thyroid nodules, 287

MIBG
iodine-123
imaging, for total and partial cardiac sympathetic denervation after surgical repair of ascending aortic aneurysm, 134
scintigraphy with, of myocardial sympathetic denervation, fatty acid metabolism, and left ventricular wall motion in vasospastic angina, 132
iodine-131, combined with myeloablative chemotherapy and autologous stem cell support for neuroblastoma, 194
scintigraphy for response of high-risk neuroblastoma to dose-intensive induction chemotherapy, 193

MIBI (*see* Sestamibi)

MicroPET R4 PET scanner
performance for rodents, 21

Microscopic
cortical dysplasia, hippocampal sclerosis associated with, neocortical temporal FDG-PET hypometabolism correlates with temporal lobe atrophy in, 297

Microvascular
integrity after primary coronary angioplasty in myocardial infarction, effects of abciximab on, 130
reactivity, coronary, dysregulation in asymptomatic type 2 diabetics, 147

Models
of kidney, 6 age-dependent multiregion, absorbed fractions and radionuclide S values for, 31

Monoclonal
antibody, Fab fragment, Tc-99m antigranulocyte, for imaging infection in different clinical settings, 233

Morphine
prolongs nuclear hepatobiliary imaging when given prior to scanning, 110

Mortality
of atomic bomb survivors, 57
cancer, risk among workers at Mayak Nuclear Complex, 60
after radiological investigation with radioactive Thorotrast, 55

MRI
contrast-enhanced, *vs.* resting Tl-201 SPECT for myocardial viability early after infarction, 136
hydro-, *vs.* FDG PET and granulocyte scintigraphy in assessment of Crohn's disease activity, 232
of kidneys, 281
3D, *vs.* other imaging modalities in arthritic finger joints, 224
vs. planar scintigraphy, SPECT, and US for thyroid volume estimation in Graves' disease, 243

Musculoskeletal
imaging, 215
lesions, benign and malignant, FDG PET of, 217
tumors, C-11 choline PET in, 227

Mycosis
endemic deep, paracoccidioidomycosis as, gallium-67 scan in defining extent of disease in, 121

Myocardium
blood flow
estimation by Tc-99m sestamibi imaging, 153
marker, tracer adenosine as (in dog), 44
reserve assessment with bicycle exercise stress in PET, 163
reserve estimation by Tc-99m sestamibi imaging, 153
in various segments characterized by rest-redistribution thallium SPECT, effect of nitroglycerin on, 124
contractile reserve, dobutamine-induced, in stunned, hibernating, and scarred myocardium in ischemic cardiomyopathy, 143
glucose use, quantification with 1-C-11 glucose *vs.* FDG PET (in dog), 45
hypoxia in, delineation using Cu-ATSM PET (in dog), 46

infarction
angioplasty in, primary coronary, effects of abciximab on microvascular integrity and left ventricular function recovery after, 130
cell death in area at risk in, in vivo detection of, 42
exercise training after, myocardial perfusion assessed by Tl-201 scintigraphy improved by, 126
myocardial viability early after, contrast-enhanced MRI *vs.* resting Tl-201 SPECT for, 136
metabolism-perfusion mismatch, oxygen-15 water PET *vs.* Tc-99m tetrofosmin SPECT showing, 155
perfusion
in diabetes, PET of, 138
imaging in Denmark, 148
-metabolism mismatch, oxygen-15 water PET *vs.* Tc-99m tetrofosmin SPECT showing, 155
SPECT, dual isotope, in women with systemic lupus erythematosus, 131
SPECT, gated, left ventricular mass measured by, 151
SPECT, stress, short-term survival benefit after revascularization *vs.* medical therapy in patients with no prior coronary artery disease undergoing, 141
thallium-201 scintigraphic assessment of, exercise training after myocardial infarction improves, 126
tomography, gated, *vs.* gated blood pool tomography for calculation of left ventricular volumes and ejection fraction, 149
tracers in clinical practice, comparison of three, 157
postischemic, repetitive supply-demand ischemia with dobutamine increases glucose uptake in (in pig), 139
remote, repetitive supply-demand ischemia with dobutamine increases glucose uptake in (in pig), 139
salvage after primary coronary angioplasty, quantitative estimation in patients with angiographic no reflow, 140
scintigraphy, simultaneous dual-isotope, clinical validation of, 150
stunned, I-125 BMIPP and F-18 FDG uptake in (in mice), 162
sympathetic denervation in vasospastic angina, 132
uptake of Tc-99m sestamibi, effect of oxygen-enriched breathing on, 137
viability early after infarction, contrast-enhanced MRI *vs.* resting Tl-201 SPECT for, 136

N

Nanocolloid
technetium-99m, lymph flow imaging after autologous lymph vessel transplantation with, 292
Neck
cancer (*see* Cancer, head and neck)
exploration, bilateral, for primary idiopathic hyperparathyroidism without preoperative radionuclide imaging or minimally invasive techniques, clinical outcomes and fiscal consequences of, 249
paragangliomas, suspected, clinical value of somatostatin receptor imaging in, 259
Necrosis
radiation, after stereotactic radiosurgery, methionine PET of, 197
Neoplasm (*see* Tumor)
Nephrectomy
side in live kidney donors, role of radioisotope renal scans in choice of, 278
Nervous
system, central, nuclear medicine, 295
Neuroblastoma
high-risk, response to dose-intensive induction chemotherapy, MIBG scintigraphy for, 193
treatment, I-131 MIBG in combination with myeloablative chemotherapy with autologous stem cell support in, 194
Neuroendocrine
neoplasms, benefit of anatomical-functional image fusion in diagnostic work-up of, 172
tumors, disseminated, long-term efficacy of high-activity In-111 pentetreotide therapy for, 40
Neurogenic
tumors, FDG PET in, 195
Neutrons
fast, in Hiroshima, measuring at distances relevant to atomic bomb survivors, 59

Nitroglycerin
effect on myocardial blood flow in various segments characterized by rest-redistribution thallium SPECT, 124
N-methyl-naltrindole
carbon-11, PET of cardiac opioid receptors with, 34
Nodules
thyroid (*see* Thyroid, nodules)
Nuclear
Complex, Mayak, cancer mortality risk in workers at, 60
medicine physicians, sister chromatid exchanges in lymphocytes of, 67

O

O_2 (*see* Oxygen)
Observer
variability and accuracy of different criteria for lung scan interpretation, 76
Octreotide
-DTPA scintigraphy, In-111, for metastatic thyroid cancer, 186
radiolabeled, inhibition of renal uptake by, lysine combined with arginine for, 261
Oncology, 167
clinical, effect of respiratory motion during PET/CT in, 2
Opioid(s)
prolong nuclear hepatobiliary imaging when given prior to scanning, 109
receptors, cardiac, PET imaging of, 34
OSEM
algorithm, for evaluation of global left ventricular function in Tl-201 gated myocardial perfusion SPECT, 161
Osseous
sites, targeting with α-emitting Ra-223 (in mice), 43
Osteopoikilosis
metastatic breast carcinoma to bone disguised by, 223
Oxygen
-enriched breathing, effect on myocardial uptake of Tc-99m sestamibi, 137
-15 water PET
vs. Tc-99m sestamibi imaging, estimation of myocardial blood flow and myocardial flow reserve by, 153
vs. Tc-99m tetrofosmin SPECT showing myocardial metabolism-perfusion mismatch, 155

P

Pain
scrotal, acute, color Doppler sonography *vs.* scintigraphy of testis in children with, 283
Pancreas
lesions, cystic, intraoperative gamma probe detection of insulinoma in elderly patient with, 255
Para-aortic
lymph node metastasis in advanced cervical cancer with negative CT findings, FDG PET for, 206
Paracoccidioidomycosis
extent of disease in, gallium-67 scan in defining, 121
Paragangliomas
head and neck, suspected, clinical value of somatostatin receptor imaging in, 259
Parathyroid
enlarged, ultrasound for preoperative localization of, 253
localization, preoperative
false-negative Tc-99m sestamibi scans in, 252
improving yield of, 236
scintigraphy, double-phase, Tc-99m tetrofosmin *vs.* Tc-99m sestamibi for, 248
surgery, separating promise from reality, 246
Parenchymal
damage, renal, in sibling vesicoureteric reflux, 271
Pediatric (*see* Children)
Pelvic
fracture, insufficiency, after pelvic irradiation in cervix cancer, 220
recurrence in previously irradiated rectal cancer patients, detection with FDG PET, 191
PEM
initial clinical results, 207
Penile
scintigraphy with Tc-99m human immunoglobulin G for distinguishing unstable and stable phases of Peyronie's disease, 284
Pentetreotide
indium-111, high-activity, in treatment of disseminated neuroendocrine tumors, long-term efficacy of, 40
Percutaneous
ethanol injection plus radioiodine *vs.* radioiodine alone in treatment of large toxic thyroid nodules, 37

Perfusion
abnormalities, reversible, during dobutamine stress Tc-99m sestamibi SPECT, comparison of late outcome in patients with *vs.* without angina having, 123
myocardial (*see* Myocardium, perfusion)
SPECT, lung, in diagnosis of pulmonary embolism, 75
/ventilation (*see* Ventilation, /perfusion)
Peritumoral
-dermal radiocolloid injection, sequential, for sentinel node biopsy for breast cancer, 212
PET
acetate, carbon-11
cardiac output assessment with, forward (in pig), 158
in prostate cancer, 202
ATSM
copper, of hypoxia in myocardium (in dog), 46
copper-60, of tumor hypoxia in lung cancer, 97
camera, brain, based on Anger-logic gadolinium oxyorthosilicate detectors, performance of, 18
of cardiac opioid receptors, 34
choline, carbon-11, in musculoskeletal tumors, 227
/CT (*see* PET/CT *below*)
exercise stress in, bicycle, for assessment of coronary flow reserve, 163
FCH, *vs.* FDG PET of androgen-dependent and androgen-independent prostate cancer, 203
FDG
cervical cancer detection with, recurrent, 205
combined with C-11 acetate, in prostate cancer, 202
in cystic fibrosis lung, FDG uptake during, 229
for differentiation between benign and malignant lesions in thorax, 90
FDG uptake in, semi-quantitative indices of, CT-based attenuation correction in calculation of, 16
-guided re-evaluation of histopathologic response in patient with high-grade sarcoma, 225
in head and neck recurrent squamous cell carcinoma, diagnostic and prognostic value of, 183
hypometabolism on, extratemporal, in temporal lobe epilepsy, as predictor of seizure outcome after temporal lobectomy, 298
hypometabolism on, neocortical temporal, correlation with temporal lobe atrophy in hippocampal sclerosis associated with microscopic cortical dysplasia, 297
impact on initial staging and therapy in locoregional advanced squamous cell carcinoma of head and neck, 181
of insulin effect on liver glucose uptake, 256
in lung cancer, non-small cell, 92
in lung cancer, small cell, prognostic value of, 178
in lung cancer, suspected, use of serial questionnaires to evaluate therapeutic efficacy of, 175
for lymph node metastasis, para-aortic, in advanced cervical cancer with negative CT findings, 206
of lymphoma, enteropathy-type T cell, 201
of musculoskeletal lesions, benign and malignant, 217
in neurogenic tumors, 195
for pelvic recurrence in previously irradiated rectal cancer patients, 191
as predictor of clinical outcome of aggressive lymphoma after autologous stem cell transplantation, 198
as predictor of response of neoadjuvant treatment for non-small cell carcinoma, 177
as predictor of response to chemotherapy in non-small cell lung cancer, 92
preoperative, of thyroid nodules, 237
semiquantitative, in prediction of brain tumor response to gamma knife radiosurgery, 196
thymic enlargement and FDG uptake on, 173
vs. CT for presurgical detection of metastasis to regional lymph nodes from esophageal squamous cell carcinoma, 189
vs. glucose, 1-C-11, for quantifying myocardial glucose use (in dog), 45

vs. hydromagnetic resonance imaging and granulocyte scintigraphy in assessment of Crohn's disease activity, 232
vs. In-111 DTPA-octreotide scintigraphy in metastatic thyroid cancer, 186
vs. PET, C-11 choline, in musculoskeletal tumors, 227
vs. PET, FCH, of androgen-dependent and androgen-independent prostate cancer, 203
vs. PET, FLT, in colorectal cancer, 190
whole body, and response of esophageal cancer to induction therapy, 188
FLT, *vs.* FDG PET in colorectal cancer, 190
FP-Gluc-TOCA, F-18 in, 258
glucose, 1-carbon-11, *vs.* FDG PET for quantifying myocardial glucose use (in dog), 45
in hemangioma, 291
imaging of somatostatin receptors, 258
instrumentation and reconstruction algorithms in whole-body applications, 12
iodine-124, evaluation of dosimetry of radioiodine therapy in benign and malignant thyroid disorders by, 240
methionine, of recurrent metastatic brain tumor and radiation necrosis after stereotactic radiosurgery, 197
/MR image fusion in soft tissue sarcoma, 6
of myocardial perfusion in diabetes, 138
pulmonary, 90
renal blood flow measurement by, dynamic, in CRF, 273
scanner, microPET R4, performance for rodents, 21
3D, ROC analysis for assessment of lesion detection performance in, 11
transmission, ordered subsets reconstruction algorithm using median root prior and inter-update median filtering for, 14
water, oxygen-15
vs. Tc-99m sestamibi imaging, estimation of myocardial blood flow and myocardial flow reserve by, 153
vs. Tc-99m tetrofosmin SPECT showing myocardial metabolism-perfusion mismatch, 155

PET/CT
abdominal organs visualized on, normal upper, accuracy of image fusion of, 169
effect of respiratory motion during, 2
FDG, for lung cancer staging, 176
FDG uptake in supraclavicular area fat during, 167
of granuloma, Teflon-induced, 238
staging of non-small cell lung cancer with, 95
of thyroid cancer, recurrent, 242
whole-body, FDG, automated 3D registration of, 5

Peyronie's disease
unstable and stable phases of, penile scintigraphy with Tc-99m human immunoglobulin G for distinguishing, 284

Phantom
physical, biventricular dynamic, validation of gated blood pool SPECT cardiac measurements tested using, 22

Pharmacy
-compounded CCK-8 *vs.* regular CCK-8, gallbladder function obtained with, 106

Phosphorus-31
magnetic resonance spectroscopy, differentiation between healthy thyroid remnants and tumor tissue after radioiodine therapy for differentiated thyroid carcinoma with, 245

Physicians
do they correctly estimate radiation risks from medical imaging? 49
knowledge of radiation exposure, 51
nuclear medicine, sister chromatid exchanges in lymphocytes of, 67

Physics, 1

Pinhole
incomplete circular orbit SPECT, mammotomography with, 24

pipzA-4
carbon-11, for in vivo evaluation of high-affinity choline uptake system, 39

Planar
scintigraphy *vs.* MRI for thyroid volume estimation in Graves' disease, 243

Platelet
glycoprotein IIb/IIIa receptor antagonist scintigraphy, Tc-99m, in deep vein thrombosis, 99

Positron emission mammography
initial clinical results, 207
Positron emission tomography (*see* PET)
Postictal
psychosis in temporal lobe epilepsy, 296
Postprandial
glucose levels, plasma, after physiologic meal in type 2 diabetics, effect of altering gastric emptying on, 117
Prediction
rules, 2 clinical, comparison among patients with suspected pulmonary embolism, 78
Probe
gamma, intraoperative detection of insulinoma in elderly with pancreatic cystic lesions with, 255
Prostate
cancer (*see* Cancer, prostate)
Psychosis
postictal, in temporal lobe epilepsy, 296
Pulmonary
(*See also* Lung)
activity on labeled leukocyte images, 100
CT, helical, 85
embolism
diagnosis, lung perfusion SPECT in, 75
diagnosis, ventilation/perfusion scan *vs.* helical CT for, 79
exclusion in clinical outcome studies, diagnostic strategies for, 83
submassive, heparin plus alteplase *vs.* heparin alone in, 81
embolism, suspected
comparison of 2 clinical prediction rules and implicit assessment among patients with, 78
CT as primary diagnostic test in, single-detected helical, 87
diagnostic strategy in, prospective multicenter outcome study, 85
with negative CT findings, outcomes after withholding anticoagulation from patients with, 88
metastases of thyroid cancer, functioning, radioiodine therapy for, effect on prognosis, 185
nuclear medicine, 75
PET, 90
Pyeloplasty
ultrasound grade of hydronephrosis and severity of renal cortical damage on Tc-99m DMSA renal scan in infants with unilateral hydronephrosis after, 275

Q

Questionnaires
serial, use to evaluate therapeutic efficacy of FDG PET in suspected lung cancer, 175

R

Ra-223
targeting of osseous sites with (in mice), 43
Radiation, 49
distribution for heavily exposed workers in first criticality accident in Japan, analysis of, 53
doses, large-body, after radioiodine therapy, 66
dosimetry (*see* Dosimetry)
exposure, doctors' knowledge of, 51
megavoltage, for pediatric tumors, second neoplasms after, 68
necrosis after stereotactic radiosurgery, methionine PET of, 197
risks from medical imaging, do physicians correctly estimate? 49
smoking and, joint effects on lung cancer risk in atomic bomb survivors, 56
therapeutic (*see* Radiotherapy)
Radioactive
Thorotrast, mortality after radiological investigation with, 55
Radiocolloid
injection
sequential dermal-peritumoral, for sentinel node biopsy for breast cancer, 212
subtumoral, lymphoscintigraphic visualization of internal mammary nodes in breast cancer with, 210
Radiography
conventional
extensive, *vs.* In-111 DTPA-octreotide scintigraphy in metastatic thyroid cancer, 186
vs. other imaging modalities in arthritic finger joints, 224
Radioiodine
effect on prognosis of functioning pulmonary metastases of thyroid cancer, 185
therapy
alone or with percutaneous ethanol injection in large toxic thyroid nodules, 37

radiation doses after, large-body, 66
in thyroid disorders, benign and malignant, evaluation of dosimetry by I-124 PET, 240
thyroid remnant ablation, rhTSH as preparation for, 244
Radioisotope
renal scans, role in choice of nephrectomy side in live kidney donors, 278
sentinel node mapping in cT1 N0 M0 lung cancer, 208
Radiolabeled
octreotide, renal uptake by, lysine combined with arginine for, 261
Radiologic
investigation with radioactive Thorotrast, mortality after, 55
staging of lung cancer improved with FDG and CT registration, 176
Radionuclide
angiography, thyroid, *vs.* Tc-99m MIBI scintigraphy and power Doppler ultrasound in differential diagnosis of solitary cold thyroid nodules, 287
renography *vs.* magnetic resonance renography, 279
S values for 6 age-dependent multiregion models of kidney, 31
therapy, depression and anxiety during isolation for, 65
voiding patterns in children with vesicoureteral reflux, 269
Radiopharmaceutical, 33
Radiosurgery
gamma knife
brain tumor response to, semiquantitative FDG PET in prediction of, 196
radiation necrosis and recurrent metastatic brain tumor after, methionine PET of, 197
Radiotherapy
for head and neck cancer, FDG PET for response to, 182
for malignancies during childhood or adolescence, thyroid neoplasms after, 62
pelvic, in cervix cancer, pelvic insufficiency fracture after, 220
for rectal cancer, pelvic recurrence after, detection with FDG PET, 191
Radium-223
targeting of osseous sites with (in mice), 43
RBC
imaging, Tc-99m, for detection of occult gastrointestinal hemorrhage, 113
Receiver
operating characteristic analysis for assessment of lesion detection performance in 3D PET, 11
Reconstruction
algorithms (*see* Algorithms, reconstruction)
Rectal
cancer patients, previously irradiated, pelvic recurrence after, detection with FDG PET, 191
Reflux
vesicoureteral (*see* Vesicoureteral, reflux)
Renal
(*See also* Kidney)
blood flow measurement, dynamic, by PET in CRF, 273
cortex damage, severity on Tc-99m DMSA renal scan in infants with unilateral hydronephrosis during follow-up and after pyeloplasty, 275
damage in women with type 2 diabetes by Tc-99m DMSA renal cortex scan, 272
failure, chronic, dynamic renal blood flow measurement by PET in, 273
function, relative, comparison by renal scintigraphy and lateralized creatinine clearance in children with bilateral vesicoureteral reflux, 268
nuclear medicine, 265
parenchymal damage in sibling vesicoureteric reflux, 271
scans, radioisotope, role in choice of nephrectomy side in live kidney donors, 278
scintigraphy *vs.* lateralized creatinine clearance, relative renal function in children with bilateral vesicoureteral reflux by, 268
uptake of radiolabeled octreotide, inhibition by lysine combined with arginine, 261
Renography
magnetic resonance *vs.* radionuclide, 279
Respiratory
diseases, chronic, exercise-induced electrocardiographic changes in patients with, 145

motion
artifacts on PET emission images obtained using CT attenuation correction on PET/CT, 4
during PET/CT, 2
Revascularization
vs. medical therapy in patients with no prior coronary artery disease undergoing stress myocardial perfusion SPECT, short-term survival benefit of, 141
Rhenium
sulfide, Tc-99m colloidal, sentinel node detection in esophageal carcinoma with, 209
Rheumatoid arthritis
finger joints, novel *vs.* conventional imaging procedures in, 224
Rib
hot spots, solitary, on bone scan, 215
ROC
analysis for assessment of lesion detection performance in 3D PET, 11

S

S values
radionuclide, for 6 age-dependent multiregion models of kidney, 31
Sarcoma
high-grade, FDG PET-guided re-evaluation of histopathologic response in patients with, 225
soft tissue, PET-MR image fusion in, 6
Scan
bone (*see* Bone, scan)
lung, observer variability and accuracy of different criteria for interpretation of, 76
ventilation/perfusion, *vs.* helical CT for diagnosis of pulmonary embolism, 79
Scanner
microPET R4 PET, performance for rodents, 21
Scatter
correction in myocardial SPET, 154
Scintigraphy
apcitide, Tc-99m, in deep vein thrombosis, 99
aprotinin, Tc-99m, in amyloidosis, 38
before and after autologous lymph vessel transplantation, 293
BMIPP, I-123, of myocardial sympathetic denervation, fatty acid metabolism, and left ventricular wall motion in vasospastic angina, 132
bone (*see* Bone, scan)
diagnosis of right to left shunt in end-stage lung disease by, 290
DMSA
of renal parenchymal damage in sibling vesicoureteric reflux, 271
technetium-99m, of renal damage in women with type 2 diabetes, 272
technetium-99m, renal, severity of renal cortical damage in infants with unilateral hydronephrosis during follow-up and after pyeloplasty with, 275
(V) Tc-99m, in active inflammatory bowel disease, 115
DTPA-octreotide, In-111, for metastatic thyroid cancer, 186
exametazime, Tc-99m, outcome of patients referred for confirmation of brain death by, 295
gallium-67
in paracoccidioidomycosis, for extent of disease, 121
in Wegener's granulomatosis, for disease activity, 230
gastrointestinal bleeding, importance of delayed images in, 112
granulocyte
with labeled antibodies, *vs.* FDG PET and hydromagnetic resonance imaging in assessment of Crohn's disease activity, 232
Tc-99m HMPAO, in inactive Crohn's disease, 115
interleukin-2, Tc-99m, in inactive Crohn's disease, 115
metaiodobenzylguanidine
I-123, of myocardial sympathetic denervation, fatty acid metabolism, and left ventricular wall motion in vasospastic angina, 132
for response of high-risk neuroblastoma to dose-intensive induction chemotherapy, 193
MIBI, Tc-99m, *vs.* radionuclide thyroid angiography and power Doppler ultrasound in differential diagnosis of solitary cold thyroid nodules, 287
myocardial, simultaneous dual-isotope, clinical validation of, 150

parathyroid, double-phase, Tc-99m tetrofosmin *vs.* Tc-99m sestamibi for, 248
penile, with Tc-99m human immunoglobulin G for distinguishing unstable and stable phases of Peyronie's disease, 284
planar, *vs.* MRI for thyroid volume estimation in Graves' disease, 243
renal
radioisotope, role in choice of nephrectomy side in live kidney donors, 278
vs. lateralized creatinine clearance, relative renal function in children with bilateral vesicoureteral reflux by, 268
sestamibi (*see* Sestamibi, technetium-99m, scintigraphy with)
somatostatin receptor, for bronchial carcinoid follow-up, 179
of testis, in children with acute scrotal pain, 283
Sclerosis
hippocampal, temporal lobe atrophy in, associated with microscopic cortical dysplasia, neocortical temporal FDG-PET hypometabolism correlates with, 297
Scrotal
pain, acute, color Doppler sonography *vs.* scintigraphy of testis in children with, 283
Seizure
outcome after temporal lobectomy, extratemporal hypometabolism on FDG PET in temporal lobe epilepsy as predictor of, 298
Semiconductor
-based gamma camera, hand-held, performance of, 26
Sentinel node (*see* Lymph, node, sentinel)
Sestamibi
as myocardial perfusion tracer, comparison with thallium-201 and tetrofosmin, in clinical practice, 157
technetium-99m
imaging with, after thyroid suppression, 236
imaging with, estimation of myocardial blood flow and myocardial flow reserve by, 153
myocardial uptake of, effect of oxygen-enriched breathing on, 137
scintigraphy with *(see below)*
vs. Tc-99m tetrofosmin, for double-phase parathyroid scintigraphy, 248
technetium-99m, scintigraphy with
false-negative, in hyperparathyroidism, primary, 251
false-negative, in parathyroid localization, preoperative, 252
limitations for localization for primary hyperparathyroidism associated with multiglandular disease, 247
vs. radionuclide thyroid angiography and power Doppler ultrasound in differential diagnosis of solitary cold thyroid nodules, 287
vs. ultrasound for preoperative localization of enlarged parathyroid, 253
technetium-99m, SPECT with
dipyridamole, for detection of cardiac allograft vasculopathy, 133
dobutamine stress, long-term prognostic value of, 127
dobutamine stress, reversible perfusion abnormalities during, late outcome in patients with *vs.* without angina having, 123
Sex
effects on SPECT imaging of stomach, 119
Shunt
right to left, in end-stage lung disease, scintigraphic diagnosis of, 290
Sibling
vesicoureteric reflux, renal parenchymal damage in, 271
Single photon emission computed tomography (*see* SPECT)
Sister
chromatid exchanges in lymphocytes of nuclear medicine physicians, 67
Smoking
radiation and, joint effects on lung cancer risk in atomic bomb survivors, 56
Soft tissue
sarcoma, PET-MR image fusion in, 6
Somatostatin
receptor(s)
imaging, clinical value in suspected head and neck paragangliomas, 259
PET imaging of, 258
scintigraphy for bronchial carcinoid follow-up, 179

Sonography (*see* Ultrasound)
SPECT
of cardiomyopathy, apical hypertrophic, 128
/CT image co-registration in abdomen with simple and cost-effective tool, 8
dual-isotope, using FDG and Tc-99m tetrofosmin after acipimox administration, feasibility and image quality of, 160
gallium-67, in temporal arteritis, 288
gated blood pool, cardiac measurements, validation using biventricular dynamic physical phantom, 22
HMPAO
of postictal psychosis in temporal lobe epilepsy, 297
Tc-99m, in early- *vs.* late-onset Alzheimer's disease, 301
images, subtraction, ictal/interictal, stratifying differences on, 300
lung perfusion, in diagnosis of pulmonary embolism, 75
myocardial, attenuation and scatter correction in, 154
myocardial perfusion
dual isotope, in women with systemic lupus erythematosus, 131
gated, automated quantitative, factors affecting left ventricular ejection fraction using, 165
gated, left ventricular mass measured by, 151
stress, short-term survival benefit after revascularization *vs.* medical therapy in patients with no prior coronary artery disease undergoing, 141
pinhole incomplete circular orbit, mammotomography with, 24
semiquantitative analysis of adrenocortical I-131 6β-iodomethyl-norcholesterol uptake to discriminate subclinical and preclinical functioning adrenal incidentaloma, 262
sestamibi, technetium-99m
dipyridamole, for detection of cardiac allograft vasculopathy, 133
myocardial uptake on, effect of oxygen-enriched breathing on, 137
stress, dobutamine, long-term prognostic value of, 127
stress, dobutamine, reversible perfusion abnormalities during, comparison of late outcome in patients with *vs.* without angina having, 123
stress, simultaneous with rest Tl-201 SPECT, clinical validation of, 150
of stomach, 119
tetrofosmin, technetium-99m
after exercise-induced electrocardiographic changes in patients with chronic respiratory diseases, 145
normal exercise and adenosine, prognostic value of, 144
thallium-201 (*see* Thallium-201, SPECT)
vs. MRI for thyroid volume estimation in Graves' disease, 243
Spectroscopy
magnetic resonance, phosphorus-31, differentiation between healthy thyroid remnants and tumor tissue after radioiodine therapy for differentiated thyroid carcinoma with, 245
SPET (*see* SPECT)
Splenosis
detection in patients with hematologic disorders, improved with combined transmission-emission tomography, 120
Squamous cell
carcinoma
esophagus, metastases to regional lymph nodes from, CT *vs.* FDG PET for presurgical detection of, 189
esophagus, sentinel nodes with Tc-99m colloidal rhenium sulfide in, 209
head and neck (*see* Cancer, head and neck, squamous cell)
Sr-89
vs. Ra-223, targeting of osseous sites with (in mice), 43
Stem cell
transplantation, autologous
chemotherapy with, myeloablative, combined with I-131 MIBG for treatment of neuroblastoma, 194
for lymphoma, aggressive, FDG PET in prediction of clinical outcome after, 198

Stereotactic
radiosurgery
brain tumor response to, semiquantitative FDG PET in prediction of, 196
radiation necrosis and recurrent metastatic brain tumor after, methionine PET of, 197
Stomach
SPECT imaging of, 119
Stress
dobutamine stress Tc-99m sestamibi SPECT
prognostic value of, long-term, 127
reversible perfusion abnormalities during, late outcome in patients with *vs.* without angina having, 123
exercise, bicycle, in PET for assessment of coronary flow reserve, 163
myocardial perfusion SPECT, short-term survival benefit after revascularization *vs.* medical therapy in patients with no prior coronary artery disease undergoing, 141
Strontium-89
vs. radium-223, targeting of osseous sites with (in mice), 43
Subtraction
SPECT images, ictal/interictal, stratifying differences on, 300
Subtumoral
injection of radiocolloid, lymphoscintigraphic visualization of internal mammary nodes in breast cancer with, 210
Sulfur colloid
Tc-99m, sequential dermal-peritumoral injection with, for sentinel node biopsy for breast cancer, 212
Supraclavicular
fat area, FDG uptake during PET/CT in, 167
Sympathetic
denervation
cardiac, total and partial, after surgical repair of ascending aortic aneurysm, 134
myocardial, in vasospastic angina, 132

T

T cell
lymphoma, enteropathy-type, FDG PET of, 201
Tc-99m (*see* Technetium-99m)
Technetium-99m
albumin, macroaggregated, scintigraphic diagnosis of right to left shunt in end-stage lung disease with, 290
annexin A5, in vivo detection of cell death in area at risk in myocardial infarction with, 42
antigranulocyte monoclonal antibody Fab fragment for imaging infection in different clinical settings, 233
apcitide scintigraphy in deep vein thrombosis, 99
aprotinin scintigraphy in amyloidosis, 38
colloid
sulfur, sequential dermal-peritumoral injection with, for sentinel node biopsy for breast cancer, 212
tin, injection, subtumoral, lymphoscintigraphic visualization of internal mammary nodes in breast cancer with, 210
tin, sentinel node mapping in cT1 N0 M0 lung cancer with, 208
colloidal rhenium sulfide, sentinel node detection in esophageal carcinoma with, 209
DISIDA cholescintigraphy, evidence of gallbladder function impairment in type 2 diabetes by, 111
DMSA (*see* DMSA, technetium-99m)
DTPA, voiding patterns in children with vesicoureteral reflux with, 269
ECD *vs.* Tc-99m HMPAO, performance in typically hypoperfused areas in Alzheimer's disease, 302
exametazime scintigraphy, outcome of patient referred for confirmation of brain death by, 295
HMPAO
granulocyte scintigraphy in inactive Crohn's disease, 115
SPECT, in early- *vs.* late-onset Alzheimer's disease, 301
immunoglobulin G, human, penile scintigraphy for distinguishing unstable and stable phases of Peyronie's disease with, 284
interleukin-2 scintigraphy in inactive Crohn's disease, 115
methoxyisobutylisonitrile scintigraphy *vs.* radionuclide thyroid angiography and power Doppler ultrasound in differential diagnosis of solitary cold thyroid nodules, 287

nanocolloid, lymph flow imaging after autologous lymph vessel transplantation with, 292
platelet glycoprotein IIb/IIIa receptor antagonist scintigraphy in deep vein thrombosis, 99
RBC imaging for detection of occult gastrointestinal hemorrhage, 113
sestamibi (*see* Sestamibi, technetium-99m)
tetrofosmin (*see* Tetrofosmin, technetium-99m)
Teflon
-induced granuloma, PET/CT of, 238
Temporal
arteritis, gallium-67 SPECT in, 288
hypometabolism, neocortical, on FDG PET, correlation with temporal lobe atrophy in hippocampal sclerosis associated with microscopic cortical dysplasia, 297
lobe
atrophy in hippocampal sclerosis associated with microscopic cortical dysplasia, neocortical temporal FDG-PET hypometabolism correlates with, 297
epilepsy, hypometabolism on FDG PET in, extratemporal, as predictor of seizure outcome after temporal lobectomy, 298
epilepsy, postictal psychosis in, 296
lobectomy, seizure outcome after, extratemporal hypometabolism on FDG PET in temporal lobe epilepsy as predictor of, 298
Testis
scintigraphy and color Doppler sonography of, in children with acute scrotal pain, 283
TET
splenosis detection of patients with hematologic disorders with, 120
Tetrofosmin
as myocardial perfusion tracer, comparison with MIBI and thallium-201, in clinical practice, 157
technetium-99m
dose, effect on left ventricular ejection fraction using automated quantitative gated SPECT, 165
imaging with, serial, of myocardial salvage after primary angioplasty in patients with no angiographic reflow, 140
SPECT with *(see below)*
vs. Tc-99m sestamibi for double-phase parathyroid scintigraphy, 248
technetium-99m, SPECT with
after exercise-induced electrocardiographic changes in patients with chronic respiratory diseases, 145
normal exercise and adenosine, prognostic value of, 144
simultaneous with FDG, after acipimox administration, feasibility and image quality of, 160
vs. oxygen-15 water PET showing myocardial metabolism-perfusion mismatch, 155
Thallium-201
comparison with MIBI and tetrofosmin as myocardial perfusion tracers in clinical practice, 157
SPECT
myocardial perfusion, effect of exercise training after myocardial infarction on, 126
myocardial perfusion gated, global left ventricular function in, OSEM and depth-dependent resolution recovery algorithms for evaluation of, 161
rest, simultaneous with stress Tc-99m sestamibi SPECT, clinical validation of, 150
rest, *vs.* contrast-enhanced MRI for myocardial viability early after infarction, 136
rest-redistribution, effect of nitroglycerin on myocardial blood flow in various segments characterized by, 124
Thorax
lesions, benign and malignant, FDG PET for differentiation between, 90
Thorotrast
radioactive, mortality after radiological investigation with, 55
Three-dimensional
echocardiography *vs.* myocardial perfusion gated SPECT, left ventricular mass measured by, 151
PET, ROC analysis for assessment of lesion detection performance in, 11
registration, automated, of stand-alone FDG whole-body PET with CT, 5
Thrombosis
deep vein, imaging characteristics of Tc-99m apcitide in, 99

Thymic
enlargement and FDG uptake, 173
Thyroid
angiography, radionuclide, *vs.* Tc-99m MIBI scintigraphy and power Doppler ultrasound in differential diagnosis of solitary cold thyroid nodules, 287
cancer (*see* Cancer, thyroid)
disorders, benign and malignant, dosimetry of radioiodine therapy in, evaluation by I-124 PET, 240
examination with I-131, thyroid cancer risk after, 63
neoplasms after therapeutic radiation for malignancies during childhood or adolescence, 62
nodules
cold, solitary, differential diagnosis by radionuclide thyroid angiography, Tc-99m MIBI scintigraphy and power Doppler ultrasound, 287
PET of, FDG, preoperative, 237
toxic, large, treatment with percutaneous ethanol injection plus radioiodine *vs.* radioiodine alone, 37
remnant(s)
ablation, radioiodine, rhTSH as preparation for, 244
healthy, after radioiodine therapy for differentiated thyroid carcinoma, differentiation between tumor tissue and, P-31 magnetic resonance spectroscopy for, 245
-stimulating hormone, recombinant human, as preparation for radioiodine thyroid remnant ablation, 244
suppression, Tc-99m sestamibi imaging after, 236
volume estimation methods in Graves' disease, comparison of, 243
Thyrotoxicosis
radioiodine therapy in, dosimetry of, evaluation by I-124 PET, 240
Tin
colloid, Tc-99m
injection, subtumoral, lymphoscintigraphic visualization of internal mammary nodes in breast cancer with, 210
sentinel node mapping in cT1 N0 M0 lung cancer with, 208
Tissue
soft, sarcoma, PET-MR image fusion in, 6
tumor, after radioiodine therapy for differentiated thyroid carcinoma, differentiation between healthy thyroid remnants and, P-31 magnetic resonance spectroscopy for, 245
Tl-201 (*see* Thallium-201)
Tomograph
High Resolution Research, single LSO crystal layer, characterization of, 19
Tomography
combined transmission-emission, improved detection of splenosis in patients with hematologic disorders with, 120
computed (*see* CT)
gated myocardial perfusion, *vs.* gated blood pool tomography for calculation of left ventricular volumes and ejection fraction, 149
positron emission (*see* PET)
Toxic
thyroid nodules, large, treatment with percutaneous ethanol injection plus radioiodine *vs.* radioiodine alone, 37
Tracers
myocardial perfusion, in clinical practice, comparison of three, 157
Training
exercise, after myocardial infarction, myocardial perfusion assessed by T1-201 scintigraphy improved by, 126
Transmission
-emission tomography, combined, improved detection of splenosis in patients with hematologic disorders with, 120
Transplantation
heart, detection of cardiac allograft vasculopathy with resting echocardiography and dipyridamole Tc-99m sestamibi SPECT after, 133
lymph vessel, autologous
lymph flow imaging after, dynamic, 292
lymphedema after, scintigraphic follow-up, 293
stem cell, autologous
chemotherapy with, myeloablative, combined with I-131 MIBG for treatment of neuroblastoma, 194
for lymphoma, aggressive, FDG PET in prediction of clinical outcome after, 198

TSH
recombinant human, as preparation for radioiodine thyroid remnant ablation, 244
Tumor(s)
aggressiveness in head and neck cancer, FDG PET for prediction of, 182
brain
recurrent metastatic, after stereotactic radiosurgery, methionine PET differentiating radiation necrosis from, 197
response to gamma knife radiosurgery, semiquantitative FDG in prediction of, 196
carcinoid, bronchial, follow-up, somatostatin receptor scintigraphy for, 179
hypoxia in lung cancer, Cu-60 ATSM PET of, 97
musculoskeletal, C-11 choline PET in, 227
neuroendocrine, benefit of anatomical-functional image fusion in diagnostic work-up of, 172
neuroendocrine, disseminated, long-term efficacy of high-activity In-111 pentetreotide therapy for, 40
neurogenic, FDG PET in, 195
pediatric, second neoplasms after megavoltage radiation for, 68
thyroid, after therapeutic radiation for malignancies during childhood or adolescence, 62
tissue after radioiodine therapy for differentiated thyroid carcinoma, differentiation between healthy thyroid remnants and, P-31 magnetic resonance spectroscopy for, 245

U

Ultrasound
Doppler
color, of testis, in children with acute scrotal pain, 283
power, *vs.* radionuclide thyroid angiography and Tc-99m MIBI scintigraphy in differential diagnosis of solitary cold thyroid nodules, 287
grade of hydronephrosis in infants with unilateral hydronephrosis during follow-up and after pyeloplasty, 275
localization of enlarged parathyroid, preoperative, 253
venous compression, in diagnostic strategy for patients with suspected pulmonary embolism, 85
vs. MRI for thyroid volume estimation in Graves' disease, 243
vs. other imaging modalities in arthritic finger joints, 224
Urea
breath tests, C-14, in children, no radiation protection reasons for restrictions on, 69

V

Vascular
nuclear medicine, 287
Vasculopathy
cardiac allograft, detection with resting echocardiography and quantitative dipyridamole Tc-99m sestamibi SPECT, 133
Vasospastic
angina, myocardial sympathetic denervation, fatty acid metabolism, and left ventricular wall motion in, 132
Venous
compression ultrasound in diagnostic strategy for patients with suspected pulmonary embolism, 85
thrombosis, deep, imaging characteristics of Tc-99m apcitide in, 99
Ventilation
/perfusion imaging, 75
/perfusion scan
interpretation, observer variability and accuracy of different criteria for, 76
vs. helical CT for diagnosis of pulmonary embolism, 79
Ventricle
left
ejection fraction, calculation with gated myocardial perfusion tomography *vs.* gated blood tomography, 149
ejection fraction, using automated quantitative gated SPECT, factors affecting, 165
function, global, in Tl-201 gated myocardial perfusion SPECT, OSEM and depth-dependent resolution recovery algorithms for evaluation of, 161

function recovery after primary coronary angioplasty in myocardial infarction, effects of abciximab on, 130
mass, measurement by myocardial perfusion gated SPECT, 151
volumes, calculation with gated myocardial perfusion tomography *vs.* gated blood pool tomography, 149
wall motion, in vasospastic angina, 132
Vesicoureteral
reflux in children
bilateral, relative renal function by renal scintigraphy and lateralized creatinine clearance in, 268
renal parenchymal damage in siblings and, 271
voiding patterns in, radionuclide, 269
Vessel
lymph, autologous transplantation
lymph flow imaging after, dynamic, 292
lymphedema after, scintigraphic follow-up, 293
Voiding
patterns, radionuclide, in children with vesicoureteral reflux, 269
V/Q (*see* Ventilation, /perfusion)

W

Water
oxygen-15, PET with
vs. Tc-99m sestamibi imaging, estimation of myocardial blood flow and myocardial flow reserve by, 153
vs. Tc-99m tetrofosmin SPECT showing myocardial metabolism-perfusion mismatch, 155
Wegener's granulomatosis
disease activity in, gallium-67 scintigraphic assessment of, 230
Women
diabetes in, type 2, renal damage by Tc-99m DMSA renal cortex scan in, 272
lupus erythematosus in, systemic, SPECT dual isotope myocardial perfusion imaging in, 131
Workers
heavily exposed, analysis of dose distribution for, in first criticality accident in Japan, 53
at Mayak Nuclear Complex, cancer mortality risk in, 60

X

X-ray
doses, very low, evidence for lack of DNA double-strand break repair in cells exposed to, 71

Author Index

A

Abe A, 26
Abletshauser C, 147
Acharya S, 62
Ahmed AR, 291
Akhurst T, 188, 191
Akinboboye O, 151
Aksakal E, 137
Albrechtsson U, 79
Alenius S, 14
Alpert NM, 176
Ang ES, 279
Annovazzi A, 115
Antoch G, 2
Aquino SL, 176
Asenbaum S, 296
Asmuth JC, 176
Audenaert K, 65
Aujesky D, 78
Aydin H, 223

B

Backhaus M, 224
Bajc M, 79
Bandhauer F, 181
Barlas D, 109
Basoglu T, 137
Bates SM, 99
Battista G, 179
Baumeister RGH, 292, 293
Bax JJ, 143
Beets AL, 162
Belakhlef A, 27
Benatar NA, 6
Ben-Horin CL, 288
Bergström KA, 30
Bernard G, 121
Bettinardi V, 14
Beyer T, 2
Bianco JA, 128
Biancone L, 115
Bilger K, 240
Bird NJ, 266
Blanco HP, 31
Blodgett T, 2
Blodgett TM, 238
Boccalandero F, 165
Boden GH, 117
Boellaard R, 19
Bogićević M, 269
Bolch WE, 31
Bonjer HJ, 248
Bottlaender M, 28
Bouchet LG, 31
Bounameaux H, 78
Bouras EP, 119
Bowsher JE, 24
Boz A, 284
Bozkurt G, 67
Brandwein M, 252
Brans B, 65
Branstetter BF IV, 238
Bronfman F, 39
Brown PH, 103
Bruce IN, 131
Buijs F, 19
Bulas D, 283
Burmester GR, 224
Buscombe JR, 40

C

Camilleri M, 119
Caplin ME, 40
Cardona S, 195
Cascio S, 271
Caviglia R, 115
Cerfolio RJ, 177
Cerulli-Switzer J, 106
Chagnon I, 78
Chapman N, 106
Chatterton BE, 295
Chertin B, 271
Choi JY, 298
Choo R, 219
Chu WW, 128
Cid E, 165
Ciliberto GR, 133
Coaguila C, 161
Cohade C, 4, 167, 169
Coleman RE, 203
Collart J-P, 75
Comans EF, 175
Conte M, 37
Cooper CS, 268
Copeland EM III, 212
Cortsen A, 154
Costa DC, 16, 190
Croasdale I, 16
Czernin J, 198

D

Dannals RF, 34
Daou D, 161
Daube-Witherspoon ME, 18
Davies G, 157
Deboer G, 219
De Bondt P, 22
De Geeter F, 149
de Groot TJ, 39
Dehdashti F, 97
de Jong HWAM, 19
de Jong M, 261
de Klerk JMH, 243
Delgado-Aros S, 119
Delpassand ES, 236
Demirel K, 287
Demura Y, 90
Dence C, 45
Deussen A, 44
Devinsky O, 300
Dey D, 5
Dhawan V, 27
Dickman PW, 63
Diehl B, 297
Dietlein M, 245, 259
Dimoulios PD, 115
Donahue JR, 223
Dörner J, 233
dos Santos Silva I, 55
Downey RJ, 188
Dresden TU, 44
Dudley NE, 249
Dusenbery KE, 68

E

Eary JF, 225
Eastick S, 126
El-Diasty T, 278
Elhendy A, 123, 127
Endo A, 53
Erdogru T, 284
Ernst YJ, 255
Eschmann SM, 120, 172, 240

F

Fanti S, 179
Faraggi M, 150
Farsad M, 179
Feezor RJ, 212
Feldman F, 217
Filmont J-E, 198
Finestone A, 49
Fischer E, 259
Fischman AJ, 173
Fisher DR, 43
Flores LG II, 35
Förster GJ, 8
Fouque D, 273
Francis DL, 190

Freimanis RI, 207
Freitag AP, 229
Fricke E, 202
Friedman JD, 141
Fröberg AC, 248

G

Gad HM, 278
Gallowitsch HJ, 237
Gayed I, 165
Geisler F, 256
Germano G, 151
Gerundini P, 12
Gilissen C, 39
Gimsing P, 38
Gladman DD, 131
Glatting G, 11
Gold DG, 68
Gonen M, 178
Gonlachanvit S, 117
Gourgiotis L, 186
Grattan-Smith JD, 281
Gratz S, 233
Graves MW, 290
Greaves CD, 71
Gunnarsson M, 69
Gunning MG, 126
Guthrie LC, 186

H

Haber RS, 253
Hachamovitch R, 141
Hahn K, 292, 293
Hany TF, 95
Harding JW, 295
Hari K, 300
Harris AM, 71
Hatayama K, 291
Havelock J, 66
Havrilesky LJ, 205
Hayes SW, 141
Heikman P, 30
Hendel HW, 38
Henderson BL, 266
Henriksen G, 43
Her D, 139
Herder GJ, 175
Herrero P, 45, 46
Hilson AJW, 40
Hindié E, 185
Hinz U, 195
Hirano T, 136
Hironaka FH, 121
Hirotani A, 145
Hodroff MA, 268
Hoekstra OS, 76
Hoffmann M, 201
Hoffmann SMA, 301
Hofmann M, 202
Hofstra L, 42
Hoh CK, 213
Holm L-E, 63
Holmes C, 301
Hong SB, 298
Horger M, 120, 172
Howarth DM, 113
Hoyos M, 108
Hsu C-W, 117
Huang W-S, 272
Huh SJ, 220
Hung YC, 206

I

Ibañez D, 131
Idris O, 151
Ikegami H, 134
Ilić S, 269
Ilson D, 188
Imperiale A, 262
Inabnet WB, 253
Inoue T, 227
Iozzo P, 256
Ishizaki T, 90
Ito Y, 153
Ituarte PHG, 246
Iwai Y, 197

J

Jager PL, 230
Janier MF, 273
Jaszczak RJ, 24
Jones DA, 105
Jones ME, 55
Jones RA, 281
Juillard L, 273
Julian JA, 99

K

Kaiser H-J, 155
Kam BLR, 160
Kaneda Y, 208
Kang MK, 220
Kapucu Ö, 287
Kapur A, 157
Karabogaz G, 67
Karp JS, 18
Kasraeian A, 212
Kato H, 209
Katoh C, 153
Katz SC, 247
Kauppinen TA, 30
Kawai K, 35
Kemp PM, 301
Kennedy JG, 223
Kim B, 220
Kim CK, 253
Kim SJ, 298
Kiratli PO, 290
Kitagawa K, 136
Kitagawa Y, 182
Kjaer A, 138, 148, 154
Kletter K, 201
Knoess C, 21
Ko K, 251
Kobayashi H, 134
Koepfli P, 163
Köksal T, 284
Konda R, 275
Konstantinides S, 81
Koo CW, 300
Koukouraki SI, 115
Koulibaly PM, 302
Koutroubakis IE, 115
Kramer EL, 247
Kramer K, 193
Kresnik E, 237
Krishnamurthy GT, 103
Krishnamurthy S, 106
Krug L, 178
Kruip MJHA, 83
Kubo S, 124
Kushner BH, 193

L

Labiris NR, 229
La Cava G, 262
Lange F, 185
Långström B, 158
LaPresto E, 297
LaQuaglia M, 62
Lardinois D, 95
Larson SM, 191, 244
Latus KA, 157
Lauer T, 44
Laumann C, 8
Leclercq MGL, 83
Lee J, 26
Lee J-K, 196
Lee KS, 189
Lees W, 113
Leide-Svegborn S, 69
Leitha T, 112
Lengerke C, 120
Le Normand L, 218
Leslie WD, 66

Lesser ML, 109
Leutmezer F, 296
Levine EA, 207
Levine JE, 194
Lewis JS, 46, 97
Liao RP, 203
Liem IH, 42
Lin C-C, 111, 272
Lin DT, 183
Lin WC, 206
Lister-James J, 99
Liu R-S, 196
Löbrich M, 71
Loncar R, 44
Love C, 100
Lui D, 266
Lundell G, 63

M

Mabuchi K, 56
Machtens S, 202
Maekura R, 145
Malveiro F, 55
Mamede M, 124
Mangiavacchi M, 133
Manos C, 217
Marchetti AA, 59
Margouleff D, 109
Mark E, 173
Marsden PK, 6
Matthay KK, 194
McCook B, 242
McFalls EO, 139
Mechanick JI, 252
Mellière D, 185
Meltzer C, 242
Merlino JI, 251
Meyer C, 138
Migneco O, 302
Mikolajczyk K, 163
Mikosch P, 237
Mindrup SR, 268
Minotti A, 251
Mintun MA, 97
Miyajima S, 132
Miyazaki T, 209
Modoni S, 37
Moka D, 245
Momose M, 134, 147
Moore HG, 191
Moretti JL, 150
Morita E, 246
Mozley D, 290
Muenz LR, 105
Mukherjee S, 177
Murad B, 139
Musumeci G, 130

N

Nahmias C, 229
Najm I, 297
Nakajima M, 209
Nakamoto Y, 4, 169
Nakamura S, 140
Neglia JP, 68
Neurath MF, 232
Neverve J, 147
Nichols K, 22
Nickel O, 8
Nielsen FS, 138
Niitsu M, 215
Nishizawa S, 182
Nobili F, 302
Noriyasu K, 153
Nowak B, 155
Numminen P, 14
Nussbaum Blask AR, 283

O

Oikonen V, 256
Ojha B, 177
Okuda Y, 145
Olianti C, 262
Olsson C-G, 79
Osman M, 167
Osman MM, 4
Ota S, 275

P

Palestro CJ, 100
Palser R, 66
Pandit N, 178
Pannu HK, 167
Perez-Bayfield MR, 281
Perrier ND, 207, 246
Petersen CL, 148
Petersen V, 92
Petronio AS, 130
Pfannenberg AC, 172
Pierce DA, 56, 57
Podreka I, 296
Pointurier I, 161
Poldermans D, 160
Pons V, 108
Poot L, 230
Preston DL, 57, 60
Price DT, 203
Przetak C, 5

R

Raffelt K, 245
Rahbek B, 154
Ravert HT, 34
Reischl G, 240
Reitblat A, 288
Reitblat T, 288
Rennie A, 51
Reske SN, 11
Richter E, 49
Rigaud J, 218
Robbins RJ, 244
Robeson W, 27
Roelants V, 75, 255
Roeske JC, 43
Rolleman EJ, 261
Ron E, 60
Rosière A, 255
Rothkamm K, 71
Roumenov D, 28
Rovai D, 130
Royal RE, 236
Rubin BP, 225
Ruffini L, 133
Rugel G, 59
Ryu JH, 88

S

Sakai K, 275
Sakuma H, 136
Sandrock D, 224
Sano K, 182
Sarafoglou K, 62
Sarlis NJ, 186
Schaadt BK, 38
Schaefer WM, 155
Scheidhauer K, 258
Schell SR, 249
Schinkel AFL, 123, 127, 143
Schipper ML, 233
Schlesinger T, 49
Schmid DT, 181
Schmidt B, 92
Schmidt M, 259
Schöder H, 183
Schottelius M, 258
Schunk K, 232
Schwarzbach M, 195
Secord AA, 205
Shalaby-Rana E, 283
Shapiro SE, 236
Sharp GB, 56
Sharp TL, 45, 46
Shaw LJ, 144
Sheedy PF II, 88

Shiang H-R, 196
Shikano N, 35
Shilnikova NS, 60
Shim YM, 189
Shimazu K, 210
Shimizu Y, 57
Shiralkar S, 51
Shokeir AA, 278
Siegel S, 21
Simonneau G, 85
Sinha N, 244
Slart RHJA, 230
Slomka PJ, 5
Sloof GW, 162
Smith A, 21
Snow M, 51
Somer EJR, 6
Sopena R, 108
Sörensen J, 158
Ståhle E, 158
Staudenherz A, 112
Stenström K, 69
Stoeckli SJ, 181
Straume T, 59
Sudoh M, 208
Sugi K, 208
Sugiura T, 140
Sun S-S, 111
Sunada I, 197
Surti S, 18
Swensen SJ, 88

T

Tadamura E, 124
Taguchi T, 210
Takahashi N, 26
Takahashi T, 132
Takeda T, 215
Takehana K, 140
Tamaki Y, 210
Tang K, 113
Tarantola G, 12
Tatsumi M, 169
Taylor CM, 71
Ten HS, 279
Thimister PWL, 42
Tiguert R, 218
Tomas MB, 100
Tornai MP, 24
Tsuchida T, 90
Tsuyuguchi N, 197

V

Valette H, 28
Valkema R, 160, 248, 261
Vandenberghe S, 22
van den Eynde F, 65
van der Heul C, 83
van Domburg R, 143
van Domburg RT, 123, 127
van Heertum R, 217
Vanhove C, 149
van Isselt JW, 243
Vanpee D, 75
van Rijk PP, 243
van Strijen MJL, 87
van Tinteren H, 175
Vehling D, 232
Vera DR, 213
Verberne HJ, 162
Vernon CB, 225
Vignogna-Barlas L, 109
Villemagne PSR, 34
Visvikis D, 16, 190
Vlajković M, 269
Vogelsang H, 201

W

Walgraeve N, 149
Walker J, 126
Wallace AM, 213
Wallhaus TR, 128
Wang GJ, 247
Watanabe H, 227, 291
Watanabe K, 132
Weber WA, 92
Weder W, 95
Weinmann P, 150
Weiss M, 292, 293
Werner C, 11
Wester HJ, 258
Westreich RW, 252
Wittram C, 173
Wong RJ, 183
Wong TZ, 205
Wong WC, 279
Wu H-C, 272
Wyss CA, 163

Y

Yamaga LYI, 121
Yamaguchi Y, 53
Yanagawa T, 227
Yang C-C, 111
Yanik GA, 194
Yap BK, 219
Yap C, 198
Yapici O, 137
Yeh LS, 206
Yeh SDJ, 193
Yeretsian RA, 238
Yoneda A, 271
Yoon YC, 189
Yücel C, 287
Yuksel M, 67

Z

Zettinig G, 112
Ziessman HA, 105
Zimmer LA, 242
Zingrillo M, 37
Zito F, 12

Order your *Year Book* today! Simply complete and detach this card and drop it in the mail to receive the latest information in your field.

The year's best literature in one convenient volume!

YES! Please start my subscription to the ***Year Book(s)*** checked below with the current volume according to the terms described below.* I understand that I will have 30 days to examine each annual edition.

Please Print:

Name ______________________________

Address ______________________________

City ____________________ State ____________ ZIP ____________

Method of Payment

❑ Check (payable to **Elsevier**; add the applicable sales tax for your area)

❑ VISA ❑ MasterCard ❑ AmEx ❑ Bill me

Card number ____________________ Exp. date ____________

Signature ______________________________

- ❑ **Year Book of Allergy, Asthma and Clinical Immunology (YALI)** $103.00 (Avail. November)
- ❑ **Year Book of Anesthesiology and Pain Management (YANE)** $109.00 (Avail. August)
- ❑ **Year Book of Cardiology® (YCAR)** $109.00 (Avail. August)
- ❑ **Year Book of Critical Care Medicine® (YCCM)** $107.00 (Avail. June)
- ❑ **Year Book of Dentistry® (YDEN)** $101.00 (Avail. August)
- ❑ **Year Book of Dermatology and Dermatologic Surgery™ (YDER)** $111.00 (Avail. October)
- ❑ **Year Book of Diagnostic Radiology® (YRAD)** $111.00 (Avail. November)
- ❑ **Year Book of Emergency Medicine® (YEMD)** $111.00 (Avail. May)
- ❑ **Year Book of Endocrinology® (YEND)** $108.00 (Avail. July)
- ❑ **Year Book of Family Practice™ (YFAM)** $95.00 (Avail. June)
- ❑ **Year Book of Gastroenterology™ (YGAS)** $104.00 (Avail. December)
- ❑ **Year Book of Hand Surgery® (YHND)** $112.00 (Avail. April)
- ❑ **Year Book of Medicine® (YMED)** $103.00 (Avail. July)
- ❑ **Year Book of Neonatal and Perinatal Medicine® (YNPM)** $112.00 (Avail. September)
- ❑ **Year Book of Neurology and Neurosurgery® (YNEU)** $107.00 (Avail. January)
- ❑ **Year Book of Nuclear Medicine® (YNUM)** $106.00 (Avail. June)
- ❑ **Year Book of Obstetrics, Gynecology, and Women's Health® (YOBG)** $111.00 (Avail. February)
- ❑ **Year Book of Oncology® (YONC)** $112.00 (Avail. November)
- ❑ **Year Book of Ophthalmology® (YOPH)** $112.00 (Avail. September)
- ❑ **Year Book of Orthopedics® (YORT)** $112.00 (Avail. October)
- ❑ **Year Book of Otolaryngology—Head and Neck Surgery® (YOTO)** $103.00 (Avail. July)
- ❑ **Year Book of Pathology and Laboratory Medicine® (YPAT)** $112.00 (Avail. March)
- ❑ **Year Book of Pediatrics® (YPED)** $98.00 (Avail. January)
- ❑ **Year Book of Plastic and Aesthetic Surgery® (YPRS)** $111.00 (Avail. March)
- ❑ **Year Book of Psychiatry and Applied Mental Health® (YPSY)** $101.00 (Avail. March)
- ❑ **Year Book of Pulmonary Disease® (YPDI)** $105.00 (Avail. April)
- ❑ **Year Book of Rheumatology, Arthritis, and Musculoskeletal Disease™ (YRHE)** $112.00 (Avail. January)
- ❑ **Year Book of Sports Medicine® (YSPM)** $106.00 (Avail. December)
- ❑ **Year Book of Surgery® (YSUR)** $105.00 (Avail. September)
- ❑ **Year Book of Urology® (YURO)** $112.00 (Avail. November)
- ❑ **Year Book of Vascular Surgery® (YVAS)** $112.00 (Avail. April)

**Your Year Book service guarantee:*

When you subscribe to a ***Year Book***, you will receive notice of future annual volumes about two months before publication. To receive the new edition, do nothing—we'll send you the new volume as soon as it is available. (Applicable sales tax is added to each shipment.) If you want to discontinue, the advance notice allows you time to notify us of your decision. If you are not completely satisfied, you have 30 days to return any ***Year Book***.